LET THEM EAT PROZAC

MEDICINE, CULTURE, AND HISTORY
Series Editor: Andrea Tone

Let Them Eat Prozac
The Unhealthy Relationship between the
Pharmaceutical Industry and Depression
David Healy

DAVID HEALY

LET THEM EAT PROZAC

*The Unhealthy Relationship between the
Pharmaceutical Industry and Depression*

New York University Press　　•　　*New York and London*

NEW YORK UNIVERSITY PRESS
New York and London
www.nyupress.org

Library of Congress Cataloging-in-Publication Data
Healy, David, MRC Psych.
Let them eat Prozac : the unhealthy relationship between
the pharmaceutical industry and depression / David Healy.
p. cm. — (Medicine, Culture, and History)
Includes bibliographical references and index.
ISBN 0–8147–3669–6 (cloth : alk. paper)
1. Serotonin uptake inhibitors. 2. Fluoxetine.
3. Depression, Mental—Chemotherapy. 4. Psychotropic drugs industry.
[DNLM: 1. Fluoxetine—adverse effects. 2. Depressive Disorder—
drug therapy. 3. Drug Industry—ethics. 4. Fluoxetine—therapeutic use.
QV77.5 H434L 2004] I. Title. II. Series.
RM332.H423   2004
616.85'27061—dc22   2004002297

New York University Press books are printed on acid-free paper,
and their binding materials are chosen for strength and durability.

Manufactured in the United States of America
10 9 8 7 6 5 4 3 2 1

Carpenter's Boat

The new wood as old as carpentry

Rounding the far buoy, wild
Steel fighting in the sea, carpenter,

Carpenter,
Carpenter and other things, the monstrous welded seams

Plunge and drip in the seas, carpenter,
Carpenter, how wild the planet is.

—George Oppen, 1962

Contents

Acknowledgments   ix

Preface: Under the Thundercloud of a Common Experience   xi

Introduction: Before Prozac   1

1   Take One   40

2   Events in Kentucky   64

3   Down the Barrel of a Lawyer   87

4   Market Force   103

5   A Pacific Fault Line   129

6   Kafka's Castle   150

7   Experiment at the End of the Millennium   174

8   The Plots Thicken   194

9   The Tort Wars   224

10   Let Them Eat Prozac   254

Epilogue: Anecdotal Deaths   284

Notes   289

Index   341

About the Author   351

Acknowledgments

I have always tried to fit my acknowledgments into a transport metaphor. At one point it looked as if the only metaphor that would do for this book was a solo skiff on a whitewater river, or a battered raft complete with bewildered souls who had lost children, parents, partners, or friends. But things changed, and this book now owes more to the efforts of others than anything else I've written. These have not been efforts to check the grammar or the facts but rather real risk-taking by many people. Among the thousands whose lives have been torn apart by SSRI antidepressants were Tim Tobin, Bill and Susan Forsyth, Linda Hurcombe, and Fiona Lindsay. Of the many who have learned what academic freedom really means, those on the same bit of river as I included Nancy Olivieri, Brenda Gallie, Helen Chan, Alison Hudgins, Rhonda Love, Peter Durie, and John Dick.

While most of us floundered, a few who had been there before knew what to do. These included Cindy Hall, Karen Barth, Skip Murgatroyd, Andy Vickery, Rhonda Hawkins, Nancy Zettler, Jim Turk, Rosemary Morgan, Peter Rosenthal, Kiké and Charlie Roach. There were others, but these stood out.

Downriver—when the going got really wild, and no one should have even thought about helping out—Tom Ban, Ned Shorter, Cyril Greenland, Trudo Lemmens, Mona Gupta, Bruce Charlton, and Charles Medawar not only thought about helping but also came on board, and without their contributions the journey would have ended far earlier.

Many people managed to throw lines to the raft at critical points, keeping it on course. These included Julie Axelrod, Ross Baldessarini, Raymond Battegay, Per Bech, German Berrios, Tom Bolwig, Arvid Carlsson, Gaston Castellanos, Jonathan Cole, Leon Eisenberg, Joel Elkes, Giovanni Fava, Max Fink, Alfred Freedman, Peter Gaszner, Abraham Halpern, Turan Itil, Gordon Johnson, Joseph Knoll, Toshihiro Kobayakawa, Brian Leonard, Isaac Marks, Robin Murray, David Nutt,

Merton Sandler, Mogens Schou, Pierre Simon, Solomon Snyder, Costas Stefanis, Fridolin Sulser, Gabor Ungvari, and Herman van Praag.

I also got huge amounts of help from Carl Elliott, David Antonuccio, Elizabeth Young, Richard Tranter, Françoise Bayliss, Richard De-Grandpre, Cedric Knight, Max Lagnado, Terry Maltsberger, Mervyn Whitford, Mariam Fraser, and Nikolas Rose, and latterly from Bob Whitaker, Vera Hassner Sharav, Andrew Herxheimer, Bill Bruneau, Andrea Tone, and Alison Waldenberg.

Many people working in the pharmaceutical industry will know that this is not a book hostile to industry but rather one that has received huge input from colleagues working in that industry. We have all been operating under the thundercloud of a common experience.

Sarah Boseley, Anne McIlroy, Duncan Dallas, Marc Edwards, and Vicky Marriott provided key coverage at critical points early in this whitewater journey, and more recently Shelley Jofre and Andy Bell have contributed hugely.

Back at base, as ever, were—among many others—Dinah Cattell, Jackie Thomas, and Tony Roberts.

I owe a special debt to the Canadian Association for University Teachers (CAUT), who picked up my case at a critical point. They owed nothing to a "foreigner" but responded to the principle, even though this lay outside their brief. I am particularly pleased that all royalties from this book will go into an academic freedom charitable fund within CAUT.

I still have no idea whether this river is about to level out around the bend of publication or if this raft will drop over a waterfall. Responsibility for a big drop is clearly not mine alone, but equally clearly, none of the responsibility lies with anyone else mentioned in this acknowledgment.

Preface

Under the Thundercloud of a Common Experience

The woman sitting in my office was a year or two younger than me. She had written some weeks before to ask if she could visit me to discuss what had happened to her husband.

Gordon, who was almost exactly my age, was a career highflier who could anticipate being promoted to the top of his profession within a few years. But, as in many walks of professional life in the 1990s, reorganization and cost-containment exercises faced him and his colleagues with uncertainties. Jane could see the pressure on him and wondered if anything could be done to help. A year previously Gordon had accompanied Jane, at her suggestion, to see their local general practitioner (GP). Gordon was not a man to seek medical help. His entire medical record consisted of a few lines. There was little in anyone's account of him to think he had a depressive illness, but his GP made a working diagnosis of depression, prescribed Prozac, and asked him to come back in two weeks. Jane could remember no warnings about hazards.

Within twenty-four hours, by her account, he was having difficulty. Even though it was the middle of winter, he complained of the heat and asked for the windows to be opened. He seemed unable to sit down. These problems continued over the weekend. A friend, Alice, left her children over to play with Gordon's children on Sunday. After collecting her children, Alice—a primary-care practitioner—mentioned to her husband that she was worried about Gordon, who didn't look himself.

Gordon's colleagues described him as obviously restless and unable to focus the following day at work. On Monday night, he stayed up changing doorknobs and doing other nonurgent small jobs until the early hours of the morning. Tuesday he went for a haircut before leaving for a meeting some miles away. On his return home, he went up to his study on the fourth floor to get his papers for the meeting. Except for further complaints about the heat, which had led him to open the study window, nothing seemed amiss to his wife that morning. She went downstairs to make him tea. Suddenly she heard a thump on the ground outside. Her husband was lying on the concrete in front of her, dying. Her question—what had happened to him?

Twenty years earlier I had begun research in psychopharmacology by looking at serotonin reuptake in depressed people. At the time, few outside the pharmaceutical industry knew a group of drugs were being developed to inhibit serotonin reuptake—the SSRIs, or selective serotonin reuptake inhibitors. Prozac was to become the best known, a symbol for a generation. I was working on just the right thing—anticipating the next wave of treatments.

Depression was then almost unrecognized, compared to our own day. Through the 1980s and early 1990s I contributed to the view that depression was grossly underdiagnosed. More awareness, the argument went, and more use of antidepressants might be much better than diagnosing people as anxious and putting them on tranquilizers. Now I was faced with the consequences. It had probably been a mistake to diagnose Gordon as depressed. Whether or not he was depressed, it was a mistake for Gordon to take Prozac. Doing so killed him.

This, then, is a story about people like Gordon, Jane, and me, and how we have been living, in the words of Tennessee Williams, under the thundercloud of a common experience. The story takes in the network of "friends" that makes the psychopharmacology and other scientific worlds go around, worlds in which the good guys could easily be the bad guys. Some of the players in this story get to play both sides, and I can't be sure I haven't simply ended up by accident on one side of an argument. The dividing lines that history interposes between the good guys and the bad guys after the event are fine ones that owe much to the fact that history is written by those who don't get caught. This is a story about a game played with certain rules.

THE RULES OF THE GAME

In the 1960s the laws governing the patenting of drugs changed. Companies could now take out patents on a compound, rather than on the method of producing it or on the use to which a drug would be put. Without this change in the rules of the game, Prozac could never have become as big a commercial phenomenon as it did. The same change made a host of new drugs inaccessible to the planet's most vulnerable populations. So it was that major pharmaceutical corporations in 2001 instituted a legal action against South Africa—for trying, as it quickly came to be portrayed, to put the needs of their people before the value of company share prices.

The same rules now apply to the patenting of genes. Biotechnology companies can patent stretches of the human genome with minimal, if any, specification of the use to which these sequences will be put. As a consequence, university or other laboratories seeking to produce a diagnostic test for a disorder find themselves liable to be sued. Biotechnology companies can charge what they want for their version of a test, and there is little incentive for them to come up with a more effective test.

Does this put academia at odds with the new health care corporations? Far from it! For twenty years now, most universities have actively encouraged their researchers to patent anything produced in or discovered in university laboratories, or have built laboratories jointly with pharmaceutical or other corporations. The products of research are likely to be sold to the highest bidder. The scientific rush to make important research findings public has been checked in many universities and hospitals by patent officers. Protesting academics are likely to fall foul of their institutions.

This privatization has been compared to enclosure in sixteenth-century England, when people lost access to what were formerly lands held in common by villages or communities. Enclosures were the basis for the capitalization of land. We now face an enclosure and capitalization of the very stuff that makes us human.

These are vast developments. Nobody could believably assess such complexity single-handedly. It would be even more presumptuous to prescribe a solution.

But when one tentacle of a beast presents itself cleanly, there is a merit in describing that tentacle in detail, so others may infer the nature of the beast. Scorn may be heaped on the blind men trying to describe the elephant, but the work of one blind man can tell those who know nothing about elephants . . . something, at least. Only the fully sighted can afford to mock the blind, and few could claim to be fully sighted about the matters raised here.

This book came about when I was grabbed by a tentacle of the beast and had a five-year chance to study it. The tentacle came tattooed with a Prozac logo. Rooms full of data pointed to the fact that the Prozac drug group could trigger suicide and violence, and that companies producing these drugs knew of the problem. This company knowledge pointed to a structural problem in the system that gives us drugs, biotechnology, and other health care product—a problem that seems likely to produce a drug or health care disaster to dwarf that of thalidomide on the Richter scale of drug disasters in the near future.[1]

The Prozac story brings interlinked problems to light, among them a creation of depression on so extraordinary and unwarranted a scale as to raise questions about whether pharmaceutical and other health care companies are more wedded to making profits from health than contributing to it. This marketing, combined with a falloff in the number of breakthrough compounds, suggests that pharmaceutical companies are now better at marketing drugs than at making them.

Those of us who are not depressed cannot step back from what has happened, for one consequence of this marketing is that it is now widely assumed that our serotonin levels fall when we feel low, and this lowering is thought to affect everything from our diets to how we educate our children and how we manage criminality. But there is no evidence for any of this, nor has there ever been. A huge gap has opened up between what is scientifically demonstrable and what people believe, pointing to a cultural phenomenon that lies well beyond the "medicalization" so worrying to sociologists and bioethicists. And in through this gap have marched a growing host of books, from Peter Kramer's *Listening to Prozac* to Andrew Solomon's *Noonday Demon*, Lauren Slater's *Prozac Diaries*, and Elizabeth Wurtzel's *Prozac Nation*. There is something here that reaches down to the level of the myths we make to live by. Our ideas of what it means to be human are at stake.

On another front, the Prozac story raises insistent questions about the regulation of big business. Many who advise regulators on the entry of drugs into the market also advise the major pharmaceutical companies. At certain points in the Prozac story, it will seem the only explanation for what has happened lies between scientifically incompetent regulation, duplicitous advice, or regulation by the pharmaceutical industry itself. On the legal front, lawyers now argue in court that one type of evidence proves nothing in the case of smoking and lung cancer and that another type of evidence is needed, while lawyers from the same companies, in the case of Prozac, can argue exactly the reverse—just one type of evidence will do very well.

Apart from these specifically moral and political matters, this story questions the input from academics at the interface between Big Business and Big Science. The training of academics is subsidized by the communities from which they come. This once seemed a reasonable option for citizens and governments, since university or other higher training produced experts at one remove from the business-industrial complex. But academics who were once the substantive movers in health care now serve as ornamental additions to business. How else can we interpret the fact that probably at least 50 percent of academic publications in therapeutics are now ghostwritten (see chapter 4), in particular those in the most prestigious medical journals? How else do we interpret a circumstance where some of the most eminent figures in the academic health-science research community appear party to the suppression of data on lethal side effects of treatments, and such behavior has become something of a norm?

These developments, laid out in detail here, should be at the very least deeply embarrassing to the academic community. To dismiss the question of who gets her or his name on a scientific article as a superficial problem, readily corrected, would be entirely wrong. It might be wrong on moral grounds, but even more important, it would allow that academic health care need not deliver better drugs or better health care. Under the veneer of modern academic authorship, the furniture is rotting.

The Prozac story reveals a lack of research so complete that academics cannot avoid questions about how well the health-science research community serves us. How far is this absence of research a direct effect of industry funding practices? Had there been independent research in psychopharmacology since 1990, Prozac could never have become the phenomenon it turned out to be. Had there been independent research, American lawyers bringing Prozac-induced suicide cases to court would not have been in the position of seeking expert witness from outside the United States, and I would not have written this story.

I would also probably now be working in Canada rather than Britain. Colleagues in the pharmaceutical industry advised me that people become legal experts only at the end of their careers. What might happen to me if I got involved? They didn't know. But for many people, what *did* happen when the University of Toronto breached its contract with me has become a symbol of a crisis in academic freedom produced automatically when pharmaceutical companies fund medical-scientific research.

I now believe it was unreasonably dangerous to leave Prozac, Zoloft, Celexa, and Paxil on the market without warnings. I believe there has been a failure by regulators and experts in psychiatry to resolve a problem to which students of medicine could have given the correct answer. Failure on this scale suggests that some new arrangement is needed to tackle the problems of drug-induced injury. And it directly implies a new and fundamental reordering of the governance and financing of health and medical research in higher education.

I believe we need a new contract between society and the pharmaceutical industry—a contract that will require access to the raw data that result when people like the readers of this book give their personal details and take risks in studies for pharmaceutical companies, doing all this for nothing, in a process that makes these companies the most profitable corporations on the planet. The issues are ones that seem to have implications across the biotechnology and other health care industries and for the interface between academia and industry.

In contrast to others who have written books hostile to physical therapies in psychiatry, I write this as someone committed to pharmacotherapy. In my opinion, getting by without physical treatments, hoping psychotherapy alone will do the job, is a romantic notion. Psychiatry is a tough and confronting business. In most people's eyes, I would count as a member of the pharmacotherapy establishment.[2] Despite occupying this inside track, I have had great difficulty bringing to light a hazard of pharmacotherapy.

This book is a history in that some of the key questions have now been answered conclusively—SSRIs can trigger suicidal tendencies. But it is still not clear what has been an honest mistake and what a conspiracy. The book remains therefore written in the first person, chronologically and through flashbacks, to avoid suggesting any one person should have known X or Y. There is the even trickier question of the motives of key figures in the drama, motives perhaps unknowable even to the players themselves. At certain places the story comes to a clear point; at others it is mired in ambiguity. In considering the possible motives of the players, my own included, it is well to remember the words of Gandhi: "He who would do a great evil must first of all convince himself he is doing a great good."

Introduction

Before Prozac

The disease that has on several occasions nearly killed me does kill tens of thousands of people every year: most are young, most die unnecessarily, and many are among the most imaginative and gifted that we as a society have.[1]

FEW COULD READ Kay Redfield Jamison's 1995 book *Unquiet Mind* and fail to agree that manic-depressive disease is debilitating and dangerous. For skeptics, the underlying statistics and science are laid out in her monograph with Fred Goodwin, then director of the National Institutes for Mental Health (NIMH), *Manic-Depressive Illness.*[2] Any remaining skeptics would be likely to recant on hearing Jamison or other international figures talk in the flesh about their illness. But for romantics, the personal testimonies of experts like Jamison can cause problems because these experts endorse treatments such as electroconvulsive therapy (ECT), lithium, and psychotropic drugs. To claim to be the survivor of a psychiatric treatment makes for glamorous television material, but Jamison and others talk about being the survivors of a psychiatric illness—one that wrecks families and careers and claims lives.

The passion of Jamison and others has brought new recognition for sufferers of mood disorders and has ensured funding for research that someday will make a difference. Yet there is a fine line to tread. Just as corporate culture can incorporate Levi's jeans and countercultural lifestyles, so also the message of someone like Jamison can be corrupted and used to sell treatments to people who should not have them—and whose lives may be put at risk by them.

As recently as 1990, there was seemingly little danger that depression could be corporatized. But about the time the Internet began to be used frequently in universities, and exam results began to prove conclusively that women on average did better academically than men, things changed. Readers who remember what it was like to live in a world without the Internet will not so easily remember what it was like to live in a world where few, if any, risked getting depression. Yet this was so only a few years ago—before Prozac.

Magazines, newspapers, and television programs are now full of stories about how extraordinarily common and seriously disabling depression is.[3] It is billed as one of the greatest and most common afflictions of mankind, second only to heart disease as a cause of disability in the world. This seems to mesh with Jamison's message that this is a serious disease. But the story of depression hides at least three disturbing surprises.

First, unlike manic-depressive illness, depression was all but unrecognized before the antidepressants; only about fifty to one hundred people per million were thought to suffer from what was then melancholia. Current estimates put that figure at one hundred thousand affected people per million.[4] This is a *thousandfold* increase, despite the availability of treatments supposed to cure this terrible affliction.

Second, the discovery of antidepressants was not recognized at the time as a medical breakthrough. Indeed, they were almost an embarrassment to the companies who found them.

The third surprise is that it was recognized from the discovery of the very first antidepressants that they might lead to suicide.

All three surprises come together in the story of Caitlin Hurcombe, told by her mother:

> The policeman, eyes averted, handed me her suicide note. There was a damp teardrop directly blurring the word "love." I thought, "Your tear hasn't dried, Caitlin, how can you be dead?"
>
> It was a Monday in April 1998 when my 19-year-old daughter balanced herself on a piano stool, covered her head with a pillowcase and hanged herself with her pony's lunge rope from a beam in the bedroom. The executioner in her head allowed her no room for error.
>
> Since her devastating death I have become an expert on suicide, on bullying, on teenagers and depression, young people and violence, on suicide prevention. Searching for a "why." All bereaved parents who have lost a loved one to suicide will experience this to one degree or another, and the common wisdom is to find a way to "let go."

Letting go of what is both irreplaceable and unforgettable is rather a tall order.

Caitlin was prescribed Prozac a few weeks before she killed herself. The inquest revealed that there was no drug in her system other than a therapeutic dose of Prozac. We had gone through a very rackety Christmas during which Caitlin learned, not for the first time, what rotters boy friends can be. Many of her friends recommended that she try Prozac for her unhappiness, not least because "you lose weight on it."

As an American expat I have too many times been duped myself by the instant cures promised by popping pills. An honest description of my feelings about Caitlin taking Prozac would be "gently skeptical." I read her an alternative medical pamphlet on the virtues of St. John's Wort over Prozac. She still wanted the Prozac and she got it. How could millions of people the world over be wrong? Danger wasn't an issue.

Her doctor said not to worry if she didn't feel better immediately, because the drug took sometimes two weeks or more to "kick in." The change in Caitlin's behavior, however, was immediate and dramatic. She danced into the kitchen after college after taking pill number one, saying she felt great. But her elation was short-lived. Her behavior turned bizarre. Break-ins at college, fierce arguments with her tutor. Ferocious poetry. Stealing a stereo from the house of a local man not coincidentally called "psycho," and saying she didn't know why. Nightmares of murdering me and of her own death. And finally on the last weekend of her life, a wild distracted skipping of college, self-mutilation, and a drunken and sordid episode in a pub.

Caitlin's life is no less precious because she gave it up. And Prozac is no less dangerous to young people just because millions swear by it. Among the hundreds of treasured letters and cards of condolence, so many said, "It's not your fault!" "Depression is a physical disease!" When first she died we tortured ourselves wondering how we could have overlooked her suffering. We thought she was just very good at masking her pain. Caitlin's counsellor concluded she was "normal," "psychologically intact." So now I know that she was a normal angst-ridden and unhappy girl-woman, finding life hard to cope with. And I believe the Prozac was her executioner.[5]

Opinions will divide on whether Caitlin Hurcombe committed suicide because of Prozac or because she was depressed. After all, Kay Jamison could easily have committed suicide before her condition was recognized. But for those who have no doubt it was the illness that caused the suicide, the story of the origins of the antidepressants offers a disturbing fact. Forty-five years before Caitlin Hurcombe hanged herself, it was known that antidepressants could produce suicides in people not depressed. In fact, we would not have had Prozac had this *not* been the case.

"NERVES BEFORE PROZAC"

During the first eighty years of the twentieth century, depression was considered a rare disorder. The vast majority of nervous states were seen as anxiety disorders. Individuals suffering from "nerves" were noted to have increased heart rates, butterflies in their stomach or other gastrointestinal complaints, headaches, sweating, and breathlessness. The influence of Freud and psychoanalysis did a great deal to popularize the existence of nerves of this kind and to shape the portrayal of this condition as an anxiety disorder that could be treated, whether by drugs or by talking therapies.

Popular thinking was also influenced by the world wars, which brought home the idea that extreme environmental stress could produce "nervous breakdowns." The most common treatment of the condition was sedation. Opiates or alcohol had been the sedative of choice through the nineteenth century. Bromides and barbiturates replaced these in the first half of the twentieth century. In the 1930s, dexamphetamine and other stimulants were marketed for people who suffered from chronic fatigue. The first of "mother's little helpers," Dexamyl, combining a stimulant and a sedative—dexamphetamine and amylobarbitone—appeared in the 1950s,[6] producing dramatic benefits for "nerves" that are still not easily explained.

People with "nerves" could access these treatments without much medical intervention, since most were available over the counter. Once medical help was sought, a prescription could be refilled regularly without further medical contact. As a result, it is harder to gauge the level of nervous problems in the first half of the twentieth century than now, but it is likely that it was no lower and no higher than today.

The launching of meprobamate under the brand name Miltown in 1955 was a watershed.[7] This drug was discovered by Frank Berger, a

Czechoslovak who emigrated to the United States before the Second World War. Drug discovery at that time had little input from academic medicine, and Berger was working on muscle relaxants in the laboratories of Carter-Wallace when he discovered that meprobamate calmed laboratory animals without unduly sedating them. Since muscular tension was a feature of anxiety, muscular relaxation without sedation might be good for anxiety states. Given that his new drug was less sedative than older drugs, Berger adopted a new term—*tranquilizer.*[8]

Miltown at first looked to be the ideal answer for everyday anxiety. It produced a pleasant, relaxed feeling that "liberated" people from their nerves, encouraging them to do things they would not have done otherwise. Because it left many people feeling *better* than well, a Miltown craze was born in the newspapers and on radio and the newly emerging television.[9]

Librium and Valium followed Miltown in the early 1960s. These benzodiazepine drugs looked as effective as Miltown but were even less likely to cause sedation or dependence. Hoffman La Roche brilliantly marketed Librium and Valium, "helping" doctors to realize that a significant proportion of the physical complaints appearing in their offices might be manifestations of anxiety. What drove ulcers, if not anxiety? No one knew what caused hypertension, but it sounded as though these patients were bottling up their anxiety. Patients with asthma or other breathing conditions were often anxious, as were patients with headaches. For all these conditions, it became widespread practice to prescribe a tranquilizer along with whatever other medication the patient was taking. Physicians were encouraged to give Valium to college students who were facing the stresses of their new environment. Housewives were regularly prescribed Valium to cope with the stresses of new suburban lifestyles. Busy executives were taking it. Sales of Valium soared in the 1970s, until at one point it was the best-selling drug on the market.

Critics began to question the appropriateness of tranquilizing on such a mass scale.[10] Would these new agents dull the natural competitiveness people need for survival in a hard world? Would people (and, indeed, nations) become less fit for survival if these drugs were overused? Problems coping at college surely were not *medical* disorders. The student revolutionaries of the late 1960s argued that it was the political system that was confusing and disorienting people, and the appropriate therapeutic intervention was to change the system rather than treat individuals. This general political charge took a specific shape when the British government took Roche to court on the issue of overpricing and won.

The benzodiazepine story came to an end in the 1980s.[11] But the undoing of the benzodiazepines came not from overcharging or from mass prescribing to mask social ills. It came when the possibility was raised, around the end of the 1970s, that these drugs that had been so relied upon might lead to dependence. This specter helped create the phenomenon of health news. Before 1980, it was unusual to see health coverage in major newspapers. In the 1980s, however, stories about benzodiazepines began to appear regularly, contributing to a regular health section in newspapers. Talk shows such as *Donahue* and *Oprah* in America and *That's Life* in England, on which individuals discuss their problems, furthered these developments. Health was a natural subject for these shows, leading indirectly to the formation of coalitions of campaigning patients on matters such as benzodiazepine dependence.

The benzodiazepines were portrayed as addictive, despite protests from clinicians that this was not the case. Animal tests of abuse liability, the establishment argued, showed benzodiazepines did not have the abuse liability of heroin, cocaine, or other classic drugs of abuse. Addicts might use "Benzos," but they had little street value. In contrast, they had a clear therapeutic niche, and most patients were able to discontinue benzodiazepines without incident. The establishment views carried little weight against a rising tide of discontent and the outlining of the concept of normal dose dependence by Malcolm Lader, a professor of psychopharmacology at the Maudsley Hospital in London, and others. Before the 1980s, addicts had been socially shunned as perpetrators of their own downfall. In contrast, benzodiazepine "addicts" were seen as victims of a medico-pharmaceutical establishment, and blame was directed at medical practitioners and pharmaceutical company executives. Doctors and drug companies became the villains of the piece.[12]

The benzodiazepines rapidly passed in Western public perception from remarkably safe medicines to one of the greatest dangers to modern society. The extraordinary nature of this development can be seen in sharper focus when contrasted with what happened in Japan.[13] Whether because of safer prescribing in lower doses, or because the Japanese are genetically less liable to dependence on benzodiazepines, or because the tranquilized state was more socially desirable in Japan than comparable states of mind in the West, there was never a problem with benzodiazepine use in Japan. When the tranquilizer market collapsed in the West, it continued to grow in Japan, despite medical reforms and a growing acceptance that benzodiazepines should not be prescribed for hypertension, ulcers, or similar conditions. In contrast, the Japanese antidepressant market remained a small one, with no Prozac available as late as 2003.

An important, though rarely mentioned, element in this story was the role of other pharmaceutical companies in bringing the benzodiazepines down.[14] When concerns were first raised about the benzodiazepines, another group of drugs active on serotonin was in clinical trials. This group of drugs, of which buspirone (BuSpar) was later the best known, was in market development, and as part of this, Mead Johnson in America and Bristol-Myers Squibb in Britain were prepared to highlight the problems of the benzodiazepines as part of a campaign to market buspirone as the first non-dependence-producing anxiolytic.[15]

Bristol-Myers Squibb sponsored symposia at conferences, special supplements in journals, and other articles by experts. They provided an opportunity for speakers to address large audiences of primary-care practitioners and psychiatrists, outlining the hazards of the benzodiazepines. This type of exercise, treading a fine line between education and marketing, is commonplace. It may do good. It may do harm. In this case it backfired. Physicians and others were skeptical of the idea of a non-dependence-producing anxiolytic. The benzodiazepine crisis had educated physicians to expect that any drug that treated anxiety would in due course be found to cause dependence. Patient resistance to BuSpar paralleled this physician skepticism: Buspirone was not as pleasant to take as the benzodiazepines. It flopped. The tranquilizer era was over, and an antidepressant era was about to start.

THE ANTIDEPRESSANT ERA[16]

Conventionally, the antidepressant story starts in 1957 with the twin discoveries of the tricyclic antidepressant imipramine, by Roland Kuhn, and the monoamine oxidase inhibitor (MAOI) iproniazid, by Nathan Kline. But the pharmaceutical companies involved, Geigy and Roche, had little interest in an antidepressant and did nothing to promote either of these drugs. Very few clinicians in office practice seemed to encounter depression. When Merck launched another antidepressant, amitriptyline, in 1961, unlike Geigy and Roche it decided it needed to market depression as well as amitriptyline. Frank Ayd from Baltimore, the first investigator to detect the antidepressant properties of amitriptyline, had published a 1961 book titled *Recognizing the Depressed Patient.*[17] Merck commissioned fifty thousand copies of the book to distribute to general physicians and psychiatrists wherever the compound was being marketed. Amitriptyline quickly became the best selling of this group of drugs, later called the tricyclic antidepressants (TCAs or tricyclics) because of their three-ringed molecular structure. But despite Merck's efforts, the antidepressants remained the poor cousins of the tranquilizers.[18]

During the 1960s and 1970s, senior figures in biological psychiatry such as Nathan Kline and Fred Goodwin in the United States and Paul Kielholz in Switzerland argued that many patients diagnosed as anxious were in fact depressed, and the appropriate treatment was an antidepressant rather than an anxiolytic. This vision led Kielholz in 1972, supported by Ciba-Geigy, to set up the first meeting of the Committee for the Prevention and Treatment of Depression.[19] The brief of the group was to establish what needed to be done to improve the recognition and treatment of depressive disorders. In the United States, Paul Wender and Don Klein set up a comparable National Foundation for Depressive Illness in the late 1980s.

The research underpinning the new thinking about depression came from social psychiatrists. In 1966, Michael Shepherd in London published the first book to suggest primary-care physicians rather than psychiatrists might be seeing the vast bulk of nervous problems, and that a great many of these problems could be viewed as depression.[20] This laid the groundwork for a host of studies in the 1980s surveying depression in the general population, which in turn formed the basis for marketing the SSRIs.[21] Far from welcoming the marketing of the SSRIs, Shepherd regarded the consequences of his research falling into the hands of pharmaceutical companies as comparable to those of the sorcerer leaving his apprentice alone in the workshop.[22]

Another development came with the creation of DSM-III. Following the introduction of the new psychotropic drugs, in the late 1960s psychiatry was faced with the development of antipsychiatry, which questioned the legitimacy of psychiatric diagnoses and practices. Psychologists posing as patients famously got themselves admitted to psychiatric hospitals, unsuspected by medical staff even though real patients easily detected the fraud.[23] The controversies swirling around psychiatry led in 1980 to the introduction of operational criteria for psychiatric disorders in a revised diagnostic manual, DSM-III. In DSM, anxiety neurosis was broken down into a number of apparently different disorders—social phobia, generalized anxiety disorder, panic disorder, post-traumatic stress disorder (PTSD), and obsessive-compulsive disorder. In contrast, the depressive disorders were collapsed into one large category—major depressive disorder.

DSM-III's new formulations emerged just as Kielholz's Committee for the Prevention and Treatment of Depression laid the basis for national campaigns such as Depression—Awareness, Recognition, and Treatment (DART), in the United States, and Defeat Depression, in the United Kingdom. Eli Lilly supported both campaigns. In the case of DART, Lilly funds went into eight million brochures titled *Depression: What You Need to Know* and two hundred thousand posters.[24] As Lew Judd, the director of the U.S. National Institute of Mental Health (NIMH) in 1987, put it: "By making these materials on depressive illness available, accessible in physicians' offices all over the country, important information is effectively reaching the public in settings which encourage questions, discussion, treatment, or referral." Campaigns like this can do great good—or they can be self-serving.

In the early 1990s, surveys by the Defeat Depression campaign found most people thought everyday depression was not the kind of condition that should be treated with pills.[25] But DART and other national campaigns were launched on the waves of an incoming tide. The 1980s saw a dramatic increase in articles about depression in both medical journals and general-readership magazines.[26] Those hostile to psychiatry may smell a conspiracy, but the real interpretation has probably to do with a vacuum opening up. Both academic and lay media were reporting benzodiazepine horror stories in contrast to the feel-good stories of previous years. There was a vacancy for stories about a new feel-good drug. News that clinicians such as Nathan Kline and Fred Goodwin had been trying to cultivate for years, previously choked of light by the canopy of overhanging tranquilizer publicity, was given a chance to grow. But no one expected it would turn out quite so easy to change medical perceptions.

The depression campaigns had a twofold strategy. One was to alert physicians and third-party payers in health care to the huge economic burdens of untreated depression. The campaigns were so successful in this strategy that a decade later no one bats an eye at claims that depression is one of the greatest single health burdens on mankind.[27] But no one asks whether treatments that are supposed to make a difference actually do produce benefits. There is plenty of evidence that antidepressants can be shown to do something in the short term but almost no evidence that things turn out better in the long run, and there are many reasons to worry that we might be making things worse. Something must surely be going wrong if the frequency of depression apparently jumps a thousandfold since the introduction of the antidepressants.[28]

The second strategy involved a series of educational campaigns to show physicians how many cases of depression they were missing—to shame them into detecting and treating depression. The tragedy of Sylvia Plath's suicide, for instance, was held up as something that could have been prevented with better recognition of depression.[29] This new emphasis has almost certainly led to diagnosis of depression for many people who do not regard themselves as being depressed or in need of treatment. In individual cases, this heightening of clinician sensitivity to depression may have saved lives; on a broader front, there is no evidence that mass detection and treatment of depression have lowered national suicide or disability rates.[30]

The antidepressant story has a further important twist. The conventional wisdom as of the early 1980s was that, unlike tranquilizers, which were feel-good agents that delivered a relatively immediate payoff, antidepressants took several weeks to work. Prescribers were educated to tell patients they could even expect to feel worse for some weeks before they began to feel better. This strategy sent the message that these were not quick-fix pills but rather medications that really corrected the problem.

But this educational information becomes problematic when these drugs are made available on prescription only from physicians trained to deliver just this message. Against a background of instructions that these pills might take many weeks to work, on the one hand, for many doctors the idea that Prozac or other antidepressants might lead to suicidal tendencies or other severe problems during the early period "before the pills begin working" seems a contradiction in terms. On the other hand, patients faced with a doctor who has not been educated about the potential hazards in the early phase of treatment risk being trapped by their relationship with their doctor. Where patients would probably discontinue an over-the-counter medication if it did not seem to suit them, regard for their doctor, who very likely will advise them to continue treatment, can convince many to continue with a treatment that might kill them.

The messages of the depression campaigns were based on treatment of people hospitalized for the types of severe depression described by Kay Redfield Jamison. For these depressions, it made sense to avoid recurrences, and long-term treatment seemed a good idea. But this was an entirely different kind of disorder from the stress and adjustment reactions and adolescent turmoil for which the SSRIs increasingly came to be administered in the 1990s, disorders that last on average less than three months.[31] Furthermore, the economics of depression put forward to justify mass detection and treatment of depression were all worked out initially on the basis of the Jamison form of depression. None of the assumptions of such models—for example, that treatment will lower suicide rates or improve quality of life—holds for the kinds of "depression" that exist in the wider society.

SEROTONIN AND DEPRESSION

For many people, one of the key factors that make it reasonable to take an antidepressant is the belief that a lowering of the brain neurotransmitter serotonin has been demonstrated in depression. If there actually were a confirmed lowering of serotonin in depression, giving drugs that raised serotonin levels might seem a good idea.

The presence in the brain of serotonin was first reported in 1954.[32] This quickly led to the hypothesis that this monoamine neurotransmitter might play some role in nervous problems. One way to investigate this possibility was to look at the levels of the main metabolite of serotonin in the cerebrospinal fluid that bathes the brain. In 1960, George Ashcroft, working in Edinburgh, found that cerebrospinal 5HIAA levels, the metabolite of serotonin, in depressives appeared to be low, leading to the first theory that serotonin might be low in cases of depression.[33]

While Europe was convinced that serotonin was a key neurotransmitter in nervous disorders, North Americans were certain that norepinephrine was more important. Julius Axelrod, working at the National Institutes of Health (NIH), had discovered an uptake mechanism for norepinephrine in 1961 and later found that tricyclic antidepressants like imipramine blocked this mechanism.[34] Axelrod dismissed European work on serotonin as unimportant—serotonin was just "a remnant of our marine past."[35]

In 1965, the NIMH's Joseph Schildkraut published his catecholamine hypothesis of depression.[36] This was the key article of the new biological psychiatry, its *Interpretation of Dreams*. Schildkraut put forward the idea that brain norepinephrine was lowered in depression and that antidepressants acted to increase its levels. Whatever the science base for this claim, crucially, this was a new language that both practicing psychiatrists and patients could understand. Talk of sexual complexes yielded to a new patter: "You have a chemical imbalance; these pills will restore your brain to normal." Magazines from *Time* and *Newsweek* to the *New Republic* and the *National Enquirer* could embrace this idea, crucial to the later success of Prozac. This key myth still flourishes in popular consciousness almost forty years later.

By 1970, however, Ashcroft had concluded that, whatever was wrong in depression, it was not lowered serotonin. More sensitive studies had shown no lowering of serotonin.[37] Indeed, no abnormality of serotonin in depression has ever been demonstrated.[38] By the early 1970s, moreover, Ashcroft and colleagues had introduced receptors into psychiatry, after which few psychopharmacologists could be heard talking about a lowering of either serotonin or norepinephrine in depression.[39] A gap opened up between the science base and public understanding—a gap crucial to the later development of media talk about lowered serotonin levels.

But if the idea of lowered serotonin causing depression doesn't come from scientific studies, where does it come from? The marketing of the SSRIs has emphasized that they increase serotonin levels: Does this not mean they were designed to increase serotonin levels in patients where it is low? The answers to these questions interlock in the story of reserpine, one of the first "antidepressants," which lowered serotonin but also led to suicide.

PROZAC PREFIGURED

The psychopharmacological era began in 1952 when two drugs, reserpine and chlorpromazine, transformed the prospects for mental illness.

Initially, there was no such thing as an antipsychotic or antidepressant, partly because both of these drugs looked like they might be useful for all nervous problems. Chlorpromazine sold in Europe under the trade name Largactil because it seemed to work for a large range of conditions. Reserpine sold as Serpasil, and its distinctive benefits probably led F. F. Yonkmann, a scientist working at Ciba, to coin the term *tranquilizer.* When meprobamate and, later, the benzodiazepines hijacked this new term, reserpine and chlorpromazine became the major tranquilizers.

Nathan Kline was the first to show that reserpine in relatively large doses could be useful for treating psychoses. There was every reason to believe that in lower doses it might be beneficial for treating anxiety or depressive disorders. This led Michael Shepherd to undertake the first modern clinical trial in psychiatry, in which he compared reserpine and a placebo in a group of anxious depressives.[40] Reserpine came out as an antidepressant.[41] The results of Shepherd's study, published in 1955, were better than later results for Prozac in similar patient groups. But the discovery of the antidepressant properties of reserpine vanished without trace, because for Ciba, the makers of Serpasil, the idea of an antidepressant was a complication rather than an added benefit, just as it was for Geigy and Roche.

Shepherd's 1955 clinical trial paper was the first of its kind. Also in 1955, another reserpine paper was the first paper in another new scientific literature. In this, Steve Brodie and colleagues at the NIH demonstrated that reserpine both sedated rabbits and lowered their brain serotonin levels.[42] This was the first demonstration of a link between brain chemistry and behavior. Brodie's study, published in *Science,* became the classic that established the field of neuroscience, and pharmacologists from around the world visited him.

Within two years, other laboratories had shown that reserpine also lowered norepinephrine and dopamine levels. Unaware that reserpine had been shown to be an antidepressant, Schildkraut made reserpine's capacity to lower norepinephrine levels the key element in his theory of depression, on the basis of reserpine's ability to trigger suicide.

The capacity of reserpine to cause suicide was not discovered within psychiatry. In the early 1950s, in addition to being used for nervous problems, reserpine was used as an antihypertensive. A number of physicians noted that hypertensive patients taking reserpine reported feeling "better than well." In 1954, Robert Wilkins, in a phrase that echoes the later Prozac story, claimed physicians were suggesting it was time to give up psychotherapy, as reserpine was good psychotherapy in pill form.[43]

But starting in 1955, a series of reports emerged of hypertensive patients becoming "depressed" on reserpine and committing suicide. In the pages of *The Lancet*, for example, immediately prior to Shepherd's report on the antidepressant effects of reserpine, papers from New Zealand and Australia report on reserpine-induced suicidality in hypertensive patients.[44] Psychiatrists argued that chlorpromazine caused similar problems.[45] Both drugs, it seemed, could make some patients feel flat and unmotivated or anxious; but in contrast to proper depression, this problem cleared up once the drug was stopped or if the patient was given a stimulant. Nevertheless, the notion that reserpine caused depression crept into the literature.

The misidentification of the problems that reserpine caused may have been one of the greatest mistakes in psychopharmacology. In the first paper to describe hypertensive patients becoming suicidal on reserpine, in 1955, Richard Achor and colleagues from the Mayo Clinic reported that reserpine caused some patients "increased tenseness, restlessness, insomnia and a feeling of being very uncomfortable."[46] Robert Faucett gave further details: "The first few doses frequently made them anxious and apprehensive. . . . They reported increased feelings of strangeness, verbalized by statements such as 'I don't feel like myself' . . . or 'I'm afraid of some of the unusual impulses that I have.'"[47] Gerald Sarwer-Foner described a subject who, on the first day of treatment, reacted with marked anxiety and weeping, and on the second day "felt so terrible with such marked panic at night that the medication was cancelled."[48]

This is not depression. These quotes are the first descriptions of a phenomenon new to physicians and psychiatrists. In 1955, in an unfortunate choice of terms, two German-speaking psychiatrists, Hans Steck and Hans Haase, labeled the problem *akathisia*.[49] Akathisia, which literally refers to an inability to sit still, was a problem first noted following brain injuries and then in the encephalitis lethargica epidemic of 1918. Encephalitis lethargica produced instant Parkinson's disease in some people, rendering them mute and stuporous, but it made others restless and agitated.[50] Akathisia was later to become a recognized hazard of antipsychotic drugs, one associated with suicide and homicide.[51] But awareness of what was involved for many years did not percolate outside a specialized psychiatric community.

The word *akathisia* remains one of the least understood pieces of medical jargon in the psychiatric lexicon, and the condition has never been properly investigated. The quotes from Faucett and others suggest that the best translation into English is probably "turmoil" or "agitation," rather than "restlessness."[52] When the problem began to show up in company trials of the SSRIs in the 1980s, it was coded under "agitation."

It is often said that a psychiatric drug can never be shown to cause suicide because patients are already at risk of suicide from the nervous condition for which they are being treated. Reserpine demonstrates the superficial nature of this response. None of the people who committed suicide on reserpine had a nervous problem—they were all hypertensive.

As we shall see, Prozac and other SSRIs can also cause suicide in individuals who have no nervous conditions, primarily by inducing mental turmoil during the early stages of treatment. Patients who develop akathisia on SSRIs are likely to be seen by primary-care physicians who have not been trained to recognize the problem. When Prozac and other SSRIs were first launched onto the market, there were no educational programs or warnings about this hazard.

One of the major differences between reserpine and Prozac is that patent laws in the 1950s meant there were up to twenty-six different reserpine-containing compounds on the market. By the time Prozac appeared, the laws had changed so that only one company could own a new compound. Thus no company had the incentive to defend reserpine as Lilly later had to defend Prozac. Arguably, because of this patent situation the problems of reserpine could be recognized, whereas later problems with Prozac could not be acknowledged without potentially putting Lilly out of business. This situation has implications for patients taking any drugs, for the psychiatrists and other physicians who treat them, and for the business practices of the corporations producing the drugs used in treatment.

The reserpine story contains all the seeds of a tragedy in the classical sense, where some flaw within the protagonist brings the hero down. In the early days of the psychopharmacological era, academia looked down in disdain at the pharmaceutical industry, often refusing to allow anyone working in the industry to join academic societies, and refusing to engage with the complex and messy problems posed by therapeutics. To this day, the conflicts between academia and industry are portrayed as a corruption of academia by industry. But an alternative is that there is a repeated failure of academics to engage with the range of scientific and moral issues involved in applied science. The SSRI drugs are among the clearest products of applied science within medicine, and their use peppers the academia/industry interface with as yet unanswered questions. Who are the flawed heroes in this tragedy—the academics or industry?

THE ORIGIN OF THE SSRIS

The scientific literature carries few full-page corrections, but in 1997 a "Correction" appeared in the journal *Life Sciences.*[53] This referred to an article published in 1995 by David Wong, Frank Bymaster, and Eric Engleman from Eli Lilly, titled "Prozac, the First Selective Serotonin Reuptake Inhibitor and an Antidepressant Drug: Twenty Years since Its First Publication."[54] The authors of the correction, Arvid Carlsson and David Wong, agreed that the 1995 article might have given the misleading impression that Prozac was the first of the SSRIs. Prozac was not the first SSRI, nor the first patented, nor the first in clinical trials, nor the first launched.

The origin of the SSRIs lies in the 1960s, when Paul Kielholz became professor of psychiatry in Basel. Given the presence in Basel of the major Swiss chemical companies, Kielholz was well placed to become a leading figure in the world of psychopharmacology. Depression was his area of interest, which he saw as underrecognized and poorly treated. Kielholz believed more had to be done than simply teach physicians to detect depression and put patients on treatment. Different antidepressants did quite different things, he argued, and it was important to select the right antidepressant for the individual patient.[55]

While the molecular structures of the early antidepressants looked very similar, leading to them collectively being called tricyclics, Kielholz argued that some of these tricyclics, such as desipramine, made people well by enhancing drive. Others, such as trimipramine, made patients well through a sedative action. And yet others had some other action on mood or emotions that appeared to be important, which he found difficult to characterize. Clomipramine was the tricyclic that appeared to have more of this mysterious action than other antidepressants.

This was a striking observation that flew in the face of Schildkraut's catecholamine theory, which claimed that all antidepressants essentially did the same thing—they inhibited norepinephrine reuptake. It took a new kind of player within psychopharmacology to resolve this mismatch between clinical and laboratory observations—Arvid Carlsson. Carlsson, from Sweden, was one of the first neuroscientists. Trained in Brodie's laboratory, Carlsson had a string of early research successes to his credit, including participation in the key study demonstrating the existence of neurotransmitter pathways in the brain. He had discovered dopamine in the brain and was among the first to suggest that it might be abnormal in Parkinson's disease, work that later led to a Nobel Prize.[56] By this time he had put forward the first evidence in what later became the dopamine hypothesis of schizophrenia.[57]

Faced with Kielholz's claims, Carlsson saw a connection between the different effects of antidepressants Kielholz proposed and the effects of these same drugs on various neurotransmitter systems. The drugs Kielholz claimed to be drive-enhancing had effects on the norepinephrine system, whereas clomipramine in particular had effects on the serotonin system.[58] This led Carlsson to suggest developing drugs that only inhibited the reuptake of serotonin. Such a drug might help clarify the nature of this mysterious other action of antidepressants and might also produce a useful agent for the treatment of depression.

But being able to detect an effect when a drug is acting on a brain system logically assumes that there is no abnormality in that system. If clomipramine corrected an abnormality in the serotonin system, all that would show up was normalization of the person being treated. Kielholz's claim, in contrast, was that drugs active on the serotonin system were detectably doing something different from other drugs. If, in cases of depression, there were an abnormality of the serotonin system, which SSRIs corrected, these should be among the most potent drugs to treat depression; but (as later became clear) there is little evidence that they work in cases of moderate to severe depression. In contrast, if Kielholz and Carlsson were right, and SSRIs do something different from other antidepressants—for instance, if they produce some kind of anxiolysis—one might expect them to be useful across a range of mixed anxiety and depressive states, rather than just for depression. This is exactly what was found.

ZELMID: THE FIRST SSRI

Following Kielholz's lead, Carlsson set to work with Hanns Corrodi and Peder Berndtsson at Astra's plant in Sweden to create an SSRI. He took the antihistamine chlorpheniramine and manipulated the molecule to come up with zimelidine.[59] Carlsson applied for a patent on zimelidine as a selective serotonin reuptake inhibitor in Sweden, Belgium, and Britain on April 28, 1971. The first patent was published in March 1972. Prozac was patented in 1974.

Zimelidine went into clinical trials comparing it with the norepinephrine reuptake inhibitor desipramine. These trials were short and not conducted on severe depression. The first results were presented in 1980, and zimelidine was launched on the market in Europe as Zelmid in 1982. The first trials of Prozac in depression were not published until 1985, and it was not launched until 1988. After vigorous promotion, Zelmid began to be prescribed widely.

Astra had signed a comarketing agreement with Merck to market Zelmid in the United States. Had this proceeded, there would probably never have been a Prozac phenomenon. Merck was the largest pharmaceutical company in the world and recognized as marketer par excellence. But just as the data on Zelmid was delivered to the U.S. Food and Drug Administration (FDA) in 1982, there were reports that Zelmid could trigger a serious neurological disorder called Guillain-Barré syndrome. This disorder, which could kill by paralyzing the respiratory muscles, led to the immediate removal of Zelmid from the market.[60]

Astra had already begun the development of a derivative of Zelmid, called alaproclate, which was being investigated for treatment of both depression and Alzheimer's disease. But alaproclate caused liver problems in one strain of laboratory mice and was dropped.[61] Shortly thereafter, Astra introduced an innovative antipsychotic, remoxipride, which seemed to have significantly fewer side effects than older agents. Several months after its launch, however, remoxipride was reported to cause aplastic anemia in a small number of people, and it too was withdrawn.

In the face of these setbacks, Astra contemplated withdrawing from the research-based pharmaceutical market to focus on over-the-counter medicines. Around 1990, it was estimated that new FDA regulations and other hurdles to drug development meant that the cost of bringing a drug to market had rocketed to $300 million.[62] No company could easily survive the loss of its flagship compounds. Astra kept going only because they had the breakthrough antiulcer drug omeprazole, the first of the proton-pump inhibitors, on its way to becoming one of the best-selling drugs on the market.[63] Despite the revenues from omeprazole, Astra was forced into a merger later in the decade. This indicates how big the drug development stakes can be. A troublesome side effect early in the life of a new compound can lead to the demise of a company. If the side effect can be portrayed as a feature of the disease being treated—for example, suicidality in the case of an antidepressant—what would a company do if the alternative were to go out of business? This is the ethical dilemma that has faced all the SSRI companies.

Zelmid's history contains two points of special note. The first is that during clinical trials and postlaunch studies, patients taking Zelmid made a greater number of suicide attempts than expected. No one knew what to make of this. Was it an artifact? The same trials indicated that some of the people who did best on Zelmid had been those most suicidal to begin with.[64] When Lilly later ran into serious difficulties getting a license for Prozac in Germany, many outsiders were mystified that German regulators came to a different conclusion about Prozac's suicide risk than had regulators in America, although presented with similar data. The Germans, however, had prior exposure to zimelidine and fluvoxamine (Luvox), whereas Prozac was the first SSRI the FDA was faced with.

The second point to note concerns the patenting of SSRIs. Although Carlsson spent two years in correspondence with senior executives at Lilly before the paper correcting the misleading impression as to who had discovered the SSRIs was published, relatively selective serotonin reuptake inhibitors had, in fact, been on the market long before Carlsson's work. To produce zimelidine, Carlsson and colleagues manipulated the structure of an existing antihistamine, chlorpheniramine, a potent serotonin reuptake inhibitor that has since been shown to share many properties of the SSRIs.[65] For example, it is effective in treating anxiety disorders and panic attacks. If companies or scientists had simply wanted to see what effects these new compounds might have, they needn't have gone to the trouble to create new drugs. But because zimelidine was a new molecule, Astra could take out a patent on it. The patent system offers the possibility of huge returns but brings responsibilities in exchange, which Astra acknowledged.

INDALPINE AND PSYCHIATRY UNDER SIEGE

Another manipulation of the antihistamines produced indalpine,[66] first developed by Gerard le Fur in a French company, Fournier Frères, later part of Rhône Poulenc. After clinical trials, indalpine was marketed in France and other European countries as Upstene, arriving just after Zelmid. It was greeted enthusiastically because it seemed to benefit patients who hadn't responded to other drugs.[67]

But indalpine ran into trouble. Clinical trials in other European countries suggested it might lower white blood cell counts.[68] This happens transiently with many psychotropic drugs and for the most part is not a serious problem, although in rare cases, if undetected, it can prove fatal. But to general astonishment, indalpine was removed from the market.

French psychiatrists were extremely upset and lobbied the company and the government. The experience of Pierre Lambert from Lyon in the south of France was typical. He and his colleagues had investigated more psychotropic drugs before launch than had any other group in either Europe or America,[69] and they believed they had seen dramatic results with indalpine. The effectiveness of the drug was symbolized for them by the apparent recovery and post–indalpine removal suicide of one of their patients. Chronically depressed, she had been transformed by indalpine. When the drug was withdrawn from the market, she relapsed. Nothing else appeared to make any difference. She kept going in the hope that the drug might be restored to the market, but when it wasn't, she committed suicide. Her suicide note asked that instead of flowers, a headstone, or anything else at her funeral, a collection should be made for medical research. Her family later donated the suicide letter and the proceeds of the collection to research.

Indalpine had been born at a time when the development sequence for compounds had not yet been set in stone, and animal studies aimed at detecting problems could continue in parallel with studies in people.

In ongoing toxicology studies after the drug was launched, some of the animals developed liver cancer. There is little reason to believe that the same would have happened in humans. But by this stage, indalpine was being prescribed far more widely than had been expected. It was therefore a statistical certainty that some of those getting indalpine would also develop liver cancers. In light of the toxicology data, who was to know whether these cancers were simply coincidental or had been triggered by the drug? These are difficult calculations for a company to make.

Another factor influenced Rhône Poulenc. A range of what were first termed ecologist or Green groups and, later, pharmacovigilance groups, some of which had been born in the antipsychiatry protests of the late 1960s, had emerged in Germany and other European countries in the 1970s. The ecologists argued against physical therapies in psychiatry. Campaigning had already led to electroconvulsive therapy (ECT) being banned in a number of countries. Psychiatry was under siege.[70] The lowering of white cells that indalpine caused made it a first drug target for these new pharmacovigilantes.

Emboldened by the demise of indalpine, the new pharmacovigilantes set their sights on nomifensine, which in a number of cases had triggered hemolytic anemia.[71] Nomifensine was withdrawn. Senior European psychiatrists were reeling at these developments. In the face of this onslaught from "fringe groups," they dug in. This was not a matter of protecting the pharmaceutical industry but of losing useful tools. There were then no other drugs like indalpine or nomifensine on the market.

The next target for the pharmacovigilantes was the best-selling antidepressant in Europe, mianserin.[72] Like indalpine, mianserin could lower white cell counts. The drug's manufacturer, Organon, received letters pointing out that mianserin could trigger this potentially fatal problem. Roger Pinder, a senior scientist at Organon, supported by many opinion leaders from psychiatry, responded that all the antidepressants then available *except* mianserin could be lethal in overdose, so that even if some people did die from white cell problems with mianserin, overall, fewer would die using it than any other antidepressant. The ecologists were not impressed—suicide, after all, was illegal. (The possibility of accidental overdose was not addressed.)

Organon's defense worked across Europe except in Britain, where the Committee on Safety in Medicines wanted mianserin withdrawn from the market. This led to a series of legal cases; Organon made it clear they were prepared to take the matter all the way to the European Court. This situation was unprecedented. In the ordinary course of events, a company faced with regulatory disapproval would simply comply. Eventually Organon won, but the disputes led to a collapse of mianserin sales in most countries.[73]

The Organon defense involved a risk-benefit calculation. When death from suicide is included in the equation, newer antidepressants may appear safer, although much more expensive and no more effective than the older antidepressants. Safety in overdose became a key card later played by Lilly in its arguments with the regulators over the safety of Prozac. This argument was new to regulators, who were being asked to contemplate a scenario equivalent to the pope being urged to allow condoms on the basis that they minimize the spread of AIDS. Unlike the pope, the regulators were faced with the dilemma that letting a drug with a known hazard remain on the market opened them up to legal actions. This was uncharted territory.

The events surrounding indalpine and mianserin put in place a set of jigsaw pieces that gave glimpses of what was later to be the Prozac story. Pharmacovigilance divisions within companies were pitted against a set of pharmacovigilantes—in Germany, the ecologists; in America, the Church of Scientology. Suicide was to become an issue in these debates. The defense of mianserin showed why companies would want to mobilize a coalition of scientists, a network of "friends," to argue the company's case.[74] The network of senior scientists that Roger Pinder mobilized on Organon's side later played a part in managing the controversy over Prozac in Europe. Lilly organized a similar network in the United States. And finally, lawsuits had become a weapon. From the mid-1980s, companies would need sophisticated legal advice on how to swim in these new waters.

THE MARKETING OF LUVOX

The first SSRI to survive on the world market was fluvoxamine, which was developed in 1973 from another antihistamine.[75] Duphar Laboratories launched fluvoxamine in 1983 in Switzerland, and in the rest of Europe between 1984 and 1986. But in Germany, fluvoxamine was held up because in clinical trials there had been a higher number of suicides and suicide attempts on fluvoxamine than on the drugs with which it was being compared. Duphar was asked to account for this.

Jenny Wakelin, working with the company, consulted with experts around Europe before coming up with the apparently clinching data. When the trials were reanalyzed, focusing specifically on those most suicidal to begin with, it appeared that fluvoxamine was more likely to reduce suicidality than the comparator drugs imipramine and amitriptyline. The lesson many drew from this was that the apparently higher rate of suicide attempts on fluvoxamine was a chance development—that, indeed, SSRIs might be even more antisuicidal than older drugs.[76] The "experts" were learning how to handle the regulators on this issue.

In the 1980s, the first patients to get a new antidepressant were patients hospitalized with depression who seemed unresponsive to other therapies—not a promising group on whom to try a new drug. Poor responses in this group, along with severe nausea in many patients, led to early clinical judgments that fluvoxamine was unlikely to make significant inroads into the antidepressant market. It never did.

But another route to salvation opened up for fluvoxamine. By general agreement, clomipramine, first made in 1958, is the most powerful antidepressant ever made.[77] This tricyclic antidepressant, with actions on both the norepinephrine and serotonin systems, was the last of the major tricyclic antidepressants to come to market. Many viewed it initially as just another "me too" drug. The FDA was keen to discourage copycat drugs and did not license clomipramine.

George Beaumont, a physician with Geigy UK, learned of reports that clomipramine might help treat obsessive-compulsive disorder (OCD).[78] Setting out to establish a niche for clomipramine in the treatment of OCD, Beaumont organized a series of studies in the early 1970s, saw a positive response to the drug, and got clomipramine licensed for the treatment of both depression and OCD in Britain.[79]

Then Judith Rapoport at the NIMH, in a randomized trial, gave children with OCD either desipramine, which has no effect on the serotonin system, or clomipramine. This study demonstrated conclusively that OCD responded to clomipramine but not to desipramine. Before then, the conventional wisdom had been that the benefits from clomipramine in OCD were because an "antidepressant" like clomipramine cleared up the mood disorder that accompanied OCD. But desipramine was also an antidepressant, and Rapoport's study had just demonstrated that it had no effects for OCD.[80] There was something distinctive about drugs that acted on the serotonin system.[81]

After publication of Rapoport's results, and in particular following her runaway best-seller about OCD, *The Boy Who Couldn't Stop Washing*, the scene quickly changed.[82] Rapoport appeared on talk shows like *Donahue* and *Oprah*; OCD, still thought to be a rare disorder, emerged from the shadows. Many who had suffered silently, concealing their rituals and intrusive thoughts for fear of ridicule or being thought insane, came forward for further studies and treatment.

Companies had regarded OCD as even less interesting than depression in the 1950s. But by the late 1980s, under the influence of Rapoport and the success of clomipramine, companies realized that OCD was a market worth pursuing. Clomipramine was finally licensed in the United States in 1990 for the treatment of OCD rather than depression. Meanwhile, Duphar set up a marketing agreement with Upjohn to develop fluvoxamine for OCD, and it made its way onto the U.S. market under the brand name Luvox.[83] Luvox was the low-profile SSRI until the killings at Columbine High School in Colorado, when it was reported that one of the shooters was on Luvox for OCD.

CELEXA AND ZOLOFT—WAR BETWEEN THE SISTERS

Citalopram and escitalopram were first produced in Europe by the Lundbeck Pharmaceutical Company.[84]

In 1971, the company hired Klaus Bøgesø as a medicinal chemist. Over the years, Bøgesø turned out to have a Midas touch at the game of drug hunting. The challenge facing him after his recruitment was to produce a selective norepinephrine reuptake inhibitor. Like other companies at the time, Lundbeck had little interest in an SSRI.

Two potential antidepressants came out of Bøgesø's first efforts— talopram and tasulopram. These were pressed into clinical trials. Both turned out to increase energy levels, and both were linked to a number of suicide attempts. This appeared to confirm one of the major theories of the time, also put forward by Paul Kielholz: that energy-increasing, or activating, antidepressants might lead to suicide. Lundbeck retreated. Suicide was the greatest hazard of an antidepressant. But Kielholz's views also suggested that nonactivating antidepressants would be far less likely to trigger suicide, and SSRIs were less likely to be activating. Following a lead from Carlsson, Bøgesø converted talopram into citalopram, the most selective serotonin reuptake inhibitor to come to the market.

The detour through talopram left Lundbeck behind its competitors. Nevertheless, citalopram became the best-selling antidepressant in a number of European countries. Lundbeck's strategy of undercutting the cost of the other SSRIs and promoting citalopram as the most selective SSRI, and therefore the one least likely to cause side effects, worked.

In the United States, the story was even more extraordinary. In January 1998, the *New Yorker* featured an article by Andrew Solomon titled "Anatomy of Melancholy," an account of the author's own depression.[85] Within a month, Solomon received two thousand letters from other depression sufferers. Clearly, he had struck a nerve. His article was anthologized in more than thirty books, and he became a spokesman in such forums as the American Psychiatric Association.[86] One of the striking points of the piece was his description of the effects of Zoloft as being like drinking fifty-five cups of black coffee, with the effects of Paxil being the equivalent of eleven cups of black coffee. Users seemed well aware of this stimulating effect at a time when both manufacturers and clinicians were denying it.

After failing to negotiate a marketing agreement with Pfizer and then with Warner-Lambert, Lundbeck gave up on the U.S. market. Finally, however, they entered into a licensing arrangement with Forrest Laboratories, a small pharmaceutical company run by a chief executive who appeared confident this drug could run, even though it would have to come from the back of the field. The chief executive was Howard Solomon, Andrew Solomon's father.[87] Launched in September 1998, a strategy of undercutting the price of other SSRIs and aggressive marketing enabled Celexa to capture so large a market share that it became front-page news.[88]

Pfizer's SSRI sertraline began life in 1977.[89] Playing around with the nuclei of some of the original antipsychotic molecules, company chemists produced a series of norepinephrine reuptake inhibitors, of which tametraline looked the most promising. When side effects halted tametraline's development in 1979, Willard Welch transformed it into a series of serotonin reuptake inhibitors, one of which was sertraline.[90]

Like Lundbeck, Pfizer was behind the competition. Sertraline hit the market in North America in 1992 as Zoloft, and in Europe from 1990 through to 1993. Pfizer emphasized technical differences between it and the other SSRIs, claiming that it had a better half-life, a cleaner breakdown route, and a lower liability to interact with other compounds in the body, and that therefore it was much safer than other SSRIs. This marketing strategy produced the appearance of science—lots of data— but very few of these data were clinically relevant. The approach was geared to making Zoloft appear "clean" compared with Prozac and Paxil.[91] The other companies responded, leading to a "war between the sisters."

Pfizer had another approach to new drugs embodied in a program called CRAM—Central Research Assists Marketing—headed up by the marketing department.[92] In the case of Zoloft, this program led Pfizer to establish PRIME-MD, a research program supposedly aimed at collecting data about primary-care depression in order to educate primary-care physicians. This, of course, made it likely that many of these doctors would go on to treat patients who had been identified as depressed, and that Zoloft would be the first drug tried. Another research program, RHYTHMS, was aimed at studying patient education and compliance. The immediate downside to such a program is that improving compliance with treatments not suited to particular patients may increase these patients' risk for suicide. The downside to the larger picture is that this type of market-driven science tends to displace real scientific efforts to answer clinical questions.

PAXIL AND THE SPECTER OF DEPENDENCE

Celexa and Zoloft have been the backing chorus for the big two SSRIs, Prozac and Paxil. Paroxetine was developed in 1978 by Jorgen Buus-Lassen and colleagues in a small Danish company called Ferrosan. Paroxetine was Buus-Lassen's second SSRI. In 1975, he had produced femoxetine, which appeared more effective than paroxetine but had one disadvantage: it was not going to be a simple once-a-day pill.[93]

Ferrosan sold paroxetine to Beecham Pharmaceuticals in 1980, which later merged with SmithKline and French to become SmithKline Beecham (SB). SB merged again at the turn of the millennium with Glaxo to become Glaxo-SmithKline (GSK), at that point the world's largest pharmaceutical corporation. Ferrosan was acquired by Novo-

Nordisk, which had little interest in psychiatry, and femoxetine died from neglect.

Paroxetine nearly died of neglect as well. Beecham was considering shelving paroxetine because it appeared less effective in clinical trials than older antidepressants.[94] A large study run by the Danish Universities Antidepressant Group later confirmed this.[95] This was at a time when the nonhospital depression market still appeared relatively small, and it was not obvious how a less effective antidepressant, even a safer one, could be expected to take a significant share in this market. As a result of company ambivalence, the clinical development of paroxetine lagged behind that of Zelmid, Luvox, and later Prozac.

Paroxetine was licensed as Paxil in 1992 in the United States and as Seroxat in 1991 in the United Kingdom. Marketers within what was now SmithKline Beecham coined the acronym SSRI. Compared to the other serotonin reuptake inhibitors, paroxetine was supposedly the *selective* serotonin reuptake inhibitor.[96] The name worked all too well. It was adopted for the entire group of compounds. Thus Paxil made Prozac and Zoloft into SSRIs.[97]

The idea of an SSRI conveys the impression of a clean and specific drug, freer from side effects than the nonselective tricyclics. However, selectivity meant different things to pharmacologists and clinicians. For pharmacologists, an SSRI could act on every brain system except the norepinephrine system, and SSRIs might in this sense be even dirtier drugs than any of the tricyclics. Clinicians were misled if they thought "selective" meant that these drugs acted on only one brain site; but this was exactly what the marketing of these drugs implied to them.

Where Upjohn had targeted OCD to carve out a distinctive identity for Luvox, SmithKline targeted panic disorder, anxious depressions, generalized anxiety disorder, and, later, social phobia. The targeting of Paxil for anxiety led to huge sales, making Paxil the closest rival to Prozac. When GSK got a license to market Paxil for social phobia, its stock rose: an antishyness pill was potentially a huge market.

Social phobia had, until the 1990s, been almost unknown in the Western world.[98] First described by Isaac Marks in the 1960s at the Institute of Psychiatry in London, social phobia presented rarely to clinics. It would be a mistake, however, to think that SmithKline somehow invented social phobia; in Japan and Korea, social phobias have always been recognized. But there is an obvious overlap between social phobia and shyness. As a consequence, there is a real risk that legitimate efforts to market a treatment of benefit for a disabling medical condition will at the same time capture a significant number of people who are simply shy—and who may be at more risk from the treatment than from their shyness. Furthermore, the term *social phobia* apparently did not suit the brave new world, and in the late 1990s it was replaced by *social anxiety disorder,* raising questions about the culture of psychiatry.[99]

While hugely successful in terms of sales, the targeting of Paxil for anxiety disorders contained a snag. Soon after its launch, primary-care physicians and others began to describe patient dependence on SSRIs through adverse-event reporting systems.[100] This happened first in Great Britain.[101] There was a much greater volume of reports for Paxil than for other SSRIs. It was first suggested that these withdrawal effects stemmed from the short half-life of the drug. It was also suggested that the fact that Paxil, more than other SSRIs, was used to treat patients who were anxious meant that any problems had to do with the personalities of these patients, who were, after all, more likely than others to develop phobias—so why not a withdrawal phobia?

Amid reports of withdrawal symptoms in the mid-1990s, Lilly convened a panel of "opinion leaders" to discuss the phenomenon of what were termed "antidepressant discontinuation syndromes" rather than dependence problems.[102] Prozac, given its very long half-life, seemed less likely to cause this problem than the other SSRIs.[103] Lilly saw a market opportunity vis-à-vis Paxil and Zoloft, their closest competitors, and began to run advertisements about discontinuation syndromes.[104]

In so doing, Lilly pointed to a general problem with the SSRIs. A key reason for the development of SSRIs as antidepressants lay in the fact that clinicians suspected all tranquilizers would, in due course, produce dependence, just as the benzodiazepines and barbiturates had done. In the early 1990s, the antidepressants were not associated with dependence. Clinicians felt comfortable denying the capacity of these drugs to produce addiction or dependence. When the Royal College of Psychiatrists launched its Defeat Depression campaign in the 1992, professional polling organizations found most people thought antidepressants were likely to be addictive. The Royal College campaign went out of its way to emphasize that antidepressants were not addictive. Until very recently, the backs of Prozac packets contained an explicit statement: "Don't worry about taking Prozac over a long period of time—Prozac is not addictive."

If by "addictive" we mean some property within a drug that will transform takers into junkies, likely to mortgage their livelihoods and futures for an ongoing supply of drugs, then the SSRIs at present do not appear to be addictive. They do not lead to a life of crime or dissolution.[105] But this does not mean SSRIs don't produce dependence. Many people experience grave difficulties in discontinuing treatment from Paxil or Zoloft. In lay terms, you can just as easily become hooked to SSRIs as on benzodiazepines. For most of us, this is the meaning of addiction.

Far from the problem being simply one of dependence that emerges on withdrawal from the drugs, the SSRIs produce what may be more appropriately termed "stress syndromes." Unlike insulin or thyroid hormone, which are replacements for a deficiency, the SSRIs are alien chemicals and, as such, are brain stressors. The consequences of this stress become apparent in some individuals on drug withdrawal, when the system attempts to regain equilibrium. But in others, the stresses can be visible during the course of treatment.

With the SSRIs, a problem called poop-out was noted early on.[106] "Poop-out" refers to the drugs losing their effect; sometimes they can be prompted to work again by increasing the dose.[107] This phenomenon first came to light in Internet chat rooms rather than through physicians informed by companies of the existence of a problem.[108] Because companies denied the problem, they could not advise on the best means of managing it. Clinicians were left to their own devices. This is hardly the kind of partnership supposed to characterize prescription-only arrangements.

The remainder of this book will deal with suicide on SSRIs, but a key feature of the Paxil story is that dependence on SSRIs is more likely to bring this group of drugs into public disrepute than the issue of suicide. Suicide is something anyone contemplating using an SSRI finds hard to envisage happening to them. But we can readily envisage getting hooked on a drug, and if this happens, we remain alive to complain about it. Public anger is likely to be fueled by growing awareness that assertions that people need to take SSRIs all their life, just as diabetics need to take insulin, were made against a background where the capacity of Paxil to produce dependence had been noted by Beecham in a series of healthy volunteer studies in the mid-1980s before the drug came on the market, and the company had been warned by senior figures in the field of this risk but, it would seem, chose to do nothing.[109]

The possibility of dependence takes the gloss off company claims that millions of us continue to take SSRIs successfully each year.

PROZAC[110]

In the 1960s, Eli Lilly's best-selling antidepressant was nortriptyline, a norepinephrine reuptake inhibitor. In late 1971, Bryan Molloy—a chemist working in Indianapolis for what was then, in terms of psychiatric drugs, a small pharmaceutical company—using another antihistamine, diphenhydramine, as a starting point, came up with a group of phenoxyphenyl-propylamines. Molloy was in this literal sense Prozac's creator. Of the fifty-seven phenoxyphenyl-propylamines he produced, the one given the code LY-94939, later called nisoxetine, turned out to have the laboratory profile Lilly was interested in. It was a norepinephrine reuptake inhibitor, and the company moved it into clinical trials.

Lilly had little interest in a serotonin reuptake inhibitor. But in line with standard practice at the time, the other compounds in the series were investigated. David Wong, a biochemist with little experience in psychopharmacology, tested all of Molloy's new series for serotonin reuptake inhibiting properties. Several of them came out as serotonin inhibitors, but LY-82816 stood out as the compound with the fewest effects on the norepinephrine system. This compound, however, was difficult to work with, as it couldn't easily be dissolved, so it was reformulated as a chloride salt, becoming LY-110140. At this point, work on LY-110140 was an academic exercise, meriting publication in a journal, the first specifically about a serotonin reuptake-inhibiting drug.[111] On this basis, Wong is sometimes described as the discoverer of Prozac.

As reports of Zelmid's progress came through, Frank Bymaster and Ray Fuller, pharmacologists with the company, looked at LY-110140's effects on behavior. They screened it for antidepressant activity. The best known screening test involved trying to block the sedative effects of reserpine on animals. All of the antidepressants then on the market blocked reserpine-induced sedation. LY-110140 did not.[112]

Another test was a rat aggression model. If a drug made rats more aggressive and more likely to attack other rats, conventional wisdom had it that such drugs had stimulant properties and might be useful in the treatment of depression. LY-110140 increased aggression in rats.

Around 1975, therefore, Lilly had a compound with a relatively unusual biochemical effect, and some poorly characterized behavioral effects, but otherwise a mystery. Carlsson's work suggested such a compound might be useful for treating nerves or depression, but most companies were adopting a wait-and-see attitude to these claims.

On September 11, 1975, LY-110140 was named fluoxetine. What was its future? There were a number of possibilities. Serotonin drugs showed antihypertensive properties in animal models, and the market for pills to lower blood pressure was much larger than the market for antidepressants. Had fluoxetine shown any clear antihypertensive action in humans, there is little doubt it would have been developed as an antihypertensive. The "behavioral effects" would then have been written out of the script in the course of a market development program emphasizing the rational engineering of a selective antihypertensive.

There were other lucrative possibilities. Early screening suggested that the drug might produce weight loss. An anti-obesity agent was certain to make vastly more money than an antidepressant. The hint that Prozac had weight-reducing properties probably drove some of the early mania, which later helped Prozac to hit the road running in 1989. This idea was still a big part of the fluoxetine development program as late as 1990, when the company hoped to license fluoxetine in a 60 mg pill under the trade name Loban for eating disorders. The vast amounts of money to be made in this market by drugs active on the serotonergic system made Redux headline news a few years later.[113]

A number of clinical investigators were invited by Lilly to a consultancy meeting in Britain in the late 1970s. One was Alec Coppen, a leading psychopharmacologist and one of the first advocates of the serotonin hypothesis of depression. They were presented with data on a range of Lilly compounds. Coppen recalls suggesting that fluoxetine might be an antidepressant, only to be met with a reply that if fluoxetine was ever developed, there was little chance it would be for depression.[114]

Lilly had good reasons to think this way, based on early clinical studies done with the drug. These were aimed at testing whether the drug was tolerable and what its behavioral effects might be in humans. The first trialist was Herbert Meltzer, who had a long-standing interest in the capacity of antipsychotics to cause side effects such as akathisia and Parkinsonism.[115] When one of his patients on fluoxetine developed muscle spasms (a dystonic reaction), Meltzer was certain the patient had accidentally been given an antipsychotic; but then other patients developed akathisia and a range of other problems more commonly associated with antipsychotics than antidepressants.[116]

Meltzer found little or no effect on depression. Other senior clinicians found something similar.[117] Most centers had patients who became agitated or akathisic. This led to recommendations from Lilly monitors that at least some patients be put on benzodiazepines while they were taking fluoxetine.[118] A far-reaching implication of this is that there is probably no clinical trial in which fluoxetine on its own has been shown to be an "antidepressant." In this patient group, benzodiazepines may well have been just as effective as fluoxetine itself.

In addition to trying to determine how tolerable fluoxetine was for patients, Lilly was trying in these early trials to establish whether there were any conditions for which it might be a suitable treatment. The company persuaded clinicians to try it out in patients with atypical psychotic disorders, as well as patients hospitalized with depressive disorders. It turned out to be ineffective in both groups: It made patients with psychotic features worse, and it has never been shown to work for hospitalized depression cases. Development of fluoxetine was at a crisis point.

Irwin Slater, a veteran of drug development within the company, was drafted to take over the clinical trials program. He tried fluoxetine out for pain syndromes, obesity, and other conditions, with no great luck.[119] Senior management were pushing to shelve the compound, but Slater and Fuller pointed out that zimelidine was almost through a clinical trials program for depression and fluvoxamine not far behind. The hierarchy relented. A clinical trial program began chasing milder depressions. Louis Fabre, later investigated by Upjohn for "recruiting patients from a half-way house for alcoholics,"[120] was approached. He gave fluoxetine to five patients; all responded. This turned the tide.

With fluoxetine rescued, the next step was to think about how to brand it. Lilly turned to Interbrand, who later claimed they invented the "discipline of naming" in the late 1970s.[121] The success of the name Prozac changed how drugs were named. James Singer, who later left Interbrand to set up his own NameBase/MediBrand, worked on the fluoxetine project.[122] Prior to Prozac, drugs had names that sounded scientific and referred in some way to the actual compound. Unlike Luvox or Zelmid, for instance, which referred to the original pharmacological

name, the name Prozac was seemingly designed to convey profession-
alism (through its "pro-" element) and the ability of the medication to
target the right area for treatment (through its "-zac" element).

Prozac's close brush with extinction may have had one long-lasting
consequence. Many clinicians have wondered why Lilly didn't bring in
low doses of Prozac. With a 5 mg dose, some of the problems that
emerged at higher doses of Prozac might have been minimized. The
conventional explanation was that Lilly had a brilliant marketing strategy, which involved selling one pill at one dose—something any fool
could give. In a later deposition, former marketer Richard Wood, who
became chief executive of the company in the late 1980s, provided a
great deal of evidence for the sales-driven "one pill fits all" formula.[123]

But another possibility lies in the alarming early history of Prozac.
In an effort to make this drug work, the company pushed the dose up
to 80 mg a day. In the mid-1980s, when FDA officials were finding it difficult to be certain that even high doses of Prozac worked, a Lilly study
demonstrated that for the new mild depression market they were investigating, 5 mg was as effective as 20 or 40 mg.[124] Joachim Wernicke
(later in charge of clinical trials in Lilly) e-mailed his colleagues:

> How much do we want to say about the 5 mg? I hedged a little, with
> the thought that we may be able to show that 5 mg is not as good on
> all measures. Some day we will have to report it if we ever want to use
> the information.[125]

In 1986, Stuart Montgomery reported that in milder depression, one pill
per week was as good as one pill a day.[126] This study vanished quietly,
even though in 2001, after Prozac had lost its patent, Lilly would market a once-a-week form of treatment.

PROZAC AND THE REGULATORS

Lilly and Prozac were ultimately saved by two changes in the clinical
trial world. In the United States, federal support for psychopharmacology research had all but shut down by the end of the 1970s. Three things
drove this:[127] the financial crisis caused by the Vietnam War; the suspicion with which the Nixon administration viewed scientists; and escalating health service costs. Removal of federal support meant the end of

independent clinical trials in psychopharmacology. Increasingly, for many investigators the only way to do research was to participate in industry-run trials.

Industry paid clinical investigators up to $5,000 per patient entered in a study and looked with favor on investigators who could recruit patients quickly. The faster the trials were completed and submitted to the FDA, the better the chances of registering a compound early in its patent life, and the better the returns on the investment. Naturally, industry would also look favorably on investigators who managed to produce the right results. This led to a situation by the end of the 1980s where some investigators were reporting on patients who didn't exist, or on "professional" patients who might have been on several investigational compounds at much the same time. In some instances, individuals other than clinicians conducted both recruitment and ratings.[128]

The second change occurred within the FDA. In 1981, Paul Leber, formerly a pathologist and then a psychiatrist, became disenchanted with clinical work in New York and moved to a job in the Central Nervous System (CNS) division of the FDA.[129] Quickly promoted to division head, Leber became a pivotal figure over the course of the next fifteen years. His first innovation all but brought the house down. Looking at antidepressant trials conducted up until then, Leber made the point that in a trial where a new antidepressant is compared to an older one and shown to be no worse than the older compound, where everybody assumed this meant that the new compound worked just as well as the old compound, it was quite possible *neither* drug was working. Proof that a new compound worked came only from trials against a placebo.

There was uproar. Many clinical trial programs did not include placebo trials, setting development back several years, at considerable cost. Worse yet, several new compounds could not be shown to work when compared against a placebo. Mianserin, the best-selling antidepressant in Europe, failed in U.S. placebo-controlled trials. This may have been because these trials were conducted in a too mildly depressed group, where it is difficult to demonstrate that *any* antidepressant is superior to placebo; but the prospect was raised that it might be increasingly difficult for new antidepressants to be registered, owing to difficulties in showing that they were superior to placebo.

This was a real problem for the emerging SSRIs, which couldn't be shown to work in hospital depression. Prozac accordingly had to make a tricky passage between the Scylla of serious depression—where it didn't work—and the Charybdis of mild depression—where mianserin had come to grief. Leber's reforms required that a new drug show evidence from two pivotal studies that it worked, and the majority of studies performed should go the same way.[130] The term *pivotal study* had crept into use as accepted code for a placebo-controlled study. As an increasing number of new antidepressants were SSRIs, and all took five to ten years to develop, Leber, the FDA, and others must have been genuinely concerned that what appeared to be a necessary reform to the system might backfire. For a time, no new drugs made it to the U.S. market, which probably contributed significantly to Prozac's impact as the first antidepressant to hit that market for what was, relatively speaking, a long time.

In the case of Prozac, there were three placebo-controlled studies. Karl Rickels from Philadelphia conducted one; it demonstrated no effect for Prozac. A second was a six-centered study, called Protocol 27, where Prozac was compared to imipramine and placebo. One of the investigators here was Jay Cohn from Los Angeles. Dr. Cohn's data were later removed at the request of FDA, as the extremely favorable results he reported were at odds with the other data generated.[131] When the remaining studies were combined, Prozac was inferior to imipramine and barely better than placebo on some scales, and no better than placebo on others. Three of the six centers failed to show it worked better than a placebo. In the final study, by Louis Fabre, there were only eleven completers on Prozac, and the study period was effectively only four weeks in duration. This study came up with a positive result for Prozac. With the Fabre study, and counting Protocol 27 as one study, the score was two to one in favor of Prozac. If the component centers of the multicenter study are counted separately, the result was four centers in favor of Prozac and four against—hardly an overwhelming majority.[132]

The plan had been to launch Prozac in the United States in 1986. The FDA finally approved it in late 1987, after over three years of scrutiny during which the agency noted serious flaws in the designs of its clinical trials.[133] A pattern of approval of less effective antidepressants had begun. Since then, it has not been uncommon for new drugs to be presented to the FDA that are superior to placebo in perhaps only two out of six trials.[134] Instead of saying that, on balance, the new drug is simply not more effective than a placebo or is of such minimal effectiveness that it is hardly worth permitting on the market, the FDA

approach is to say that any trials comparing a new drug to an older antidepressant in which the older drug appeared no different to a placebo
were failed trials. That is, the trial rather than the new drug has failed.

These ambiguities can be seen clearly in the license application for
Zoloft, where only one of five studies indicated superiority over
placebo.[135] A further study claimed superiority for Zoloft when some
patients who had their treatment discontinued "relapsed," but in this
case, what was termed "relapse" may have been withdrawal from
Zoloft. Zoloft did worse than amitriptyline and failed in two hospital
depression studies.[136] As Paul Leber ended up putting it:

> How do we interpret . . . two positive results in the context of several
> more studies that fail to demonstrate that effect? I am not sure I have
> an answer to that but I am not sure that the law requires me to have an
> answer to that—fortunately or unfortunately. That would mean, in a
> sense, that the sponsor could just do studies until the cows come home
> until he gets two of them that are statistically significant by chance
> alone, walks them out and says he has met the criteria.[137]

For those who believe that approval of a drug by the FDA means that it
is in some sense good for you if taken properly, the situation is even
more problematic than the above scenario might suggest. "Two positive
studies" doesn't mean the drug works for depression in two studies. It
means there are two studies in which the drug can be shown to have an
effect in depression—can be shown to do *something*. Whether it is a
good idea to take any of these drugs is not addressed. In other words,
these trials do not offer evidence the drug works in the sense that most
people mean by the word *works*—that is, evidence that this drug clears
the problem up.

Companies marketing their products do not have to reveal anything about the very weak evidence on which registration was based.
The new compound can be sold with all the glossy slogans of rational
engineering, hints of added benefits for weight loss or whatever, and
celebrity endorsements. Since the end of the 1980s, companies have not
had to bother with any questioning by independent investigators about
just how good their compound really is, as there are increasingly few independent investigators left in psychopharmacology.[138]

Adopting the principle in trials for mild to moderate depression
that a drug is an antidepressant if in some instances it is possible to

show a difference to a placebo, it would almost certainly be possible to show that stimulants such as dexamphetamine, methylphenidate, and even nicotine are antidepressants. Using these rules, in a population of mild to moderately depressed patients, the benzodiazepines would come out as antidepressants. The fact that no one has done such trials owes everything to a business calculation: These older drugs are off patent, so no company stands to make money from them.

There is a key point to take from all this. We are accustomed to the notion that our regulators are looking after us, that they are acting in some sense as consumer watchdogs. But this is not their role. The role of a regulator is to adjudicate on whether, for example, a yellow substance in front of him or her meets minimal criteria for butter; to ensure, for example, that it is not lard injected with color. Regulators are not called upon to determine whether this butter is good butter or not, or whether butter is good for your health. Consumer watchdogs must do that. Within medicine, the physician is supposed to be the consumer's watchdog—which, given that they rarely consume the product, makes for an ambiguous and commercially unique situation.

The legal situation is even more complex. If the mandate of the regulators is to let drugs onto the market that are proven to have an effect, what the FDA have been doing is defensible. If the brief, as per the wording of the statutes in most countries, is to license drugs that are effective, then the case of the SSRIs is much less certain.

LAUNCH

Prozac was launched in the United States and Canada in 1988. In Britain, a launch was planned for 1984 but did not materialize until late in 1989.[139] At the time, Britain was seen as quick to approve drugs, while the FDA was widely criticized for taking much longer than other regulators. Prozac bucked this trend.

In line with a strategy developed in 1983, the early sales pitch in most countries emphasized that Prozac lacked the supposedly nasty side effects of the older tricyclic antidepressants but was as efficacious as these drugs and came in a convenient once-daily dosage.[140] Borrowing from the mianserin story, there was an emphasis on safety in overdose. Market surveys before launch repeatedly asked people like me whether the fact that this new drug did not cause weight gain would influence our prescribing. Right from the time of its launch in America, patients were lining up asking for Prozac by name, an experience new to American psychiatrists.

Over the course of the next few years, every company with an SSRI ran clinical trials comparing their drug with the older tricyclic antidepressants. When all clinical trials were analyzed together, the SSRIs were no more effective in outpatient depressions than were the older agents.[141] As for the tolerability profiles of the SSRIs compared with the older drugs, the dropout rate of patients from clinical trials was almost equal—it would take over thirty patients assigned to either set of drugs before there would be one less dropout in the SSRI group. This was the case even though these trials were almost exclusively designed by SSRI companies, so that in over 30 percent of trials, the SSRI had been pitched against the tricyclic generally thought to have the most side effects—amitriptyline.[142] There was therefore an extraordinary contrast between the marketing hype and the trials underpinning it. When these studies were analyzed, the greatest predictor of outcome lay in the sponsorship details of each study.[143] Later in the 1990s, it became clear that a large number of trials with less favorable results for the SSRIs were simply not reported, and that the results on quality-of-life scales used in many of these trials were almost universally left unreported.

The trump card for the SSRIs has been that a greater number of patients are likely to be put on and remain on what is thought to be a "therapeutic dose" of the drug than is likely with other agents. But even here, the puzzle is that no more than 40 percent of patients take their drugs for more than few weeks.[144] Something goes wrong with the other 60 percent. This "something" tempts clinicians to blame patients and tempts the "experts" in the field to blame the average clinician, who supposedly hasn't stressed to the patient the importance of remaining on treatment for six months or more. Nowhere in the literature is there any concession to the possibility that SSRIs may not suit up to 60 percent of those put on them.

By the time Prozac got its license, the crisis over the benzodiazepines had become severe. The psychiatric and primary-care worlds were receptive to the idea that behind every case of anxiety lay a case of depression. No one was inclined to question the idea that antidepressants were a more scientifically rational treatment for the nervous states presenting in the community than anxiolytics, especially when no one then expected an antidepressant to produce dependence. Add in the fact that, compared with older antidepressants, these new drugs were safe in overdose, and there seemed to be no good reason not to prescribe them.

The plans had been to launch fluoxetine in Germany in 1984, but it took six more years for "Fluctin" to reach the market there. Probably very few people outside Eli Lilly knew of the German regulators' view on fluoxetine as of May 1984:

> Considering the benefit and the risk, we think this preparation totally unsuitable for the treatment of depression.[145]

I

Take One

TONY L, one of the first patients I put on Prozac, was turning 50. He had a successful professional life and an attractive family. But both were being torn apart by a combination of stresses at work and home and by his nervous disorder.

When Tony first came to see me, he appeared depressed or obsessive-compulsive or both. Either way, taking the edge off his OCD or his depression might help.[1] My preference was to use behavior therapy, but I told Tony there was a new group of antidepressants acting on the serotonin system that might possibly be useful for both depression and OCD, enabling us to cover two problems with one drug. He took a prescription for 20 mg Prozac.

Several days later, having overcome his indecision about taking pills, he started treatment. On the third day, he felt "wonderful" but found it difficult to sleep, complaining that his mind was frighteningly "like a video on fast forward."[2] The next day he felt "miserable and helpless." Although it was increasingly difficult to focus on things, he could not stop thinking, with no particular content to these out-of-control thoughts.

Tony suspected the Prozac had caused the problem and discontinued treatment, only to find the symptoms continued. I took phone calls from him and reassured him that while his problem might have been drug-induced, it should clear up. I saw him five days after he'd stopped the pills. At that point he was better, although still unwell.

I assured him there were other drugs we could try. One was Luvox, which I had no reason to think would cause serious trouble. Uncertain, Tony delayed a month before starting this new drug.

After the first dose of Luvox, Tony felt agitated and nauseated. Feeling better the next day, he took a second dose but was unable to sleep that night. He seemed to be in a rerun of his Prozac experience. In both instances he felt "dangerous." After the second dose of Luvox he wanted, for example, to "get into my car and drive a long distance at high speed whilst sorting out the problems of Western civilization as I went." Again his mind felt "like a video on fast forward." He had "a distinct feeling of my brain and my body being separated with my mind set to hurt and my brain overactive."

The following morning he felt dreadful and unable to do anything—"helpless, ill, mentally restless, beyond despair, and suicidal." He halted the pills immediately, but this reaction lasted for a week. During the week, he noticed finding it difficult to "gauge the passage of time . . . I looked at the clock frequently that night and it appeared repeatedly to show the same time."

Tony's reactions were a puzzle. I got hold of his old medical notes. While a student at university, he had briefly been seen for a nervous reaction. At the time, he had been prescribed the tricyclic antidepressant imipramine, which also inhibits serotonin reuptake. This appeared to cause an unusual fuguelike state. It began to seem this man had a peculiar reaction to drugs acting on the serotonin system,[3] but I had no idea why.

His preference for pills over behavior therapy showed he was not antipills. One possibility was that Tony had a general problem with all psychiatric drugs, either some physiological sensitivity or a neurotic reaction. After his disastrous response to SSRIs, we put him on a monoamine oxidase inhibitor (MAOI), which has the opposite effect on the serotonin system, and this worked quite well for him.

Unfortunately, Tony did not get the benefits that taking SSRIs can offer in OCD, which might have made a difference to his future. It is now clear that if he'd been coprescribed a benzodiazepine, trazodone or propranolol, these drugs might have minimized his adverse reactions. Treatment might have been able to continue until his body had adjusted to the SSRI. Alternatively, if a lower, 5 mg dose of Prozac had been available, he might have found the reactions disturbing but tolerable until they wore off.

These are not insignificant points. This man's professional and family life were later torn apart irrevocably. His "instability" on the drugs may well have colored the reactions of his colleagues or his family to him. It may even have colored his own assessment of himself, leading him to give up on many things when he should not have done so. At the time, the idea that the injuries caused by a drug like Prozac might be both direct and indirect escaped me completely. It was a problem that was to revisit with a vengeance nearly ten years later.

TEICHER, GLOD, AND COLE

When I saw Tony, I was unaware that Prozac had already been reported to make people suicidal. I was in the process of moving jobs from a university post in Cambridge to one in Wales when the first paper by Martin Teicher, Carol Glod, and Jonathan Cole from Harvard appeared in the *American Journal of Psychiatry* in February 1990.[4] This outlined the cases of six individuals who had become obsessively preoccupied with thoughts of suicide and in some cases had made suicide attempts after going on Prozac. The authors fingered the Prozac these patients had been given.

I first became aware of the article that summer, when visiting the Department of Pharmacology in Galway. Brian Leonard, my former head of department, asked me what I made of it. I suspected he had been asked by Lilly to give them a reaction. For both of us, the primary interest in the Teicher report lay in the fact that drugs supposed to increase serotonin levels were not supposed to lead to suicide.

A series of articles by Herman van Praag during the 1970s and 1980s put forward the idea that individuals with low levels of serotonin metabolites in their cerebrospinal fluid were liable to impulsive acts.[5] On this basis Prozac might even be better than other drugs for patients who were suicidal. Although I was skeptical of van Praag's proposal,[6] it was difficult to know where the Teicher phenomenon might fit into this story.

Teicher was a biologically oriented psychiatrist with a background in preclinical research, testing out hypotheses by giving drugs to animals. He had done significant work on circadian rhythms and had a general interest in psychopharmacology. Glod was a nurse tutor who later went on to an academic position. Cole, a professor of psychiatry at McLean Hospital, had been responsible in the early 1950s for the first randomized controlled trials on chlorpromazine and had considerable experience in assessing and managing the problem of antipsychotic-induced side effects such as tardive dyskinesia. This was a man who knew all about the hazards of scare stories about drugs in the public domain—a man to whom the American Psychiatric Association turned to contain public hysteria. Their article described six patients who came to their attention during 1988.[7]

- First was a 62-year-old woman, Mrs. A, a patient of Cole's, with a 17-year prior history of depression, who had been put on Prozac as part of a clinical trial for Lilly. On the eleventh day of treatment with a 60 mg dose of Prozac, she had "forced obsessional suicidal thoughts consisting of intense and obsessive wishes to kill herself and described by Mrs. A as 'uniquely bad' . . . she felt 'death would be welcome.' She also felt like jumping out of her skin, but had no signs of motor restlessness." Her Prozac was stopped and she improved considerably after three days. As Cole later put it, he'd seen patients who were suicidal before but never anything quite like this.[8]
- Second was a 39-year-old man with a long history of depressions. He had previously done well on an MAOI; after a relapse, he was switched to Prozac. After three weeks on a 20 mg dose he appeared to be more depressed and preoccupied with "violent self-destructive fantasies." After Prozac was discontinued, imipramine and doxepin (both serotonin reuptake inhibitors) were tried but did not appear to help. According to Teicher, this man's suicidal thoughts persisted until the MAOI was restarted, and he developed similar suicidal thinking again when reexposed to Prozac a year later. Just what happened this patient was less than completely clear, as I was later to find out.
- The third case described was a 19-year-old student who seemed partly phobic and partly psychotic, with hints of an eating disorder as well as depression. She had previously had a variety of medications and occasional suicidal thoughts. Over the course of two weeks on a mixture of Prozac and the antipsychotic perphenazine, she became paranoid, depressed, irritable, and developed "disturbing self-destructive thoughts." Her Prozac was increased and her perphenazine reduced because she showed signs of akathisia, but she became more depressed and preoccupied with thoughts of death. When her Prozac was increased further, she became actively suicidal. After a further increase in Prozac to 80 mg per day, she became violent and self-mutilating. When Prozac was finally discontinued, her self-destructive urges eased and she subsequently improved markedly.
- Fourth was a 39-year-old woman described as having a borderline personality disorder. Her depressed moods responded to an

MAOI but she suffered side effects. She had a previous history of suicide attempts that appeared to be cries for help. Two weeks after being put on 20 mg of Prozac per day, she became significantly more depressed, with persistent thoughts of suicide. Although she herself began to blame the drug, she wished to continue taking it, apparently because other people had responded to it. After she began to drink alcohol some weeks later, while on an 80 mg daily dose of Prozac, her Prozac was stopped. Two weeks later she made a suicide attempt that did not appear to be a call for help. When interviewed after the suicide attempt, she made it clear that she had been having persistent severe suicidal ruminations, that she felt unreal, and that she had a belief she could neither fight nor control her suicidal impulses. The suicidal thoughts diminished over three weeks, and when she went back on the MAOI, she got much better.

- Fifth was a 39-year-old woman whose past depression had been successfully treated with MAOIs. She had had persistent suicidal thoughts before but no suicide attempts. After starting on 20 mg Prozac per day, her dose was increased to 40 mg per day, at which point she began to have suicidal thoughts for the first time in years—fantasizing about purchasing a gun, something she'd never done before. On 80 mg of Prozac per day, she complained of out-of-body and other symptoms. When her Prozac was stopped, the suicidal thoughts cleared up. She later said that while on Prozac she had embraced thoughts of suicide in a way she had never done before. There was something different about this kind of suicidality.

- The key case in the series was a 30-year-old woman with a history of bipolar and multiple personality disorder, who had first been suicidal at the age of 17. MAOIs seemed to help her; tricyclic antidepressants did not. Teicher put her on a combination of medications, but she remained anxious, depressed, suicidal, and withdrawn. When Prozac was added to the mix, she appeared to get worse, with increased feelings of anxiety and splitting. She began to self-mutilate, planned lethal overdoses, and put a loaded gun to her head. One of her internal personalities began to shout at her to commit suicide. At this point her Prozac was discontinued, but it took a month for her suicidality to clear up.

Subsequently, it became clear that Teicher and his colleagues had other cases. These included a 15-year-old boy with OCD who had actually committed suicide after two weeks on Prozac.[9]

This was a complex group of patients on a range of medications other than Prozac, and with a range of diagnoses in addition to depression. Some had been suicidal before. Why implicate Prozac? These senior investigators, who had seen depressed and suicidal patients before, believed they had never seen anything quite like this. However much suicidality there had been in the background of some of these patients, something new seemed to emerge with treatment. All appeared to be reporting a recognition that "Gee, I've been suicidal before but never anything quite like this. This was ridiculous."[10]

Publication of the Teicher article prompted a firestorm of criticism. These were cases being treated in a specialized center for suicidal and complex patients. There might be no implications for normal clinical practice. The alternative possibility—that the problem might be even *worse* in normal clinical practice, that less severely ill patients might have been at even greater risk—was apparently never contemplated by either Teicher or his critics. Another complaint was that these patients were on multiple other medications: How, therefore, could Prozac be blamed? Again, the alternative—that these other medications might have been *protective*—was never considered. Nobody knew that Lilly had put patients in its clinical trials on some of these other medications to minimize Prozac-induced problems.[11]

THE PUZZLE DEEPENS[12]

I filed the Teicher article for further reference. A few weeks later, a community worker brought a patient with a peculiar story into the hospital. He had been a senior manager in a public utility company. After his retirement, 63-year-old Alan L. had moved with his wife to Wales. He was a very English stiff-upper-lip type, of the friendly rather than severe variety. Alan had a history of depression, which did not include suicidal thoughts. Thirty years before, he had been prescribed a combination of an MAOI and benzodiazepines and remained on them after recovery. During the 1980s benzodiazepine fuss, he reduced and discontinued these without much difficulty, continuing with the MAOI.

When he retired to Wales, his mood slipped and he sought help. But his new primary-care physicians and psychiatrists didn't know him.

A decision to change his medication was taken, and things began to slip out of control. He had to be admitted to the hospital. He was subsequently seen regularly in an outpatient clinic, where his antidepressant was changed frequently. During 1988 and 1989, he was given flupenthixol, Parstelin, alprazolam, thioridazine, viloxazine, and maprotiline,[13] along with Valium. Nothing seemed to work very well, but he had no suicidal ideas during this period. Then, in January 1990, he went on dothiepin, which, unlike the other drugs with which he had been treated, has some serotonin reuptake-inhibiting properties. A week after this, he took a minor overdose of sleeping pills.

He developed a classic melancholic depression with early morning waking, mood variation so that he was worse in the morning and improved in the evening, poor concentration, loss of appetite, and loss of interest. In the hospital, he responded to electroconvulsive therapy. He was discharged on amoxapine and tranquilizers and did well at home for four months. But in August, he began to wake again early in the morning and found his mood swinging. His concentration slipped and he became apathetic. His amoxapine was changed to trazodone, with little effect.

Then he was put on 20 mg of Prozac. According to his wife, his spirits lightened during the subsequent week. He became more active but also tenser and more restless. Sixteen days after starting Prozac, he got out of bed at 5:00 a.m. and went walking in the rain. He came back five hours later with sand in his shoes, seemingly unable to give an account of where he had been. Detailed questioning later at the hospital revealed that, intensely preoccupied by suicidal thoughts, he had set off determined to kill himself by throwing himself into one of the many quarries around the area. He later told us that the only thing that had prevented this happening was his inability to find a suitable locale.

Five days later, he again woke early and walked into the sea fully clothed. The coastline where he lived is very shallow and he had to walk out several hundred yards to get to armpit depth. By that time, he had begun to have second thoughts and retraced his steps, with difficulty, sustaining cuts on his feet and arms in the process. We admitted him to the hospital.

My initial hunch was that Alan had ended up with too much time on his hands and had to spend too much of it with his partner in Wales, where they had no network of friends or activities. Alan declared his love for his wife, but my hunch was that he resented her, and if he were able to express this, things might improve. He appeared very tight-lipped whenever she was on the ward, and she seemed the kind of woman who did the talking for her man. Once she left the ward, he would brighten up and become more active. I disliked her on the basis of what I saw happening. But Alan did not agree that there were any difficulties in his marriage.

One option in this kind of situation is to undertake an Amytal interview, using the barbiturate to relax the person in the hope that his barriers to the disclosure of sensitive information drop.[14] Following an injection of Amytal, Alan was asked to imagine himself in the front garden of his house. He was then asked to give a detailed description of the scene: "Is the sky blue? Are there clouds? Is it windy? Is it cold? Are there flowers or shrubs in the garden? What kind? Now turn around and face the house and describe it—the color of the curtains, the color of the doors, the color of the window frames, the size and shape of the house and so on." The challenge is to get the person living as much as possible in this mental scene.

Alan was then walked up to his front door and asked to ring the bell and see who answered. I expected it to be Alan's wife. He was asked to describe her in detail while I observed his expression closely. The hope was that, if the interview process had succeeded, his "true" emotions would show themselves clearly when faced with the person who answered the door. He seemed happy to see his wife.

There are clinical fallbacks when the situation develops in this manner. If the psychiatrist was convinced that the wife was to blame, he or she might interpret the simple fact of so little animosity or resentment as evidence that the patient must be so resentful that he had blocked it out of his consciousness. My belief, however, is that what an individual thinks or feels is available to consciousness, but he or she may have difficulty articulating it. Such difficulties in articulation should betray themselves to some extent in body language. Very little will ever be repressed completely outside awareness. In Alan's case, whatever hostility was present when we saw him with his wife dissolved in this more relaxed situation.

But another, quite unexpected story unfolded. While being walked around his house, Alan began to discuss fantasies of killing himself before coming to the hospital. Where before he admitted to only two suicide attempts and described these as completely out of character, he now described getting the sharpest serrated carving knives in the house and contemplating cutting deeply into his wrists. He described fantasies of holding the earth wire, commonly at that time attached to the pipes of the cold tap under the sink in the kitchen, while at the same time plunging a steel knife into a nearby live socket. There were other suicidal thoughts, none of which he had communicated to us. He was visibly upset. He insisted that these thoughts were out of character. It was difficult to know what to make of it.

At this point, Alan had been off Prozac for five weeks. It became clear that he was not as severely depressed as had first been thought. He was started on 75 mg of imipramine at night, with the dosage increased after one week. Around day ten, he was noticeably more tense, restless, and anxious. He appeared to move about more but also to be less able to sit down and talk. There was no apparent suicidal ideation, but he later put this down to being safe in the hospital. He was less clear on how he might have been feeling had he been at home. The coin dropped. We were seeing him slowly develop some form of drug-induced condition before our eyes—a condition for which akathisia seemed the best word.

His imipramine was discontinued. He was switched to phenelzine, an MAOI. Three weeks later he was much better and was given weekend leave. He came back after the weekend beaming, and shortly afterward he was discharged, fully recovered. Seeing Alan and his wife together, it was now clear that they were a very happily married couple.

Witnessing this change before my eyes made a difference. Alan's history made it clear that treatments that acted on the serotonin system did not suit him. He had always done well in the past on MAOIs and now had responded to them again. The mistake had been to take him off his MAOI. On Prozac, and later imipramine, he had developed something akin to akathisia but without visible pacing. He was unable to stay with a conversation or sit beside other patients or staff in a relaxed fashion. He was visibly hunched up in a way he hadn't been before.

All of a sudden, the reports by Teicher and colleagues seemed far more interesting. They, too, had described patients who had responded poorly to Prozac but who subsequently responded to MAOIs; they, too, seemed to be describing a state rather like akathisia.

NOTIFYING LILLY

I approached the local Lilly representative and described my clinical problems. Hiram Wildgust, a regional manager for Lilly, paid me a visit. Hiram was a widely liked, ever-visible presence for Lilly at UK psychiatric meetings during the 1990s.

I was keen to find out if Lilly had further details that might be relevant to what I was witnessing. The responses from the company indicated that after 2.38 million prescriptions in the United States, there had been fifty-one cases of reported "euphoria," thirteen of "CNS [central nervous system] stimulation," and eleven of "hyperkinesis."[15] My comment at the time was "It is not exactly clear what these terms mean as they have been applied by company medical officers attempting to categorize what may be a diverse range of reactions."[16] My hunch in the case of our first subject was a substance-induced dissociation. A number of sensitive individuals, in response to a wide variety of agents, can react with amnesia, depersonalization, derealization, or explosive automatic reactions. But nothing in Lilly's database seemed to fit either Tony's or Alan's case. I gave Hiram copies of the first draft of the cases to read. No comments came back.

In the summary of an article later sent to *Human Psychopharmacology*, I suggested that what had happened in both instances was a matter of drug-induced side effects. The risk with these side effects, as opposed to the traditional side effects of the older antidepressants (such as dry mouth or difficulties passing water), was that they could be misattributed by the individual to personal failings or to a worsening of the illness. A misattribution like this might lead someone to spiral down. I still believe this dynamic contributes something to the clinical picture, but I am less inclined to believe that the extra distress people feel is simply because of their misattributions. I think there is a much greater element of direct drug-induced dysphoria.

THE CONTROVERSY TAKES SHAPE

Meanwhile, things were boiling up in Boston. Maurizio Fava and Jerrold Rosenbaum from McLean's twin, Massachusetts General Hospital, published a survey undertaken prior to the publication of Teicher's study.[17] They approached fifty-nine psychiatrists working in the

Clinical Psychopharmacology Unit and the General Psychiatry Practice Service of Massachusetts General Hospital and received replies from twenty-seven. They asked for details on the number of depressed patients treated during 1989 who had received MAOIs, tricyclics, Prozac, lithium, or other antidepressants. They received reports on 1,017 patients. The question was whether any patients who had not been previously suicidal had become suicidal on any of the therapies. The answer, according to Fava and Rosenbaum, was that suicidal ideation was no more likely to emerge on Prozac than on tricyclics, MAOIs, or other antidepressants.

The same data were reanalyzed by a number of different people, including David Graham from the FDA,[18] the American College of Neuropsychopharmacology,[19] and, later, Teicher and Cole.[20] All concluded that the most reasonable interpretation of the Fava and Rosenbaum data is that Prozac was approximately three times more likely to be associated with the emergence of suicidality than other treatments. Lilly, however, uses the Fava and Rosenbaum article to this day, without any acknowledgment that it is quite possible to interpret its data as supporting the argument that Prozac induces suicidality.[21]

Meanwhile, a series of other authors filed papers on Prozac and suicide. William Wirshing, Ted van Putten, and others, reporting in July 1992 from Los Angeles, gave details of five women patients.[22]

- The first was a 39-year-old woman who became obsessionally suicidal after two weeks on 20 mg of Prozac. She, too, had prior history of a poor response to imipramine and a good response to an MAOI.
- The second, 24 years old, became restless but not suicidal after two weeks on 20 mg of Prozac. Alprazolam was added to Prozac, and for three months she did reasonably well, until she subsequently became both markedly restless and obsessionally suicidal. An increased dose of alprazolam helped her, but it was only when the Prozac was discontinued that the restlessness and suicidality cleared up.
- In the case of another woman, when her dose was increased to 40 mg per day, she began to feel like jumping out of her skin and began ruminating on suicide. Her restlessness was relieved with lorazepam and a reduction in her Prozac. When she was reexposed to a 40 mg dose, her restlessness returned.

- The fourth woman had a long and complicated history and was on an antipsychotic that made her akathisic but not suicidal. When 20 mg of Prozac was introduced, she initially improved and asked for the dose to be increased. On 40 mg, however, she became "unbearably" akathisic in a way that was "100 times worse than anything I've experienced before." She became suicidal. Her akathisia and both the auditory hallucinations and suicidal ideation that had developed while she was on Prozac melted away once it was discontinued.
- The final patient initially felt "better than I can remember" on 20 mg per day of Prozac. But when the dose was increased to 40 mg per day, she became agitated, frantic, insomniac, and restless. She began to think of killing herself to gain relief. The problem cleared up after her Prozac was stopped. She was later able to continue with 6.6 mg of Prozac per day.

These reports were important for a number of reasons. Van Putten was regarded as a leading expert on drug-induced akathisia and its harmful consequences; that his name was associated with a series of reports that Prozac had led to suicidal ideation, and had done so by producing a form of akathisia, was significant. This study also provided persuasive evidence of patients who had developed a problem on Prozac that improved when treatment was discontinued, only to worsen again when they were reexposed. As Paul Leber of the FDA put it: "This month's *Archives of General Psychiatry* contains a letter describing in reasonable detail 5 patients who experienced akathisia and suicidal obsessional ruminations that seem to be causally linked (e.g., challenge, dechallenge, rechallenge) to the use of Prozac."[23]

In 1991, Mark Riddle, Robert King, and colleagues, working at the Yale Child Study Centre, reported on six children, aged 10 to 17, who were treated with Prozac for OCD.[24]

- After five weeks of treatment, one of the subjects experienced "very real" violent nightmares about killing his classmates, from which he found it difficult to awaken. He had to be hospitalized, where his Prozac was discontinued and over several weeks he settled down. When he was later restarted on Prozac, his suicidal ideation returned.

- One 14-year-old girl on Prozac began to ruminate about suicide and to bring a knife to school. When her Prozac was increased, her suicidality got worse.
- Another 14-year-old girl became suicidal and agitated on Prozac. She was switched to imipramine, which didn't help. When she was changed back to Prozac, she became violently suicidal. She had to be transferred to a longer-term unit, where she remained significantly suicidal until all antidepressants were stopped.
- Yet another 14-year-old girl, who had initially responded well to 20 mg of Prozac per day, made a first suicide attempt after several months of treatment. In the hospital, her Prozac was increased to 40 mg per day, and over the following two weeks she became agitated—pulling out her hair, biting her nails, hitting her legs, and requiring restraint.

This paper described the development of intense suicidal ideation in these patients on Prozac, which recurred on reexposure to the drug. Increased dosages led to the emergence of the problem, where lower doses did not. The pattern was one of a Prozac-induced disturbance emerging during the first few weeks of treatment or shortly after an increase in dose. The fact that these cases involved children being treated for OCD is of significance, given that Lilly's later defense was that it was the disease depression, rather than Prozac, that was to blame for suicides.[25]

A final series of three cases came from Anthony Rothschild and Carol Locke.[26] Rothschild and Locke had felt it was safe to rechallenge three patients with Prozac, to see if they would have a repeat suicidal reaction.

- The first patient was confined to a wheelchair. Two weeks after first starting Prozac, she had become extremely agitated. In an effort to gain relief, she had jumped from the roof of a building, sustaining multiple fractures of her arms and legs. Eleven days after restarting Prozac, she again developed "severe" anxiety, restlessness, and an inability to sit still. She described the panicky agitation as identical to what she had felt prior to her previous suicide attempt. "I tried to kill myself because of these anxiety symptoms. It was not so much the depression." When the

Prozac was stopped, her agitation resolved within seventy-two hours.

- Another man had jumped from a cliff for similar reasons. Reexposed to Prozac, he again became restless, paced, and became insomniac. "This is exactly what happened the last time I was on Prozac, and I feel like jumping off a cliff again." This time, instead of stopping the Prozac, Rothschild and Locke gave him propranolol. There were grounds to believe that propranolol, which blocks S-1 receptors, might relieve the problem. Within twenty-four hours, it did.

- The third patient had also jumped off the roof of a building the first time she went on Prozac. When rechallenged with the drug two weeks later, she "began complaining that she'd move her legs back and forth and pace constantly to relieve anxiety. On examination she'd constantly shift her legs while seated and would get up from the chair many times to walk around the office. She stated that this restlessness was driving her 'crazy' and that she was feeling like she did during her last suicide attempt." For this patient also, the addition of propranolol led to a "complete remission of the restlessness, anxiety and suicidal feelings."

By this time, the case against Prozac was compelling.[27] That the problem worsened with higher doses is a strong indicator of cause and effect. That it cleared up on halting the drug and reappeared on reexposure followed the FDA's recommended method for determining causality. This was also the in-house method that all drug companies, including Lilly, used to assess causation. The mechanism by which Prozac produced these problems was, in fact, sufficiently well worked out that predictions could be made about what antidotes might help. Finally, the problem had been reported in people who were not depressed, undercutting what was later to be Lilly's main defense: "It's the disease, not the drug."

In the summer of 1991, at a British Association for Psychopharmacology (BAP) meeting in York, I presented details of our Prozac cases. Stuart Montgomery, then chairman of the British Association for Psychopharmacology, was in the audience.[28] He challenged the validity of my descriptions in such a hostile manner that a number of those present approached me afterward to comment on it. Others were supportive. Eugene Paykel, professor of psychiatry in Cambridge, suggested that *agitation* might be a more appropriate term than *akathisia* for what was involved. Two months later, in September, Montgomery was one of the independent experts brought in by the FDA to consider the question of Prozac-induced suicidal ideation.

At the time, I was about to become the secretary of the British Association for Psychopharmacology. Several months later, I organized a regional BAP meeting in Wales. Stuart came to chair it. Over a meal, he informed me that the cases I had reported had been of concern to Paul Leber of the FDA, who had been present at the meeting in York.

CONSULTANT FOR LILLY

In 1991, Hiram Wildgust invited me to join a consultancy panel for Lilly. It had become common practice in the late 1980s for companies to convene panels of opinion leaders when drugs were launched. Advice might be sought, for instance, on the merits of educational campaigns, such as a campaign to increase the recognition of depression. Members of a consultancy panel are often told that because their opinions on drugs in the company's pipeline will be canvassed, confidentiality agreements are required.

Participants are usually told that one of the advantages to the company is that if problems surface for a drug, the company can approach members of the panel for their views on how to handle particular issues. They might also direct the media to willing panel members— media training was on offer. The arrangement allowed both the company and the clinicians, when approached by the media, to say these experts were not being paid to take a position. A particular beauty of the arrangement is that if only one person in a consultancy panel takes a company line, the company can trot out the others—who will be some of the senior figures in the field, including journal editors and heads of department—to swear that this kind of arrangement does not compromise their judgment and that any suggestion otherwise is offensive.

Panels might have ten to twelve members. The participants enjoy the opportunity to travel from wherever they live to somewhere central, to meet for a meal in a restaurant they might never be able to afford, to stay in a luxury hotel, and to engage in conversation with colleagues. The meeting the following day will be relaxed. Added to this is a fee that in the early 1990s varied between $1,000 and $1,500 for the day, depending on the company involved.

With a certain amount of nervous interest, I agreed to participate. My hunch was that at some point I would be grilled about our study on suicidality. But it was never mentioned. On one occasion, the purpose appeared to be to inform us about the Church of Scientology. I had to miss this meeting, but I wrote asking for background materials. As editor of the British Association for Psychopharmacology's newsletter, I was making efforts to persuade Duncan Campbell, an investigative journalist who had written about the hazards of fringe groups for medicine, to write a piece for us. The Animal Liberation Front had shortly before planted a bomb under the car of a psychopharmacology researcher in Bristol, severely injuring him, and neuroscientists were nervous that groups like the Church of Scientology might become a real threat.

After publication of the article on SSRIs and suicide in *Human Psychopharmacology,* I received calls from the Citizen's Commission on Human Rights, an organization linked to the Church of Scientology. My secretary was told that it was very important that the caller get hold of me—literally a matter of life and death. I refused to take any of the calls. The Church of Scientology was not a group with whom I would wish to have any association. Indeed, their espousal of the "Prozac is a problem" position made me, and I'm sure others who saw problems with Prozac, more sympathetic to Lilly's position.

THE EMPIRE STRIKES BACK

When the question of suicide first hit the media, spokespersons for Lilly stated that they had analyzed clinical trial samples of several thousand patients for evidence of anything like this—and found none. The data behind this claim finally surfaced in the *British Medical Journal* on September 25, 1991, in an article by Charles Beasley and colleagues from Lilly[29] that purported to be a meta-analysis of Lilly's clinical trials, examining evidence from 3,065 patients. Over 1,700 of them had gone on Prozac, with the remainder on comparative antidepressants or placebo. There was no evidence, the article claimed, that people taking Prozac as a group became any more suicidal than those taking imipramine or placebo.

The entire analysis hinged, however, on one question from the Hamilton Rating Scale for Depression, item 3. This is a five-point item that is scored in response to the question:

> *This past week, have you had any thoughts that life is not worth living, or that you'd be better off dead? What about thoughts of hurting or even killing yourself?*
> Item 3
> 4 Has made a serious suicide attempt
> 3 Has clear suicidal ideas or gestures
> 2 Wishes he were dead or any thoughts of possible death
> 1 Feels life is not worth living
> 0 Absent

When this item was analyzed, the average scores of patients taking Prozac fell as much as the scores patients on imipramine and more than the scores in patients taking placebo. There were two messages: that Prozac was good for treating suicidality in depressed people, and that there were scientific data for 3,065 patients on one side, and anecdotes on the other. Which was a disinterested observer to believe? This message went right to the heart of the professional identity of a nervous profession. Lilly's strategy worked, even though the article's flaws should be obvious to any college student.

Raters in trials rate in a global way. If a patient is improving, raters whiz through an interview, often completing the scale afterward in a manner that indicates a general improvement in the overall score. If some aspects of the patient's condition are improving—which they might be even when the patient is becoming more suicidal—raters often won't bother asking the suicide question. They go on their overall sense of the patient's functioning. This rating by halo effect was almost inevitable in a study not designed to address the question of the emergence of suicidal ideation. Clinicians who weren't looking for this problem weren't going to find it and rate it.

Item 17 on the Hamilton Scale, for instance, is about sexual functioning. Based on this and spontaneous reporting in clinical trials, Lilly's early claims were for a rate of 5 percent sexual dysfunction on Prozac. But subsequent studies with scales sensitive to drug-induced sexual dysfunction found rates of 70 percent.[30] This indicates how a problem can be completely missed through inadequate means of investigation.

These points seemed so obvious that I wrote to the *British Medical Journal*.[31] In addition to pointing out the problems with the Hamilton Rating Scale, I pointed out that in a group analysis of the kind Lilly had performed, if a significant number of people improve, their scores will drown out the noise being produced by patients who have worsened. The method Lilly had used was not appropriate to the question. It would be much more appropriate to do challenge-rechallenge studies.

Charles Beasley from Lilly replied, expressing surprise at my characterization of item 3 of the Hamilton Scale as an insensitive measure of suicidality.[32] There was no indication from Beasley's reply that in 1986 company personnel had, in fact, agreed with my point.[33] He went on to affirm that using rechallenge to determine the causality of rare events was scientifically appropriate.

Beasley didn't reply to the other letter written to the journal, from Ian Oswald.[34] A distinguished professor of psychiatry from Edinburgh, Oswald had been involved in a BBC *Panorama* documentary that gave a gripping account of possible hazards with the hypnotic Halcion. During this investigation, it became evident that a number of studies on Halcion had nonexistent patients. Other studies involving prisoners produced ambiguous results in the light of later patient claims that Halcion had made them psychotic.[35] Similar reactions were noted in the prisoners. Did the prisoners have psychotic disorders or a vulnerability to psychosis, or were they manipulative? It was difficult to be certain.

Finally, there appeared to be errors in a key Upjohn study. Upjohn's view was that these were simply transcription errors. The BBC program suggested otherwise. These issues converged in the case of Ilo Grundberg, who, while taking Halcion, had shot her elderly sleeping mother nine times in the head. Oswald's assessment was that she was depressed with delusions. Others referred to the stress she was under. Ms. Grundberg blamed the Halcion for what she did. Upjohn settled out of court, reputedly for a large amount of money. Had the problems with Upjohn's study played a part in motivating them to do so?

Oswald alerted the Medicines Control Agency in the United Kingdom that some of the information on which the registration of Halcion depended was not accurate. This necessarily led to a suspension of Halcion's license in Britain; if anything were to go wrong in the future and plaintiffs took cases, the government itself might otherwise have been liable. A political storm ensued. The controversy ended up in the courts a few years later, when Oswald and Upjohn laid countercharges of libel.[36]

In his letter about Prozac, Oswald wrote that a recent television program cited Lilly as claiming that data from controlled trials of more than 11,000 patients showed no significant increase in the likelihood of suicidal acts by patients treated with Prozac.[37] The Beasley paper referred to only 3,065 patients. Oswald noted that the high-powered statistical tests Lilly used were only as good as the data. If these data were not being collected properly in the first place, the statistical tests were worthless.

His closing shot was: "The *BMJ* is a journal of distinction and, dare I say it, perhaps also of some innocence. At a time when in the United States the manufacturer of fluoxetine is facing litigation, the corporate defense attorneys will be pleased by the journal having published a piece authored wholly by the manufacturer's employees." This was strong stuff.

ELSEWHERE IN TOWN

On May 6, 1991, *Time* magazine ran an eight-page article on "The Thriving Cult of Greed and Power."[38] The magazine cited Cult Awareness Network as saying, "Scientology is quite likely the most ruthless, the most classically terroristic, the most litigious and the most lucrative cult the country has ever seen." The article outlined a history of the foundation of Scientology by L. Ron Hubbard, a former science fiction writer whom a California judge had labeled a pathological liar, and claimed the organization had applied for status as a religion in a move widely seen as a strategy to avoid paying taxes. This led to a running conflict and series of legal cases with a range of organizations and with the Internal Revenue Service. Other countries were split on whether to allow church status to the movement.

From the start, Hubbard's 1950 *Dianetics: The Modern Science of Mental Health* had put Scientology on a collision course with psychiatry. Scientologists were opposed to a range of psychiatric treatments, from ECT to Ritalin, and were regularly seen protesting outside American Psychiatric Association meetings. The Church founded the Citizens

Commission on Human Rights (CCHR) in 1969 to take these issues forward. According to *Time,* lawsuits were one of its chief weapons. In 1990, several years after Hubbard's death, CCHR filed a citizen's petition with the FDA, asking what it was going to do about Prozac. Over fifty lawsuits regarding Prozac were filed. Was this an orchestrated campaign? In fact, very few of the lawsuits appear to have had anything to do with the Church of Scientology.

The *Time* article was way over the top.[39] Even Saddam Hussein was portrayed less badly. My copy of this article came from Lilly. The American Psychiatric Association, meanwhile, had swung behind Prozac, applauding the FDA's rejection of the Scientology petition on August 1, 1990, and emphasizing a message that was beginning to appear with increasing regularity: It's the disease, not the drug.

In 1994, the American Psychiatric Association Press published the book *Psychiatric Practice under Fire.*[40] The first chapter dealt with the Scientologists' attack on Prozac. Other chapters outlined the attack on ECT, the emerging problems posed by managed care, attacks on the benzodiazepines, and the negative influence of excessive bureaucracy and regulation in general. The Prozac chapter, written by Rosenbaum from Massachusetts General, took a by now standard approach, castigating the Scientologists. There were three messages. First, Prozac was the most researched drug in history. Second, the problem was the disease, not the drug. And third, the real tragedy of the Prozac story lay in all the people who would commit suicide because they were being denied access to an effective treatment. These three assertions were becoming the chorus lines in the background of the Prozac story.

On April 19, 1991, before *Time* ran its piece, the *Wall Street Journal* came out with a piece quoting (among others) Rosenbaum that "the public's fear of Prozac as a result of this campaign has itself become a potentially serious public-health problem as people stay away from treatment."[41] The same day, Melvin Sabshin, medical director of the American Psychiatric Association, wrote to members: "Many of you have written to express concern about attacks on psychiatry and treatments such as ECT, Ritalin and Prozac from the Citizens Commission on Human Rights.... Today's *Wall Street Journal* carried a lengthy front-page article detailing these attacks. Our Division of Public Affairs worked with the reporter in the development of the article."[42]

The FDA convened an advisory committee for September 20, 1991.[43] Ten outside experts met to hear representations from a variety of citizens and patient groups, together with evidence presented by Lilly company employees and other senior figures in U.S. psychopharmacology. The atmosphere was tense. Daniel Casey, a widely liked psychiatrist, chaired the meeting wearing a bulletproof vest.

The patients' testimonies came first. A majority echoed the scenarios described by Teicher and others. They called for the relabeling of Prozac or even its outright removal from the market. Its problems might be rare—3.5 percent of takers was the figure bandied about—but who would want to risk being one of that 3.5 percent? Against them were ranged voices from organizations such as the American Psychiatric Association, the National Depressive and Manic-Depressive Association, and the U.S. Pharmacopeia Drug Information Service. Lilly was given the largest section of the meeting to present what were essentially the data from the Beasley meta-analysis. Part was presented by Jan Fawcett, professor of psychiatry in Chicago, who had written extensively on the role of sudden upsurges of anxiety in the provocation of suicide and the desirability of concomitant sedation early in the treatment of depression. Another part was presented by Charles Nemeroff, a professor of psychiatry at Emory University in Atlanta.

Paul Leber and Bob Temple of the FDA acknowledged the dramatic impact of the patient testimonies. The problem for FDA officials was that few of them had ever treated anyone. They were dependent on the experts in the room—some of whom appeared to have significant conflicts of interest.[44] David Dunner, for instance, another respected psychopharmacologist, had trials in train with Lilly worth $200,000. These panelists had been given waivers regarding conflict of interest on the basis that this was a meeting supposedly about *all* antidepressants and the responsibilities of *all* companies, even though Lilly was the only company to attend. Stuart Montgomery had been flown over from England to the meeting, but neither Cole nor Teicher was invited to participate.

The dilemmas were acute. As Leber put it, how did they know that relabeling all antidepressants as potentially dangerous wouldn't lead to fewer people being treated? It might just be possible to do the "right" thing and yet end up with more suicides as a consequence. The room had heard some awful stories, but how much of this was due to bad psychiatric practice rather than a bad drug? Would changing the labeling of the drug lead bad practitioners to do any better? Was it the FDA's job to improve standards of clinical practice?[45]

What Leber couldn't say on the record was that even though the regulators recognized that Lilly's analysis did not resolve the issue, once a drug was on the market, the FDA was fairly powerless.[46] Citizens and others seem to think they have a guardian in the FDA, but the agency is small and critically dependent on information from manufacturers and a handful of consultants. If the FDA intervenes after a drug is on the market, there is a chance that subsequent deaths due to lack of availability of a treatment will be blamed on the agency's action. The agency could even be threatened with legal action. If a company chooses to ignore a problem, there is little the FDA can do.

The motion put to a vote on the panel at the September meeting was whether there was credible evidence that antidepressants increased the risk of suicide. The panel voted against advising the FDA that the evidence supported this position. They were not asked to vote whether there was evidence that antidepressants do *not* increase the risk of suicide in some people, in which case the vote would also have had to be "No, there is no evidence." Was this an innocent wording of the motion? Despite these votes about antidepressants as a group, an FDA press release that day suggested the vote exonerated Prozac.

Despite the vote, Leber nevertheless advised Lilly that it should conduct a large prospective blind test-retest study, with input from Teicher. Lilly representatives met with the FDA on several occasions and discussed what studies the situation called for. There was general agreement that the best bet was a prospective rechallenge study in which patients who had had difficulties of the Teicher type with Prozac would be randomized to either Prozac again or an antidepressant active on the noradrenergic system.[47] The protocols for this study were drawn up by Lilly, the investigators approached, and the clinical trial materials prepared, but the study was never conducted. Lilly and the FDA agreed further that a scale sensitive to the emergence of suicidal ideation should be developed and incorporated into future trials. The scale was developed but never used.

Does the FDA position make sense if seen in the light of documented understandings that proper studies would, in due course, be carried out? Leber had said at the meeting, "The sponsor, Eli Lilly, was asked . . . to examine data from previously conducted controlled investigations and was also asked to develop plans to conduct new studies, including clinical trials and epidemiological studies, studies that could provide more direct answers to the questions that have been raised in the open session earlier."[48] Casey left the meeting telling reporters and other companies that further research needed to be done. But the meeting in September 1991 became a defining moment, one that somehow let Lilly off the hook. No further research was ever done.

One of the most striking observations came from Bob Temple of the FDA. On the one hand, he was faced with expert assessments that depression was a terrible illness, leading to high suicide rates, and a welter of statistical data from Lilly showing how Prozac was devoid of any deleterious effects; on the other hand, he was impressed by the patient testimonies. Temple spotted a pattern. The experts, he pointed out, were talking about chronic hospital depression. The patients in the meeting, however, some of whom had survived highly lethal suicide attempts, appeared to be a group with no previous psychiatric history. In some cases, they had been put on Prozac for an eating disorder or to stop smoking. Was there something there, he asked?[49] No one answered.

STALEMATE

Almost immediately upon publication of their study in 1990, Teicher and Cole were visited by Beasley and David Wheadon from Lilly, who reassured them that nothing in the development work on Prozac pointed to drug-induced suicidality. Some time afterward, Teicher was called in to discuss Prozac with Joe Coyle, head of the Department of Psychiatry at Harvard.[50] Coyle was the first of the new generation of neuroscientists to become head of a psychiatric department. The summons to Teicher seemed to indicate Coyle was under pressure to squash talk of problems with Prozac.[51] When Teicher made it clear that he had the support of other senior colleagues within Harvard, Coyle declared himself satisfied.

Teicher attended the FDA hearing on antidepressants and suicide in September 1991 but was not allowed to make a presentation. The transcript of the meeting outlines an interest he declared.[52] He was in discussion with a company called Sepracor. The shapes of certain molecules mean that some drugs come in mirror-image forms, called isomers, whose actions can be quite different. Unlike the other SSRIs, Prozac and Celexa were mixtures of two isomers. Sepracor specialized in separating out the isomers of drugs.

Later in 1991, at an American College of Neuropsychopharmacology (ACNP) annual meeting, a session was given over to the Prozac question. The Lilly side came armed with handouts. Teicher again presented his material.[53] The reception was hostile. A string of senior figures in American psychiatry lined up at the microphone to criticize him. There was support from the floor, however, from clinicians who insisted they had seen the same phenomenon.[54]

The session gave rise in March 1992 to a statement, made on behalf of the ACNP by John Mann,[55] that there was no evidence at that point to prove Prozac increased rates of suicide, but that physicians had a duty to warn their patients about possible hazards. It called for further research—which never happened. Mann had previously published an article that reviewed the possible ways in which the mechanics of the serotonin system might give rise to the problems outlined by Teicher.[56]

The ACNP statement caused concern among companies. Pfizer, about to launch Zoloft, convened an expert panel to assess the implications. At one of these panels, Casey, who had chaired the FDA hearings on Prozac, suggested Pfizer needed to establish whether Zoloft could cause akathisia and could induce suicidality.[57]

In another article, published in 1993, Teicher and Cole went further and claimed explicitly that Prozac could cause suicidality.[58] They outlined six mechanisms whereby this might happen. Shortly after this, Martin Teicher appeared to fade out of the Prozac story.

2

Events in Kentucky

JOSEPH WESBECKER'S FATHER died in 1943, leaving the 1-year-old to be brought up by his 16-year-old mother. His poor and difficult childhood included time in an orphanage. In his 20s, he began work as a printing-press operator in the Standard Gravure plant in Louisville, Kentucky. Working his way up the trade to a journeyman's card, he married and had two sons. When the printing industry ran into difficulties in the 1970s, pressure increased on Wesbecker and his colleagues as more work was asked of fewer employees. When Mike Shea bought Standard Gravure, using money from the workers' pension fund to defray the purchase cost, employees began carrying guns to work, and threats became commonplace. Wesbecker's marriage broke down.[1]

Wesbecker began to see psychiatrists and was diagnosed as having depression. After a suicide attempt, he was put on a number of different medications. In the summer of 1988, his physician, Lee Coleman, prescribed the recently released wonder drug Prozac. Wesbecker stopped Prozac after two days, claiming it didn't suit him. He went on disability in the spring of 1989. He had begun to dread his job and was concerned about going back. Then his disability payments were cut.

On August 10, 1989, Coleman suggested trying Prozac again. When he saw Wesbecker a month later, Coleman found him much more agitated and volatile. Coleman wanted to stop the drug and made a note to this effect, but Wesbecker, who had fifteen days of pills left, refused to stop. It had helped, he claimed. When Coleman asked how, Wesbecker said Prozac had helped him to remember an incident at work where he had been required to perform an act of oral sex with one of the foremen while his coworkers watched. According to Wesbecker, this event—imaginary, as it turned out—had been the price of getting off a printing press he hated.

Coleman later testified, "I knew that Prozac in some people could cause nervousness—can cause agitation, can cause sleep problems, plus I had started him on it three or four weeks before. When you start a new medication and something different happens, you tend to suppose that it's the medication that is causing it within that period of time."[2]

A number of Wesbecker's friends later reported that over the next few days he was agitated, his sleep was poor, his appearance was unkempt, and he was pacing endlessly. On the evening of September 13, he went for a meal with his ex-wife Brenda, who said, "He was just more nervous. He paced more. While we were eating, he got up two or three times and went to the bathroom in the middle of the meal. He didn't finish all of his meal. I didn't either, because he just kept doing that. I finally said, 'I'll just get a go box.'"[3] His son James said that on the morning of September 14, "he really wasn't the same person."[4]

Later that day, Wesbecker went to the printing presses with an AK-47 and other guns and walked through the plant, killing eight people and severely wounding twelve before shooting himself dead.

Did Wesbecker's Prozac play a part in the events of September 14? On the one hand, he was at risk for suicide, and the printing press was an accident waiting to happen. On the other hand, his history shows prior intolerance to Prozac and evidence of decompensation when he was reexposed to it. The almost psychotic development, where he talked of nonexistent sexual abuse during his final course of treatment, was of a type that had been reported in other settings, that had been found in Lilly's trials with Prozac,[5] and that has since been reported in certain patients on Prozac.[6] Something similar led to the discovery of the first tricyclic antidepressant, imipramine.

FACING A JURY

Almost from its launch, Prozac generated legal actions. By 1990, fifty-four cases were pending. By the mid-1990s, Lilly faced a series of civil suits, 160 of which were consolidated in a Federal Multi-District Legislation (MDL) case. The California firm of Kannanack, Murgatroyd, Baum, and Hedlund had fifteen cases, one involving Del Shannon, the singer of the 1960s hit single "Runaway." The drug was also cited in a number of crimes.

A group of attorneys involved in these cases met in 1992 and agreed that the first case to go to trial should be clear-cut and winnable. Leonard Finz, Leonard Ring, and Paul Smith were the most prominent lawyers involved. One of the clearest cases was Paul Smith's *Biffle* case in Texas, and one of the most difficult was the *Wesbecker* case in Kentucky. Smith sent a letter to the other lawyers outlining the agreement to move forward with *Biffle* first.[7] "Obviously, it is my preference to get this case tried at that time, especially in the light of the fact that Judge Finz has the Kentucky litigation set for trial immediately behind this and that case is the weaker case."

Martin Biffle had been on Prozac only for a matter of days. The drug was present in his body at autopsy after his suicide. His prescribing physician was willing to testify that he had not been suicidal prior to being given Prozac, and a series of friends and coworkers were agreed that none of them would have expected him to commit suicide. The Biffle trial was scheduled for the end of 1993. But it took until the end of 1994 before a case reached court—and then it was the *Wesbecker* rather than the *Biffle* case.[8]

The lead attorney for the plaintiffs in the *Wesbecker* case in Louisville, Kentucky, was Leonard Ring. But one month before the trial was scheduled to take place, Ring had a heart attack that compromised the blood supply to his brain. Nancy Zettler, his junior counsel, felt unable to take on the case alone. She sought help from Paul Smith, who, in addition to taking the *Biffle* case, had become the lead attorney in the MDL cases. Zettler and Smith got an extension on the case and spent half a year taking depositions from fifty-six people, mostly from Lilly, which took eighty-three days and filled almost twenty-one thousand pages of print.

When Zettler first applied to Lilly for internal documents, she was told there was nothing on the computer. It turned out four million pages worth of documents in hard copy had been downloaded from the computer. She was told she could have them.[9] This is common practice in cases involving large corporations. A reasonable expectation might have been that plaintiffs' lawyers would call off the hunt, but Zettler and a colleague, Monica Putnam, set about going through the documents. Their willingness to do so may have contributed to the increased likelihood that documents will be routed through a company's lawyers, with the company then withholding them on the basis of attorney-client privilege. The documents from the *Wesbecker* case therefore shine a unique light on some of the normally hidden operations of large corporations.[10]

Zettler and Putnam hit on a strategy to ease their task as they worked through the material. They persuaded trial judge John Potter that Lilly should provide the relevant documents for each of the company's employees three weeks before that employee was due to be deposed.[11] Smith and Zettler finally took twelve boxes of documents that Lilly claimed were covered by attorney-client privilege to Judge Potter for a decision. He decided in favor of the plaintiffs.

Among those deposed were David Wong and Ray Fuller, involved in making the drug, and Charles Beasley and John Heiligenstein, who ran the clinical trials programs from the late 1980s and were responsible for assessing reports of adverse events. Zettler and Smith also deposed other key people such as Paul Stark and Dorothy Dobbs, clinical trial monitors, and Catherine Mesner, a clinical research associate. A range of other people from Lilly's clinical division past and present included Irwin Slater, Robert Zerbe, Dan Massica, David Wheadon, Joachim Wernicke, and Max Talbott from regulatory affairs in Lilly. Clinicians from Lilly Germany were brought over, including Hans Weber and Nick Schulze-Solce. Zettler and Smith also deposed the bosses, from heads of sections such as Leigh Thompson and Gary Tollefson up to Vaughn Bryson, Melvin Perelman, and Richard Wood from the boardroom and chief executive level.

Lilly employees denied being trained by lawyers but gave standard responses to the effect that randomized controlled trials were accepted as the gold standard in the field, and that there were no trials to show Prozac had negative effects. Depression was said to be a terrible disease that could lead to suicide. Prozac was frequently described as the most studied drug in history. The responses raise the possibility of brainwashing rather than coaching.

The depositions have either a Jesuitical or pedantic tone. Key players, asked whether they had seen a certain document, would say no, perhaps because the document with which they were presented was a photocopy of something they had seen, rather than the actual thing. They would deny remembering anything without crystalline recall of the event. Charles Beasley couldn't remember the number of studies in the meta-analysis on which he had spent more than a year.

Here is an excerpt from Nancy Zettler's deposition of Catherine Mesner:

Q. Did you ever see any meeting minutes generated from any of the division meetings that you attended regarding Fluoxetine?

A. I don't remember.

Q. Catherine, you understand that you're sworn to tell the truth?

A. Yes.

Q. You understand that to a certain extent saying you don't remember when you do have a vague memory is not telling the truth?

Larry Myers (for Lilly). . . . . She's not going to be governed by a definition that you apply, Nancy.[12]

John Heiligenstein, after extensive difficulties remembering, was asked by Paul Smith:

Q. So it's your testimony . . . that in this phone conversation between yourself and four scientists at Eli Lilly and Company and the medical examiner who was responsible of the autopsy in connection with Joseph Wesbecker's death, you can remember nothing about that phone conversation other than the medical examiner was frustrated about the Scientologists being involved.

A. Yes, yes, sir.

Q. Have you ever had trouble with your memory Doctor Heiligenstein? . . . Have you ever seen a physician for problems with your memory?

A. Have I ever seen a physician for problems with my memory. Yes, as I recollect.

Q. When did you first see a physician for problems with your memory?

A. Probably sometime in 19—, I didn't see it specifically for that. (After spelling out that he had consulted for possible adult ADHD and was prescribed Ritalin.)

Q. Have you ever been criticized by any of your colleagues for memory problems?

A. It's ironic because I think for the most part I've only received compliments for my memory.[13]

The plaintiff's attorneys had a further obstacle. Even though they had been offered a room full of documents, sensitive documents had been routed through the legal department or even to outside attorneys

and were then withheld. Catherine Mesner was asked about the challenge-rechallenge study Lilly had undertaken to do:[14]

> Q. Would you have turned over the final copy of the protocol
>   and any other documents you had in your file related to the
>   rechallenge study to the legal department in Lilly in one of
>   these quarterly document collections?
> A. Yes.
> Q. Were those documents that were returned to you either in
>   original or in copy form?
> A. Usually I received a copy back.
> Q. Do you have a specific recollection of receiving a copy of the
>   final protocol in the rechallenge study back from the legal
>   department?
> A. No, I don't remember.

Smith's folksy, humorous style in these depositions disarmed some of
his witnesses more than they intended. Zettler was far more combative.
Between them, they were deposing witnesses for a series of trials, including Smith's MDL cases and other cases[15] in addition to the Fentress
(Wesbecker) case. Other attorneys sat in on some of the depositions, including William Downey of Kannanack, Murgatroyd, Baum, and Hedlund.

   One of the fascinating things about the depositions and subsequent
trial is how much time Smith, clearly intrigued by the implications,
spent on the question of the interface between neurochemistry and free
will. But with no science background, he was unable to see that the
rudimentary state of neuroscience in the 1990s, let alone the 1970s when
Prozac was made, permitted little or nothing to be said about any such
interface.

   Smith and Zettler completely missed the issue of how relatively ineffective Prozac was for depression. No one asked the simple question:
If Prozac was a better serotonin reuptake inhibitor than older antidepressants, and if serotonin was lowered in depression, why wasn't
Prozac bringing about recoveries in hospital depressions quicker than
older drugs? They focused on early clinical reports that patients with a
combination of psychotic and affective symptoms (schizoaffective) had
done particularly badly on Prozac, because some reports had labeled
Wesbecker as schizoaffective. But in their efforts to land a punch on this

target, they missed the fact that Prozac couldn't be shown to work at all in severe depression.

Smith and Zettler ran into yet another obstacle when they tried to call an expert witness. It seemed all the psychopharmacologists they approached were either retained by or consultants to Lilly—or were just unwilling to get involved. Jonathan Cole was unavailable because seriously ill for much of 1993 and 1994. Martin Teicher seemed uncomfortable with all the documents unearthed and too nervous to get involved,[16] claiming that a lot of pressure had been brought to bear on him.

In the end, the plaintiffs went with two experts. One was Nancy Lord, who had both medical and legal qualifications and who had worked in the pharmaceutical industry with Abbott Laboratories on the development of a hypnotic. Lord knew a lot about how clinical trials should be conducted.

The other expert was Peter Breggin, a notable critic of psychopharmacology who was closely associated with one of the famous antipsychiatrists of the 1960s, Thomas Szasz, a professor of psychiatry from New York. Breggin's 1991 *Toxic Psychiatry*[17] is powerful rhetoric that many psychiatrists find unsettlingly good on the marketing of psychiatric disorders and a medico-pharmaceutical complex. But at the heart of the book is an argument for the moral superiority of psychotherapy to pharmacotherapy that few biological psychiatrists could endorse. In 1994, Breggin brought out a new book, *Talking Back to Prozac*,[18] based on his role as an expert witness in the *Fentress* and other cases, but this also ends with a romantic argument about the superiority of psychotherapy over drug treatments.

A few years before the *Wesbecker* case came to trial, Lilly had hired a new chief executive. Through the 1980s the company had experienced a number of setbacks and had also developed a reputation for weak moral values. Profits were sliding. Chief Executive Vaughn Bryson was ousted in a boardroom battle, and the company turned to their first outsider as chief executive, Randall Tobias. Tobias came from AT&T and had no background in pharmaceuticals. He aimed to downsize the company. Furthermore, he had heard a message: Depression was costing the workplace millions of dollars. Businesses and other organizations should know that in the longer run, diagnosing depression and getting treatment for their employees could save them money.[19]

FENTRESS ET AL. VS. ELI LILLY[20]

After five years, the Wesbecker case finally came to trial in Louisville on September 28, 1994. Lilly made it clear from the outset that the company would fight rather than settle this case. Wesbecker offered the perfect opportunity to play the "disease, not the drug" card. Here was a man with an extensive psychiatric history, including a suicide attempt five years earlier, working in a plant that was an accident waiting to happen. Lilly argued he came from a family with three generations of nervous troubles. In building their argument, Lilly's attorneys deposed four hundred people, making Wesbecker, as one witness put it, "one of the most studied serial killers in history."

At trial, Smith and Zettler faced various disasters. After an impressive performance on examination from Smith, Breggin was faced with Joe Freeman, the attorney for Lilly. Freeman let Breggin launch into his hobbyhorse—how psychotherapy was to be preferred to pharmacotherapy. A psychotherapeutic approach let people build better principles for living.

Freeman then confronted Breggin with material he had written in 1980: "Have you written 'that permitting children to have sex among themselves would go a long way toward liberating them from oppressive parental authority'?"[21] Breggin stumbled forward into a left uppercut: "Did you accept money for putting these ideas in writing and selling them to the general public of the United States of America?" Freeman went on to quote: "The difference between believing in the divinity of Christ and believing in oneself as Christ is merely a difference in religious point of view." Holding a copy of *Penthouse,* he challenged Breggin to explain why he had written an article for that magazine blaming American and British psychiatrists for the Holocaust. It might have been possible to explain these points to a jury with enough time, but not on the witness stand. These guys didn't take hostages.

Lee Coleman also failed Smith and Zettler. State jurisdictions vary, and according to Kentucky rules, Lilly was not debarred from retaining Coleman. So although he had previously been one of the main proponents for the argument that it was Prozac that caused Wesbecker's symptoms, he effectively became a witness for Lilly. Questioned by Smith about his earlier views, he testified that his views had changed after he had been made aware of further material by Lilly.

The real success for Smith and Zettler was Nancy Lord:

When I looked at the Lilly data, I didn't find it was adequate to study this drug. The data was flawed for a number of reasons. First of all, the protocols were not well designed. . . . Not only did they permit the use of concomitant medications, but they permitted the use of psychotropic concomitant medications. . . . If someone came on to a trial and got, say, insomnia, they couldn't sleep, or they became jumpy and agitated, instead of having them withdraw and counting that person as someone who couldn't handle the drug, they simply gave them Dalmane to go to sleep, which had a lingering anxiolytic effect during the next day.[22] [. . .]

It looked like they did everything possible to kind of tone down the problems with the drug rather than give them a rigorous, systematic and comprehensive evaluation to define what the problems were and then put it in the package insert so that doctors could be warned not to use the drug in certain types of patients, or to use it more carefully.[23] [. . .]

In my opinion, this drug has not been approved. It's been approved with sedatives, but taking fluoxetine all by itself has never been studied.[24]

Some patients in trials were recorded as having severe agitation, but in the summaries of side effects this became nervousness or was not recorded as a drug side effect, "as the investigators were instructed not to record as adverse experience symptoms of depression."[25] Patients who dropped out for "patient decision" were not followed up to establish whether demands on their time or agitation on the drug had led to their dropout. A number of patients who had clearly become worse on Prozac were deemed to be treatment nonresponders rather than sufferers from side effects of the drug. This pattern had begun from the very first trials, with patients who became severely agitated, suicidal, and psychotic being classified as treatment nonresponders. Yet, when Lilly was approached by investigators wondering how to handle emerging side effects, one of the options suggested was to reduce the dose of Prozac—an option that concedes a causal link to Prozac.[26]

Today, the statistical analysis of clinical trials would be done according to a plan put in place before the trials began, but this didn't happen with Prozac. Investigators in many cases were allowed to break the blind and put patients who had done well on Prozac onto maintenance treatment with it, or switch those who had done poorly on, for instance, imipramine to maintenance treatment with Prozac. Maintaining a group of patients in this way on Prozac makes it possible to claim that when the company controlled for length of exposure on the drug, there wasn't a hazard. In this case, what was happening was that patients with the early-onset side effects linked by Teicher and Cole to Prozac were diluted by the addition of a selected group of favorable responders to Prozac.[27] There may have been nothing deliberate about this kind of selection, just simple inexperience or incompetence on the part of the company personnel running the trial.

Lord brought out an equal and opposite problem that happened when patients did poorly on Prozac. The pattern was that after a certain number of weeks off Prozac, all possible drug-induced difficulties were coded under whatever other drug the patient might then be on. On the surface, this might seem reasonable. After all, if a patient has been some months off Prozac and is having difficulties, should these be put down to previous Prozac? But in fact, it is far from reasonable. The rate of suicidal acts on placebo or other antidepressants in Prozac trials is less than five per one thousand. The rate on Prozac is ten per one thousand patients. But if the records of one thousand patients are tracked after they go off Prozac, only those who have problems are recorded, and five of these commit a suicidal act and are added to the non-Prozac group, then this instantly pushes up the non-Prozac rate to approaching 10 in 1,005—a rate identical to the Prozac rate. The sicker the patients are or the more likely they are to have drug-induced side effects, the more likely they are to stay in contact with the services and be recorded this way.

It was difficult to know what impact Lord's devastating but highly technical testimony might have had on a jury. It was relatively easy for Lilly to appeal to the fact that the FDA had approved this drug, with the implication that FDA officials must have considered all these points and were nevertheless content to approve Prozac. Smith and Zettler couldn't expect a jury of laypeople to find the FDA guilty, but Lord's testimony did a great deal to set up the key event of the *Wesbecker* case.

Judge Potter had ruled that evidence on another Lilly drug, Oraflex, was inadmissible, as this was not the drug on trial. Oraflex was the brand name for benoxaprofen (Opren in Britain), a new painkiller, which had been released in mid-1982 in the United States after being on the market in Britain and elsewhere for some years. It was an expensive aspirin that produced adverse effects, which aspirin didn't. Direct sunlight caused a rash and made fingernails separate from their nail beds. Despite these ominous signs, the drug got approval and was released in a wave of hype that emphasized it was particularly safe. There was a rapid increase in sales until it turned out that in the prelaunch investigation of Oraflex, a large number of older people developed a range of seriously disabling liver and kidney problems along with their rashes and peeling fingernails. A number of deaths occurred.[28]

Lilly denied the drug could be causing these side effects. The issue was settled when an independent laboratory demonstrated a dangerous accumulation of the drug in older people. Oraflex was withdrawn and Lilly prosecuted for failing to report to the FDA the full details of its clinical trials program and reports of toxicity abroad. In Britain, over one hundred deaths were attributed to Oraflex, and over four thousand individuals suffered serious side effects. In the United States, forty-nine deaths were attributed to it, and a jury awarded one plaintiff $6 million. When Lilly finally settled in the United Kingdom years later, claimants got $3,000 on average.

Lilly had another disaster with diethylstilbestrol (DES), a hormone preparation used in the 1950s and 1960s to prevent miscarriages. In 1971, it was discovered that DES could be connected to the development of vaginal cancer in the daughters of women who had taken it during pregnancy, leading to a set of legal actions that lasted two decades.

During the Wesbecker trial, Zettler and Smith had tried to call to the witness stand Beasley and Max Talbott. Zettler had noted that Beasley, when deposed, was perspiring through his suit in what was a cool room. Talbott had cried off his first deposition date and spent long periods of time in the restroom before and during the second date. Lilly argued that the court could not require the attendance of these witnesses, who worked outside a five-hundred-mile radius from Louisville, and refused to send them. Instead, Lilly sent Leigh Thompson, who had been in charge of coordinating the company's responses on the Prozac suicide issue.

Thompson praised Lilly's methods of collecting clinical trial data as the model for the field. Other witnesses followed this line, despite the testimony of Nancy Lord. When one of Lilly's experts, Robert Granacher, stated that he would have confidence in any drug approved by the FDA, Smith finally intervened. Lilly, he argued, had opened itself up to detailed questioning on its standards for conducting clinical trials—as, for example, in its trials with Oraflex. Despite his earlier ruling, Potter agreed. It seemed the gloves were about to come off. But Smith suddenly asked for time in adjournment and then declared that the case for the plaintiffs was closing. A surprised Potter asked both sets of lawyers if money had changed hands. They denied that it had. One of the jurors later notified the judge that she thought she had heard talk suggestive of a settlement. Asked by Potter to comment on how this juror might possibly have come to this point of view, neither set of lawyers appeared to have any idea.[29]

The jury recessed and came back with a nine-to-three verdict in favor of Lilly, the barest minimum Lilly could get by with. They did so after hearing the judge sum up in a manner that left some of them convinced he had "instructed us to find Wesbecker at fault, so that Prozac had nothing to do with it."[30]

Judge Potter. Has everybody got their copy? Okay. The first page is the full title of the case, which lists all of the plaintiffs and the defendant. Second page, "The Court instructs you as follows: Instruction no. 1, Fault of Eli Lilly and Company.

"A drug is defective if it is improperly tested or not accompanied by suitable warnings or instructions to the prescribing physician.

"A drug is unreasonably dangerous if a prudent drug manufacturer, being fully aware of the drug's effect and operation, would not put the drug on the market or would do so with additional warnings or instructions.

"You will find Eli Lilly at fault if you are satisfied from the evidence as follows:

"(a) That Lilly manufactured and sold the drug Prozac;

"(b) That Prozac as manufactured and sold was in a defective condition and unreasonably dangerous;

"(c) That Mr. Wesbecker ingested Prozac prior to September 14th, 1989; and

"(d) That such defective condition was a substantial factor in causing Joseph Wesbecker's actions on September 14th, 1989.

"Otherwise, you will not find Lilly at fault. If you find Lilly at fault, proceed to Instruction No. 2. If you do not find Lilly at fault, enter your verdict on Verdict Form A and proceed no further.

"Instruction No. 2: Fault of Joseph Wesbecker.

"On September 14th, 1989, Mr. Joseph Wesbecker had a duty not to injure or harm any plaintiff in any manner.

"The Court instructs you that Mr. Wesbecker violated this duty and that you will find him at fault."

Potter had instructed the jury that they could find Lilly at fault if Prozac was a substantial factor in causing Joseph Wesbecker's actions. But then he had gone on to instruct them to find Wesbecker at fault.[31] Had Potter's summary stressed that all parties agreed Wesbecker carried out the actions, but the question was how much Prozac might have contributed, he would have conveyed a different impression. Concerned that he might have inadvertently misled the jury, after the trial Potter offered Zettler the possibility of a retrial.[32]

The press wrote up the outcome as a vindication of Lilly and Prozac. Chief Executive Randall Tobias was reported as saying, "The members of the jury, after hearing the scientific and medical facts . . . came to the only logical conclusion—that Prozac had nothing to do with Joseph Wesbecker's actions."[33] Lilly's public relations officer, Ed West, indicated how the verdict would be seen: "If it becomes apparent it's very difficult to win big money in Prozac suits, this probably sends out a message." West added a statement from Tobias: "The verdict demonstrates the futility of blaming medications for harmful and criminal acts."[34]

Why did the jury vote this way? The trial transcripts suggest that if a single factor led to Lilly getting out of the case intact, it was the destruction of Wesbecker's character. They scored no hits on the science of depression or suicide or for their clinical trial procedures, which had so nearly been their undoing. But the jurors were left with the impression that Wesbecker was a bad man and that he had a choice as to his behavior.

It turned out the Wesbecker case had indeed been settled *before* the jury's verdict. Rather than face evidence on Oraflex, Lilly had offered what was later described as an "astonishing" sum of money. Pretrial estimates were that Lilly stood to be hit for anything between $150 and $500 million if they lost. Added to that would be the incalculable consequences of a guilty verdict. The settlement terms offered a high/low split, so that whatever the jury verdict, the plaintiffs got substantial sums of money—a large amount if the plaintiffs won and a lesser but still significant amount if the defense won. Smith's share made him a wealthy man.[35] An angry Potter filed a motion to have the not-guilty verdict quashed and replaced with "dismissed with prejudice as settled." The case went to the Kentucky Supreme Court, which found that "there may have been deception, bad faith conduct, abuse of the judicial process or perhaps even fraud."[36]

As Potter later put it, "In my opinion, it was not proper because I do not think you should secretly pay money to the other side to have them pull their punches. In basketball it's called shaving points, in boxing it's called pulling your punches. . . . I think the public has the right to expect that a trial is a *bona fide* contest and not some sort of show that one side puts on with the consent of the other to influence public opinion. It was done to discourage other plaintiffs and to help settle the pending lawsuits for less money than they might have been settled for otherwise. Between these two parties they got what they wanted but I think a bigger issue is whether the system was somehow corrupted a little bit and I believe it was."[37]

MEANWHILE

I was unaware of legal developments in the United States when, in 1994, I was approached to write a review for a new journal, *CNS Drugs*, on "The Fluoxetine and Suicide Controversy."[38] I sent my draft for comment to some of my contacts in Lilly, took note of the comments that came back, and sent the review off. It was an innocent review, even stating, ironically, that of course "these data from several thousand patients, and the evidence that fluoxetine reduces suicidal ideation, must on any scientific scale outweigh the dubious evidence of a handful of case reports." Notwithstanding this piece of irony—which was to cost me dearly—the article came down firmly on the side of saying that Prozac did cause suicide. But the problem, as I saw it, was one that could be managed with the proper warnings.

I was forwarded a copy of a formal response from Joanna Nakielny of Lilly.[39] Did I want to reply? I assumed at the time that this letter would not have come simply from Joanna, but I was unaware of the levels of medical and legal scrutiny my article had been subject to and the care that had gone into crafting a reply. It later became evident that the article had crossed the Atlantic and that there had been input from high up in the medical division of the company. A standard response must have been drawn up at some point, because several years later, when Alyson Bond from the Institute of Psychiatry wrote a further review on some of the complications of SSRIs, Charles Beasley responded almost immediately to her article, and his response covered almost identical ground to Nakielny's.[40]

The Lilly messages claimed there was no evidence that Prozac caused akathisia, no evidence that akathisia led to suicide, and no evidence that Prozac led to suicide. In its response to both Bond's article and my own, the company contrasted the handful of anecdotal reports with the weight of scientific evidence from its own meta-analysis. Beasley referred to the 1991 study by Fava and Rosenbaum, as well as a 1996 study by Warshaw and Keller that I was to meet again. Alyson Bond was surprised at the weight of the reply from Lilly.[41] Her article had not been aimed at reigniting the Prozac-and-suicide story.

At the end of 1994, after he had recovered from illness and surgery, I interviewed Jonathan Cole at an American College of Neuropsychopharmacology meeting as part of ongoing research on the history of psychopharmacology. Cole had been present from the establishment of the field and coordinated the early investigations of psychotropic drugs.[42] Our interview was about the evolution of the field during the 1950s and 1960s, not about Prozac, but I did ask if he regretted coauthorship of the Teicher paper. He did not know I had anything to do with the matter and said he didn't regret his role, concluding that Prozac still caused serious side effects[43] and that he would be happy to testify anywhere to that effect.

Should Prozac be accompanied by a warning? He supposed most clinicians would warn patients to take appropriate steps to minimize the risk. Against this background, the need for a warning seemed to him uncompelling.

I was not convinced. Bostonians may have known about Prozac's disadvantages, but elsewhere . . . ? Neither Cole nor I knew about the Wesbecker verdict handed down two days before our conversation.

Two weeks before the Wesbecker trial started—several months after my review article on Prozac and suicide—I had an invitation to meet with Joanna Nakielny and Gordon Coutts from Lilly, along with Tim Cassady, a company attorney from the United States handling European affairs. The invitation was to advise them on medico-legal issues. Despite having just published the review for CNS Drugs that year,

I felt no animus toward Lilly. The side effects, as I saw them, were ones that could be handled with appropriate warnings. I had no idea the corporation might be fighting for its life on just these issues.

We met on September 12 in London. The Lilly group outlined possible clinical scenarios, none of which seemed likely to have been caused by Prozac. If this was the kind of action they were facing, they had my support. They were interested in my views; I gave them. I suggested comparing akathisia to the irritable or snappy state that anyone might get into after one cup of black coffee too many. I could recognize in myself that I might shout at my children and regret it after an extra cup of black coffee. But should someone beat a criminal charge because they'd had too much black coffee? There seemed no way a jury would ever excuse someone on this basis.

The group were interested in my views on Peter Breggin. I gave fairly standard psychiatric views. When Breggin's *Toxic Psychiatry* came out in 1991, I arranged for it to be reviewed by the *British Association of Psychopharmacology Newsletter*. The most succinct review, by David King from Belfast—"Too toxic to read"—was unprintable.[44] Debbie Harrison of Lilly had, in fact, written the most favorable review.

THE JICK STUDY

The key event of 1995 was a publication in the *British Medical Journal* at the start of the year (which meant the article was in press during the Wesbecker trial). This was an epidemiological study by Hershel Jick and colleagues.[45] There was drama in the figures, the choice of words, and what one might read between the lines. Based in Boston, Jick and colleagues had investigated the computerized databases of British primary-care physicians. They had been able to assemble information on over 172,000 patients who had been prescribed a range of antidepressants, including Prozac. The figures for suicides on Prozac were substantially higher than the figures for any other antidepressants—2.1 times higher than those for dothiepin. Dothiepin was regularly denounced in vehement terms by the makers of the SSRIs as the archetypal older lethal-in-overdose antidepressant. It was also, in 1995, the best-selling antidepressant in Britain.

Because dothiepin was prescribed far more than all the other antidepressants, the figures for suicide associated with its use became the reference figure against which the figures for Prozac and other antidepressants were compared. Dothiepin came out midway among the antidepressants. Compared with other antidepressants supposedly safe in overdose, such as mianserin, trazodone, flupenthixol, and Prozac[46]—all of which might have been given to patients who were more suicidal— dothiepin seemed much less dangerous. Were the figures high for Prozac and these other drugs because they were being given to riskier groups? When efforts were made to control for this bias, the figures for mianserin, flupenthixol, and trazodone all fell, suggesting that these drugs were, in fact, being given to patients at greater risk. The figures for Prozac, however, remained the same.

A number of other drugs came out as even safer than dothiepin. One was lofepramine, an older antidepressant safe in overdose. The figures in the Jick study for lofepramine, which was a norepinephrine reuptake inhibitor, mapped onto the figures in a large Swedish study, which also found it to be the safest antidepressant.[47] The oddity of this was that according to 1980s thinking, norepinephrine reuptake inhibition should have made lofepramine an activating drug and more likely to lead to suicide.

Thinking on antidepressants and suicide in the 1980s was dominated by the same ideas of Paul Kielholz that had led to the synthesis of the SSRIs.[48] Kielholz's thinking had stemmed from a trial with imipramine he had conducted in 1957, in the course of which there had been two suicides. Before imipramine, the traditional wisdom had been that people on their way into or out of a depression were most at risk of suicide. This led Kielholz to the idea that any antidepressant might increase the risk of suicide simply by increasing the number of exits from and subsequent reentries into depression.

Kielholz later moved on to the idea that activating antidepressants, like the MAOIs, might be riskier than other antidepressants. In the 1960s, phenelzine had been the best-selling antidepressant, and it was this drug that Sylvia Plath had been on when she committed suicide a week after starting treatment.[49] The idea that activating antidepressants were riskier dominated the field before Prozac.

When Jick and colleagues looked at rates at which people committed suicide in the month after being prescribed a new drug, the figures for Prozac increased even further. This fit exactly with the Teicher profile that Prozac led to suicide by causing agitation during the first few weeks of treatment.

But you can only cut a piece of cloth so far. Older age is known to make suicide more likely. Men are more likely than women to commit suicide. And previous suicide attempts predict later suicides. When the Jick study controlled for all these factors at the same time, the results for Prozac were still 2.1 times greater than the rates of suicide on dothiepin. But this doubling of the suicide rate was no longer statistically significant. No one therefore could say that the Jick study had proven beyond all doubt, in all circumstances, that Prozac caused people to commit suicide. But the paper unquestionably gave a strong enough signal that Prozac could trigger suicide to warrant at least a follow-up study. Perhaps the most interesting feature of the Jick study is that it could easily have been repeated, but nothing happened.

HOMEGROWN AKATHISIA

A major part of my research around 1995 involved investigating the cognitive effects of psychotropic drugs to see whether different drugs have different effects on memory or attention. A tranquilizer such as Valium gives an experience completely different from an antidepressant like Prozac; no one who had either of these blind could confuse them with each other or with a placebo. Astonishingly, however, when it comes to giving computer-delivered cognitive tests, it may be impossible to detect which drug a person is on, or even to confirm that the individual is not on a placebo. Alternative explanations for these findings are that inside the brain these different drugs all act the same way, or that our psychological tests are useless. The challenge was to find some test that could discriminate between drugs so obviously dissimilar.[50]

In 1993, Steve Tipper, the world's leading expert on tests to demonstrate negative priming, had moved to Wales. There was good reason to believe that the differences among drugs should be detectable on his test, a much more subtle one than many conventionally used for this kind of work. We organized to recruit sixty volunteers from the medical and nursing staff of the psychiatric unit as well as clinical psychologists, psychology students, and others. They would be randomized single-blind to a once-off dose of 5 mg of droperidol, an antipsychotic; 1 mg of lorazepam, a benzodiazepine tranquilizer; or a placebo. These drugs were chosen primarily because they came in liquid form and could be concealed in orange juice. Doses were low enough to leave us worried that some people might show no effect.

A steady stream of subjects came through my office, took their orange juice, and sat down in front of the computer screen to do a set of very boring tests. They then had to hang around for three hours before repeating the tests. In the final analysis, the negative-priming test did show differences between the drugs. But the results were to remain lying in a drawer, not written up, because something else right in front of my eyes took priority.[51] The volunteers getting droperidol were having difficulties.[52]

I watched, fascinated. Drinking their juice in the morning, they looked normal and healthy, but an hour or so after taking the drug, they looked pallid and somehow shrunken. In some cases, they looked like they'd just contracted the flu, an impression reinforced by running noses. In most cases, they looked restless. This was not akathisia with obviously restless feet; it was a restlessness whose sufferers might opt to move around without being fully able to explain why. Unlike foot-tapping restlessness, which can sometimes happen without the person being upset by it, these volunteers were uncomfortable. During the three-hour period between the tests, they moved regularly around the unit or to and from their cars. They went for walks to "clear my head." But when I asked them how they were feeling, the invariable response was "fine."

We later convened a focus group for those who had been on droperidol to get a better idea of what had happened to them. To a person, they had felt dysphoric, unsettled, and disturbed even while telling me they felt fine. They found it difficult to put their unexpected experiences into words. It was not like anything that had happened to them before. Some had said nothing because they didn't want to make fools of themselves, assuming they might be on the placebo and worried that complaints might simply demonstrate their suggestibility. Others felt awful but couldn't believe the drug was causing this. They had begun to think about some of the worst moments in their life. Highly personal memories of previous unhappy times—broken relationships or loneliness—seemed to be flooding back. And if they had previously held themselves responsible for these unhappy times, they seemed to hold themselves responsible for feeling the way they did now as well. This happened to Richard Bentall, one of the world's leading experts on what leads people to attribute events that happen to them to themselves rather than to the situation they are in. Richard seemed powerless to apply to the situation what on one level he scientifically knew to be true. His heart overwhelmed his head. He was reduced to tears within an hour.[53]

Phil Thomas, a senior university colleague, became irritable and belligerent. Gwen Jones Edwards, a consultant psychiatrist, became restless and unsettled. The drug transformed her skin and posture so that she looked like a "schizophrenic." She felt everything was an effort one minute and then experienced waves of restlessness the next. One minute she would be okay doing something, and the next minute she was paralyzed. And it kept on going. A week after taking just one pill, she was still feeling strange, and at several points during the week she became suicidal.

Gwen later described her experiences on the national UK radio program *All in the Mind,* and wrote an article for a patient magazine describing the experience very vividly.[54] She sent the first version of this article to the journal *Human Psychopharmacology,* but the reviewer dismissed this subject as neurotic, arguing that reactions this long after a single dose were not possible. However, I had correspondence from Merton Sandler, a professor of chemical pathology and one of the early psychopharmacology pioneers, who in the late 1950s had suffered adverse effects from a single dose of reserpine for four weeks. It made him paranoid and belligerent.[55] So Gwen's reactions were not unusual. What was interesting was how the field had forgotten that reactions like this, lasting as long as this, could indeed happen after one-time use of psychotropic drugs.

This study changed my approach to the hazards of Prozac. Dotted around the literature are reports from psychiatrists who themselves became dysphoric or suicidal after taking antipsychotics.[56] Comparing drug-induced agitation or turmoil to the effects of too much coffee no longer seemed right. Other researchers working with healthy volunteers had seen similar effects in their colleagues but had not emphasized the point, for fear of jeopardizing all healthy volunteer work.[57] In the course of developing antipsychotics from the 1950s to the 1970s, it had been common practice for clinicians and scientists working with pharmaceutical companies to try these drugs themselves. They knew all about drug-induced akathisia and dysphoria and how awful it could be. A changing ethical climate in the 1970s made it difficult to conduct scientific experiments on vulnerable populations such as prisoners, the mentally handicapped, or others whose consent could not be freely given. Students and company employees were also thought to be vulnerable, as it might be argued they felt forced to take the drug.[58] As a result of these changes, company personnel in the 1990s had much less firsthand knowledge of their drugs.

Nevertheless, there is a solid literature on antipsychotics making patients suicidal or homicidal. No one denies that this can happen. Indeed, Lilly and other companies from 1997 were to sell their new, atypical antipsychotics on the basis that they caused less akathisia and were therefore less likely to make patients suicidal than older antipsychotics. Given that Prozac had been noted right from the start to cause dysphoria and agitation, it was hard to see how Lilly or anyone else could deny it might also lead to suicide or homicide.

ON THE BRINK OF ENGAGEMENT

In the mid-1990s, the British media began to pay attention to the increasing use of Ritalin for children. In my last year as secretary of the British Association for Psychopharmacology, I put forward the idea of a consensus conference to establish the basis on which it would be legitimate to prescribe psychoactive drugs to children. This took place in January 1997 and involved American, British, Canadian, and European academic child psychiatrists, along with Paul Leber and Barbara van Zwieten, senior regulators from North America and Europe. In contrast to Ritalin trials, all of which showed the drug worked, none of the trials with antidepressants in children published by 1997 seemed to show they were helpful.

An intriguing feature of the meeting was that North American psychiatrists were happy to prescribe large amounts of psychotropic drugs to children, including antidepressants, whereas in Britain the majority of child psychiatrists still boasted that they had rarely, if ever, prescribed Ritalin or an antidepressant. This didn't seem to be a matter of clinical trial evidence. If everyone had been following the evidence, both countries would have been using Ritalin, but neither would have been giving antidepressants. This was a cultural matter.

As the convener of the meeting, I had to negotiate a path that would work for both the advocates of Ritalin and Prozac and the psychologists present who were hostile to drug therapies for children. The acceptable answer all around was to put the interests of the child first and to monitor whatever treatment was offered, whether pharmacotherapy or psychotherapy. All options should be genuinely on the table, and if children were not responding to one approach, there should be a genuine review of their cases to make possible switches from pharmacotherapy to psychotherapy and vice versa.[59]

Somewhere around this time I got around to reading John Cornwell's *The Power to Harm,* a gripping inside account of the *Wesbecker* case published the year before. It took several more years before I knew of dramas Cornwell had missed.

For instance, shortly before the *Wesbecker* trial began in 1994, Marilyn Tobias, the wife of Lilly's new chief executive, committed suicide. She had been taking Prozac shortly beforehand. Leigh Thompson, the up-and-coming Lilly golden boy who was aiming at a place on the board, and who had done more than anyone to save Prozac, vanished after the trial. As the Halcion story suggests, when company personnel become a liability, they move on.[60]

Cornwell left unanswered the question of why *Wesbecker* was the first Prozac case to be tried. It turned out that Paul Smith, the lawyer who had wrestled a corporate giant to the floor on the worst possible of cases, had settled the *Biffle* case in September 1993, but this case was not cited anywhere as settled until after the *Wesbecker* trial—some sixteen months later. Not knowing about the *Biffle* settlement had inhibited anyone else from pushing forward any of several other clear cases to trial in the interim. Was it circumstance or design that led to the *Wesbecker* case's being the first—and very nearly the only—case to actually end up in court?

Smith's depositions in the case appear brilliant to the historian or sociologist trying to understand how the pharmaceutical industry worked in the 1980s and 1990s. But not all lawyers would see them this way. For all the revelations he extracted, he let Lilly provide justifications for what had happened that would seriously compromise the ability of other lawyers to tackle the issues. Many lawyers would have cut to the chase, as Nancy Zettler was more inclined to do. Finally, the terms of the *Wesbecker* settlement required Smith to win or lose: a verdict of eight to four and a mistrial would have given him nothing. Against this background, the comments of neutral parties that his performance in summing up for the plaintiffs was very weak, scream out for an explanation.[61]

Immediately after the *Wesbecker* case, Smith brokered settlements in a series of outstanding cases—for instance, fourteen of the fifteen Kannanack, Murgatroyd, Baum and Hedlund cases. These deals made Smith wealthy but later led to legal actions from colleagues.

Nancy Zettler had an outstanding Chicago case involving "Corky" Berman. She was perhaps the only person who knew enough after *Wesbecker* to construct a case to take to the Department of Justice. But nothing happened: she was burned out after *Wesbecker*, and her case remained unsettled. Until it went to trial or settlement, this case would inhibit her from taking any action to the Justice Department, in case an adverse ruling compromised her clients. The *Berman* case remained pending until October 2002.

For me, discovery of these things lay in the future. In the meantime, notwithstanding the Jick study, by 1995 the Prozac fire had died back to its embers. I accepted an invitation from Lilly to attend the April 1996 American Psychiatric Association meeting in New York. I had been asked to give a view on a murder case in Britain involving Prozac and had argued that there was no cause to implicate the drug. Other cases had come my way, but none that had led me to implicate Prozac. After one case I had not been able to support, I was contacted by the lawyer involved, Graham Ross, who complained that if he had seen the statement on the bottom of my 1994 article on fluoxetine and suicide, indicating that I was a consultant to Lilly, he would never have referred the case to me. The clear implication was that I was biased against plaintiffs. Despite this statement of my links to Lilly, a set of lawyers who knew all about these links were about to send me a case quite different from anything I had seen before.

3

Down the Barrel of a Lawyer

A LETTER ARRIVED in May 1997 from a California legal firm, Baum, Hedlund, Aristei, Guilford and Downey, outlining the case of a man on Prozac who killed his wife and then himself. Surprised that an American legal firm had approached me, I reacted dismissively at first. But since I was to attend an American Psychiatric Association (APA) meeting two weeks later in San Diego, only fifty miles from the Baum, Hedlund office, I contacted them.

The APA was rapidly expanding to international status. In 1996 the World Psychiatric Association meeting attracted six to ten thousand delegates, while the APA meeting registered sixteen thousand or more. A large proportion were foreigners brought by pharmaceutical companies. Zeneca, whose antipsychotic Seroquel was heading toward launch, was bringing me.

I had an ulterior motive. Researching the history of the antidepressants, I had seen that the conventional history was wrong. Max Lurie, an unknown from Cincinnati, had made the first discovery of an antidepressant in 1953. I tracked down all Luries in the Cincinnati area in 1996 and finally got through to Max. He doubted that anyone would find his 45-year-old memories reliable and turned down my request to visit him. A year later, I got back in touch with Max, and he agreed to meet.[1]

I let the lawyers know I would fly to Cincinnati from San Diego, and if they wanted me to look at material, I would bring it on the plane to Cincinnati and meet with them the day after that. Most legal briefs I had seen were no more than a few inches thick. But the material waiting for me in the Hilton Bay Hotel on the evening of May 24 filled two photocopier-sized boxes. The first box included a bundle sealed in black paper, labeled "Photographs," which I quickly closed. There were diaries kept by William and June Forsyth. Then there were hundreds of pages of depositions from relatives, friends, medical staff, and others. Finally, there were statements from experts for Lilly outlining why

Prozac was not to blame in either death. There was too much to take to Cincinnati, so I selected the medical depositions.

By the time I met the lawyers, I had learned that William Forsyth had been a man in his sixties under some stress. Relations with his wife had been mixed for a few years. He had gone on Prozac and ten days later had butchered her and killed himself. It had come as a shock to those involved, even the treating doctors, one of whom speculated that some intruder must have done it. The intruder possibility was ruled out by the police investigation. Another of the treating doctors stated that murder-suicide had been beyond the realm of possibility.

William Downey, a partner in the firm, showed up along with Cindy Hall, a paralegal, and a man called Andy Vickery. Downey took the lead. He was pretty clear that the evidence strongly implicated Prozac. The bit of the evidence that I had seen didn't seem so clear-cut to me.

Cindy Hall was deadpan. She fielded technical questions about what pieces of information might be in which deposition. She didn't seem to trust me. Vickery seemed a bored hanger-on. He, I was told, would be the trial attorney should the case go that far.

The conversation bobbed around. I told them that if I were Lilly, I'd describe akathisia as similar to being wired with coffee, and I'd invite a jury to consider whether they would excuse a murderer just because he had drunk too much coffee. I outlined my involvement as a consultant for Lilly, but they didn't seem concerned. They made it clear that they wanted me to decide if I could say with reasonable medical certainty that Prozac had been a causal factor in the Forsyth case.

Reasonable medical certainty was then a new idea for me. I can now quickly decide whether I can get to reasonable medical certainty on a case and don't have philosophical agonies about it, but there, in the San Diego sun, I had no idea what it meant. I was still grappling with the concept two weeks later.

For the attorneys, it meant being 51 percent certain that Prozac had contributed to the deaths of the Forsyths. After it became clear that I wasn't going to be able to reach 51 percent that afternoon, the conversation began to wind down. Downey suggested I read some of the children's testimonies on my way home.

Fishing out a checkbook, he also retained me. I didn't think I'd given any indication I was likely to be involved in the case. They told me that they had to file in ten days. I didn't think I'd be able to make up my mind that quickly. I already knew that the daughter, Susan Forsyth, was involved in a Prozac Survivors Support Group and the son, Billy Jr., had traveled to Lilly's plant in Indianapolis and put leaflets on cars in the parking lot that told Lilly employees their company had produced and was marketing a drug that killed people. Lilly accused Billy Jr. of trespassing and painted all Prozac survivor groups as having links to either Peter Breggin or the Church of Scientology. This was not a case Lilly wanted to settle, and nothing about these aspects of it inclined me to sympathize with the Forsyths.

I didn't just have to make my mind up about William Forsyth; I had to work out what I was doing in this situation. There were people at the APA meeting it might be worth talking to—people like Tony Rothschild, whom I had met six months previously, at an American College of Neuropsychopharmacology meeting. Rothschild had cowritten one of the more interesting case studies of Prozac. I had just published my book of interviews with senior figures in the field, *The Psychopharmacologists*,[2] and he was one of the first people I'd met who had a copy. He introduced himself at the ACNP meeting and let me know how much he enjoyed the book.

Rothschild expressed surprise that there were more Prozac cases but not that lawyers had contacted me rather than him. When I asked my three lawyers why they got in touch with me, they had said that the profile of this case seemed to fit the profile of Alan L. I'd described. But why hadn't they asked Tony Rothschild? They had written to him, they said, but got no answer. Tony wasn't surprised they had chosen me; a lot of things had gone on, he said.[3]

What to do? I spoke with two colleagues from industry and outlined the problem. But the discussion wasn't about whether they thought Prozac could trigger this kind of carnage; the problem was how would my industry contacts react if I got involved in the case. Would other pharmaceutical companies take an attack on one of their number as an attack on all of them?

These two seemed to think that if the case was clear-cut on clinical grounds, I should go ahead. But they also hinted that this was the kind of thing older men did at the ends of their careers, when they couldn't be hurt. How would a company hurt someone? These two didn't seem to know.

I read Susan and Billy Forsyth's depositions on the way home. Contrary to what I had expected, they were persuasive, describing respectable parents and a relatively stable marriage, and bewilderment at the tragedy.

WILLIAM FORSYTH'S STORY[4]

William Forsyth was born in Michigan in 1929 and moved to Los Angeles with his mother as a child. In 1955, at Scott Air Force Base in southern Illinois, he met June, who was then in first-year English. They married on the base six weeks later and were posted to West Germany for two years.

After returning home in 1957, the Forsyths moved to Los Angeles and began a car rental company. They had two children, Susan and Billy Jr. By 1986, William Forsyth was a wealthy man, with investments in apartment complexes. He was approached by Los Angeles airport, which wanted to buy the land on which his automobile business was based. He sold and retired.

Billy Jr. moved to Maui in 1981, and the senior Forsyths began to visit Maui regularly when they became grandparents. During 1989 and 1990, they built a home on Maui at Kanapalli Hillside and, in 1990, moved to Maui full time. This was June's dream. Billy Jr. had an attractive lifestyle there, using his boat to take anglers out deep-sea fishing and tourists to watch the whales off Maui. Bill Sr. enjoyed going out on the boats. The children and their friends described Bill and June's relationship as good, with no hints of violence or danger.

Bill had less involvement in his son's business than expected, but June became active in a Christian church, made new friends, and became more assertive. Retirement was an opportunity for a new life; instead of merely supporting her husband in business, she was free to look after herself. She explored co-counseling aimed at deepening her relationship with Bill, now that they were together so much more. She would have preferred him to be as keen on the new church as she was. But he wasn't. Both were more church-oriented than a comparable European couple. I had initially been inclined to accept Lilly's lawyers' view that June's pressure became oppressive and irritating for Bill. But as I read further, I found it increasingly hard to sustain that interpretation.

It seemed from their questioning of Susan and Billy Jr. that the Lilly approach was to portray William Forsyth as a man with a long history of nervous problems, one who had never really coped with retirement and who was being oppressed by his wife and son. At one point the idea was even floated that his son and wife might actually have been conspiring against him to take away his money. Certainly, William Forsyth was having some difficulties as 1992 turned into 1993, but as I read the record, he seemed a man at a loose end rather than one who was oppressed. There was no evidence of any ill will between him and his wife. He appeared happy to go to church and was even committed to it.

He had spells of anxiety in 1992 and communicated his discontent to his wife, his son, and others. Twice during the year he left Hawaii and returned to southern California, where he still had business interests. At one point it seemed he might even leave the marriage. But there had been no violence, and he stayed away only a few weeks.

While in southern California on one of these trips, William Forsyth sought out a marital counselor, Tom Brady, and arranged for June to come over and visit Brady with him for seven sessions. This seemed to make a difference. Brady's assessment of the case was interesting. A man used to conflict in marriage, he did not see the Forsyths as a relationship in serious difficulty. There were differences between them and adjustments to be made, but this was a relationship that had endured and would continue to endure.

While in California, waiting for June to join him for their first session with Dr. Brady, an apparently nervous William Forsyth went to a primary-care physician who prescribed a tranquilizer, Xanax.[5] His nerves got worse. Back in Hawaii, William Forsyth visited Dr. Riggs Roberts, a psychiatrist in private practice. In December 1992, Riggs Roberts diagnosed William Forsyth as being depressed—not a serious depression; not suicidal; not needing hospitalization. Riggs Roberts continued the Xanax and started Bill Forsyth on nortriptyline—Lilly's norepinephrine reuptake inhibitor from the 1960s.

Thirty years previously, Bill Forsyth had been drinking to excess. He stopped, joined Alcoholics Anonymous, and had not, it seemed, touched alcohol for thirty years. He was unhappy about now taking pills. But he was also a man to do what his doctor told him to do, and during the course of the following weeks, he probably took his pills as prescribed. They made some difference, but it was not clear from the records just how much difference. Things still were not right, but it was not clear whether the problems at this point stemmed from difficulties with June or with his prescribed drugs aggravating rather than relieving his symptoms. Riggs Roberts made medication changes, adding trazodone (Desyrel), a sedative anxiolytic drug sometimes used to treat depression.

Perhaps locked into a medical model of what was going on, with no great reason (as I read the record) to believe that a drug was going to make a big difference, and certainly not because the gravity of the situation demanded it, Riggs Roberts decided on another approach. He suggested Forsyth try Prozac. He gave him a supply of 20 mg pills, of which he was to take one per day. The next day Forsyth felt great and telephoned Riggs Roberts to say he was 200 percent better. Riggs Roberts told him that he was experiencing the Prozac miracle.

But the miracle was short-lived. The following day Forsyth felt terrible—so bad that he informed his wife and son that he needed to go to the hospital, fast. Astonished, Billy Jr. called Riggs Roberts to inform him of what was going on. Roberts was surprised and tried to talk Billy out of taking his father to the hospital, but William Forsyth was insistent, and Billy had already arranged to take him to the Castle Medical Center on Oahu.

There, William Forsyth was admitted by a resident staff member who noted that he did not seem to have the kind of condition that warranted admission. That Mr. Forsyth was so anxious to be admitted was doubly surprising, given that he had never been a psychiatric patient in his life and probably never could have imagined being one. He was admitted under the care of Dr. Randolph Neal, who saw him the next day. Dr. Neal was also surprised by the admission. There were no notes made by the medical staff to indicate that they thought William Forsyth was suicidal. His Prozac had been stopped on the first day after his admission to Castle but was restarted the following day.

The records reveal a man who attended some groups and activities but appeared unable to settle down in a relaxed fashion to participate in anything. He left activities early and spent a good deal of time on his own.

Six days after admission, he indicated he wanted to go home. The Castle doctors were now uneasy about Forsyth leaving, but without any clear idea why. The Medical Center policy preferred that patients discharging themselves give notice, a common practice, although not usually legally binding. The simple requirement of giving notice often deters someone, and as it turned out, Forsyth didn't leave the next day. But nor did he settle down. Ten days after he had begun on Prozac, he left the hospital.

June came to collect him. They went home and had a meal together that evening. Billy Jr. visited and later described his father as looking shaky, gray, and nervous—a man vastly changed from several weeks before. That evening the family agreed things had gone wrong the previous week, but that they could overcome the difficulties if they pulled together. Billy and his wife, Kim, were expecting their fourth child in less than two weeks, and William got on tremendously well with his grandchildren. The third of March was a new day. They would go out whale spotting with Billy Jr. This was something to look forward to, and in the course of the following days they would sit down together and plan a more exciting and involved future.

When his parents didn't turn up by the time of the final boat trip of the day, Billy Jr. became concerned. He went by their house in the early evening. He found his parents lying in, as a police officer described it, "more blood than [he] had ever seen." William Forsyth had stabbed his wife fifteen times, then fixed a serrated kitchen knife to a chair and impaled himself on it.

BEING DEPOSED

By the time I got home, I had come to think this was the kind of case where Prozac *must* have been a contributing factor. There was no suicide note; there were no signs of premeditation. Forsyth's behavior was inexplicable in terms of what had gone before. I asked colleagues whether they could they see any other way to explain what had happened, or any hazards of participating in this kind of case. No one had any other explanations. No one knew what getting involved in the case might mean.

I wrote to the Medical Protection Society to check that my insurance would cover participation in the case—a formality, I thought. The reply regretted that coverage did not extend to legal cases in the United States and advised me not to get involved; there was always a risk that the plaintiffs might take an action against an expert who they felt had jeopardized their chances of winning.

I explained this problem to Baum, Hedlund. The answer came back was that this was a remote technical possibility—although, worryingly, one case did offer a precedent. Bill Downey wrote me a letter of indemnification. With this in hand, I penned my report, indicating that I believed on the balance of probabilities there was no other explanation for what happened: Prozac had disturbed the equilibrium of William Forsyth's mind so that his death and the death of his wife followed as a consequence of that disturbance. I sent the report off. Nothing happened. I began to think that it might all have gone away.

A month later, I was told I would have to be deposed. I had no idea what a deposition was. (They don't happen in Britain.) At this stage, I knew nothing about the extensive depositions in the *Wesbecker* case. But I knew enough to know being interrogated by lawyers might be scary. I had gotten around to reading Cornwell's account, in *The Power to Harm*, of Peter Breggin being all but mugged on the witness stand.

The deposition was set for a well-worn Hilton Hotel at John F. Kennedy Airport. I was just checking in when Bill Downey and Cindy Hall appeared. I pleaded for guidance on what was likely to happen and some indication as to how I should handle it, but no pointers were given, nor any hints offered as to what tack Lilly might take. I was led to believe that when another of Downey's experts, Ron Shlensky, a forensic psychiatrist, had been deposed by Lilly a short time previously, Lilly's lawyer Andy See had focused on scientific methods in general and randomized controlled trials in particular, which, according to See, were the gold standard in the field for demonstrating cause and effect. This seemed to be something new for everyone and no one seemed to have a clear fix on what the right answers were. According to Downey, Shlensky had ducked and weaved on the issue. I was uncomfortable. If I ended up against the ropes, they weren't offering any quick duck-and-weave classes.

We started at 8:00 the next morning in a small hotel meeting room. At one end of a long table that could have accommodated twenty people comfortably, Andy See—who worked for Shook, Hardy and Bacon—sat with heaps of papers laid out in front of him and crates of documents lined up beside the table. I sat opposite, with the court stenographer between us. Downey and Hall were also seated around the table with cartons of documents.

Very early on, we ran into difficulties.[6] See asked if I had done research on the issue since my involvement in the case. How could I? I'd been involved only for eight weeks; no one could do research on the subject in that period of time. So my answer was "no." See all but folded up his documents and left. Then it turned out that research for a lawyer was something very different from research for a medic. Research meant "Had I read something?"

Then See raised the matters of randomized controlled trials and the nature of science. Isn't it important to adhere to the highest standards of scientific methods? Are randomized controlled trials thought to be the gold standard in the clinical field? His next step would be to ask where the randomized controlled trials were to show that Prozac caused suicide; the trick was not to slip down this slope. I refused to accept any of See's points, and tempers began to fray on both sides of the argument. There were quite a number of repetitions of "If you'll just answer my questions, we will get done because we all want to get done." It had been agreed that he had only until 4:00 p.m. to ask whatever he wanted or score whatever points he could, since I had a plane scheduled for 5:30. At one point he advised me that there were certain things he had to get through and that I'd have to come back if he didn't. It was difficult to know from looking at Bill or Cindy what they made of it all.

See confronted me with my 1994 words about data from several thousand patients counting for more in any scientific balance than a handful of anecdotes. Even with written evidence from follow-up letters that this was meant ironically, he wanted me to agree that my statement was meant literally.[7] I responded, "I wrote this article without thinking we were going to be going through the nitty-gritty. I didn't write it as a legal piece. As I keep saying to you, I wrote it within a certain scientific convention about how you handle these issues"—a scientific convention that dictated scientists *suggest* that the earth *might possibly* be round, rather than state unequivocally that it is.

See handed me a letter written to the *American Journal of Psychiatry* by a Dr. Cynthia Hoover. Following Teicher's initial study, Hoover had written in to the *Journal* reporting a similar case.[8] But the letter See was now showing me was from a year later, when the same patient had gone on imipramine and become suicidal. Clearly relishing the situation, Andy See put it to me, "In Dr. Hoover's letter to the editor she states that because of the subsequent history of the patient . . . the occurrence of suicidal ideation in this patient while he was taking fluoxetine was merely coincidental. . . . Doesn't Dr Hoover's subsequent report point up the problem of relying upon case reports of individual patients in order to come to conclusions about causation?"

But Hoover had missed the fact that imipramine also had significant serotonin reuptake-inhibiting properties. What she had unwittingly done, pretty much as we had done with Alan L., was provide a test-retest report. This strengthened rather than weakened the case against Prozac.

At one point, the issue of homicide-suicide came up. Had I researched it? No. With regard to any person with major depression, is it not possible, See suggested, to predict whether that particular person will commit the act of homicide-suicide? This was relatively easy. Homicide-suicide was so rare in Britain that it would make the national news, and therefore I could predict it wouldn't happen without some factor beyond the usual course of events—such as Prozac. A few months after getting home, I was consulted on the 1996 case of Reginald Payne, who, on the tenth day of a course of Prozac, murdered his wife, Sally, in bed and, after leaving a note on the fridge warning his son not to go upstairs, threw himself off a two-hundred-foot cliff. The case had appeared in the national newspapers, although I had missed it at the time. I was later to hear about another, similar American case: Brynn Hartman had gone on Zoloft and, on the tenth day of treatment, shot her husband, Phil, and then herself.

At 4:20 p.m., it was suddenly all over. Bill and Cindy congratulated me in the elevator on the way down; but surely they said this kind of thing to all their witnesses? For them, this had been a routine chore; for me, it was a first. As we parted for our respective planes, I asked Bill what would happen to the case. He said it would probably settle. After the elation of survival, this was a letdown. The case had seemed to me increasingly clear-cut. And *some* case needed to be won in order to make a difference. Had I only begun to feel it was winnable because the adversarial system forces us to take positions and then start justifying them? Bill wasn't sounding like a crusader. For him, a settlement was a win: The clients got something, if not an apology, and of course the law firm got money. Cindy, as it turned out, was a crusader who believed passionately that Lilly was in the wrong, but she concealed this completely from me. Bill, unbeknownst to anyone, wasn't going to live to see this case to its end. A cancer of his esophagus killed him. I never saw him again.

I flew home. Nothing disastrous had seemed to happen. When I read the deposition later, my greatest embarrassment about it was that the stenographer had evidently found my accent very difficult.

GENERAL CAUSATION

Andy See had confused me by raising the question of what he called general causation. I assumed he was referring to whether I thought Prozac might make even healthy volunteers suicidal. I replied that I hadn't thought about trying this, but it would be an interesting idea, which alarmed him. He clarified that what he meant was "Have you submitted for peer review the methodology that is the reasoning process behind using the categories of data or other information that you say you have relied upon to form your opinion in this case?" I didn't think I needed to—lots of textbooks covered this one. He disagreed.

In response to efforts by Lilly to get me removed from the case after the deposition, I put together a general causation statement outlining the basis of my views that Prozac could induce suicidality. This meant revisiting questions of cause and effect. How did one prove a drug caused an adverse effect? Getting a grip on these issues led me to write an article, which I sent to David Nutt, editor of the *Journal of Psychopharmacology*. Some editors wouldn't have the stomach for something like this; a more enterprising editor could have fun by sending it to one reviewer he knew to be vehemently opposed to the idea that there might be anything wrong with Prozac, and also to a more receptive reviewer.

I got back a brief supportive review and another review with three pages of criticisms that came as close to abuse as one ever gets in the review process.[9] But the covering letter from the journal made it clear that I didn't have to give up on this one. After considerable revision, drastic shortening, and a covering letter to show how I was taking the criticisms into account, I resubmitted the article. It went back to the second reviewer, who responded:

> This paper remains apparently unchanged . . . they still do not have the courtesy to the reader to fully report the findings of Beasley *et al* . . . , they continue to confuse agitation and akathisia . . . the authors' grasp

of the literature is modest and their grasp of data is apparently absent
. . . this paper lets down the authors, the journal and, frankly, the scientific community.[10]

Nevertheless, after further revisions, David accepted the paper.[11]

During revisions, I revisited the Jick study.[12] See's focus had been on the relative risk of Prozac as compared with dothiepin. Prozac appeared to be 2.1 times riskier. A figure of 2.0 is the conventional threshold at which epidemiologists conclude there may be something that warrants further study. A risk greater than 5.0 is very worrying. In the case of cigarettes and lung cancer, the risks are 15 times greater for smokers than for nonsmokers. Legally, the level of the relative risk with Prozac was an important issue.

The Jick figures translated into 189 suicides per 100,000 "patient years" (that is, per 100,000 years of patient treatment), rising to 272 per 100,000 patient years for those on their first month of Prozac treatment. The conventional standard is that depressed people have a 15 percent risk of committing suicide at some point during their lives. This translates into a figure of roughly 600 suicides per 100,000 patient years. Against this background, one way to read the figures for Prozac was that perhaps it wasn't as good as other antidepressants in lowering the risk that stemmed from depression but that it nevertheless did lower that risk. Eli Lilly emphasized that depressed patients were seventy-nine times more likely to kill themselves than people who weren't depressed. These figures could be used to argue not only that Prozac did not cause a problem but that there was a compelling moral case for ensuring that people who were depressed got treatment, in order to save lives.

Then it dawned on me: The Prozac figure should be compared not with the figure traditionally cited for people who were depressed but with the figure for primary-care depression—people who had never been hospitalized for their depression. These were the people who would get Prozac, because the drug was not being used in hospital depression. This was the issue that Bob Temple from the FDA had flagged at the FDA hearings on Prozac.

With resident Claus Langmaack, I looked more closely at the 1970 classic paper in the field by Samuel Guze and Eli Robins from Washington University, St. Louis, published in the *British Journal of Psychiatry*. This was the source of the magical figure of a 15 percent lifetime risk of suicide in depression—six hundred suicides per one hundred thousand patient years.[13] But the Guze and Robins paper was a two-page article summarizing the results of fifteen studies of depressed patients followed up for risk of suicide from the pre-antidepressant German and Scandinavian literature. It was easy to believe that these hospitalized melancholics and severe manic-depressives had a 15 percent lifetime risk of suicide. But these were *not* the patients being given Prozac.

A publication from a research group in Southampton, which had added more recent studies to the original Guze and Robins studies, estimated that the lifetime risk of suicide in depressives was 6 percent.[14] But even this applied only to hospitalized patients. What was the figure for nonhospitalized patients? Claus and I could show that if the hospital rate of suicide was applied to all patients now being diagnosed as depressed, instead of five thousand suicides in Britain per year from all causes, there would have to be nine thousand suicides from depression alone. Obviously, then, the rate had to be lower for community depression. But what was it?

A paper just out offered an answer. "Jed" Boardman and colleagues had collected 212 suicides and unexplained deaths, over a five-year period, from the nearly half a million people living in the North Staffordshire area.[15] Medical records enabled them to identify those who had been in contact with the mental health services prior to their death. This made it possible to model much more accurately what the rates for depressed patients not in contact with mental health services might be. Jed and I came up with a figure of less than 30 suicides per 100,000 patient years for primary-care depressives. Comparing this with the Jick figure of 272 per 100,000 patient years for patients in their first month of treatment with Prozac gave a ten times greater relative risk on Prozac.[16]

Our modeled figure was in line with the only other figures available. A group of general practitioners in Holland had followed up depressed patients over a ten-year period and determined a figure of thirty-three suicides per one hundred thousand patient years[17]—remarkably close to ours. But even more interesting was a study from Lundby in Sweden.[18] This gave Lilly its figure that depressed patients were seventy-nine times more likely to commit suicide. But Lilly had selectively compared the figure for *hospitalized* patients from this study with the figure for people who were not depressed. This resulted in a seventy-nine times greater rate for depressed people.

The Lundby report was a unique study looking at a small Swedish district over a thirty-year period. The drawback was that only several thousand people were involved in the study; the great advantage was the huge time frame involved. It gave a figure for the suicide risk for patients who were depressed but had never been hospitalized. This was before the creation of modern depression, before the transformation of cases of Valium into cases of Prozac. A patient in the Lundby study could have been off work for six months and still be registered as mildly depressed. The suicide rate for this form of mild depression was *zero*— raising the possibility that mild depression might even confer some protection *against* suicide.

A later study from Gregory Simon and Michael Von Korff looked at suicides among depressed patients who were being treated by a health maintenance organization in Puget Sound. In this study, figures from the early 1990s showed nonhospitalized depressed patients committing suicide at a rate of forty-three per one hundred thousand patients. But patients not given drugs for their depression had a rate of suicide of *zero* per one hundred thousand patients, reinforcing the suggestion that mild depression could be in some way protective.[19]

This sobering possibility raised many issues. One was the selective use of figures from the Lundby study by Lilly. Lilly hadn't cited the figure for mild depression. This was an easy mistake to make if you were operating from a bunker in Indianapolis, but the entire psychiatric community appeared to have let this one slip by. We had become complicit in persuading primary-care physicians and other mental health workers to recognize and treat depressive disorders. We did so as part of efforts to detect depression, which sought justification in claims that treating depression would lower national suicide rates. There was no indication that anyone seemed to realize the figures we all so readily bandied about simply didn't apply.

DISQUALIFYING HEALY

Meanwhile, Lilly had sent a series of requests and supplemental interrogatories to the plaintiffs' attorneys. These were all variations on the following theme: Admit that no clinical trial or epidemiological study demonstrates a statistically significant difference in risk of akathisia or suicide or homicide between patients taking Prozac and those taking any other antidepressant. Even before waiting for a reply, Shook, Hardy and Bacon argued, in an application for summary judgment, that the plaintiffs had failed to make an acceptable general case that Prozac could lead to suicide and/or homicide. Judge Alan Kay overruled it.

Both Judge Kay and Lilly at this stage were focusing on the Jick study. Lilly had provided a declaration from Herschel Jick that his study did not prove Prozac caused suicide—a statement I could have made if I were Jick. What was more alarming was the drift away from recognizing, as Jick himself had done in an earlier paper, that in this area, test-retest methods rather than epidemiological studies were the way to prove cause and effect.[20]

Lilly came back at the issue with a declaration from Tony Rothschild that his test-retest study proved nothing, and with further declarations from Jick. Judge Kay had to be admired for keeping his nerve. I didn't know when I might be knocked out of the whole thing. One of the Forsyths' experts had already been disqualified, so this was no mere formality.

Gut-wrenching and draining motions for reconsideration of the original denial of summary judgment followed, based on claims that my evidence against Prozac was not adequate. Each arrived by courier or by fax and required a quick turnaround.

In the midst of these, Lilly filed another motion to disqualify me on the basis that they had consulted me on legal issues in 1994. This was the meeting with Lilly's attorney (described in Chapter 2), who declared he had understood the meeting to be confidential and accordingly had shared privileged information. "The facts presented compel Dr. Healy's disqualification as an expert for plaintiffs." Not only was this motion filed three months after the cutoff date, it was simply wrong. I would have loved to have received information from Lilly in 1994, but none had been forthcoming. Judge Kay dismissed the motion.

Lilly continued to file motions right into the week before the case was due to start in Hawaii in March 1999, leaving me unsure whether anything would ever happen. As I left Britain en route to the trial via an American Psychopathological Association (APPA) meeting in New York, I still didn't know if the trial would go ahead.

I had been asked to lecture on the history of the antidepressants at the APPA meeting in New York, a meeting whose subject was the treatment of depression.[21] In the two years since I was approached in the

4

Market Force

IN FEBRUARY 1997, two months before I heard about William Forsyth, I began working with another drug, reboxetine. Often when one group of drugs causes trouble, a new group is required to bring the problem to light. The hazards with barbiturates became clear to everyone only when there were benzodiazepines to market. Similarly, dependence on benzodiazepines became a health care crisis when there were new drugs active on the serotonin system to market. Reboxetine, marketed by Pharmacia and Upjohn, had no actions on the serotonin system.

The Upjohn pharmaceutical company had run into a worldwide barrage of negative publicity with its hypnotic Halcion, but it suffered especially in Britain, where it faced one of its most determined critics, Ian Oswald. Halcion was withdrawn from the British market, and in 1994, Upjohn and Oswald became embroiled in one of the longest libel trials in British legal history.[1] In its wake, a new, merged company, Pharmacia and Upjohn (P&U), was formed.

A forerunner of Pharmacia, Farmitalia Carlo Erba, had reboxetine sitting undeveloped on its books for a long time. Reboxetine was structurally similar to fluoxetine, but a small tweak of the molecule made it a norepinephrine reuptake inhibitor rather than a serotonin reuptake inhibitor—an NRI, as the company hoped to call it.[2] Although animal tests as early as 1984 suggested this might be an antidepressant,[3] the drug languished because neither Farmitalia nor Pharmacia had experience in psychiatry. Conventional wisdom recommended against trying to market a single drug from a class. Most successful compounds in all areas of medicine come to the market as a group of compounds, which together help to create a new market. The SSRIs are a good example. But if any company could pull off the trick of marketing a stand-alone psychotropic drug, it was Upjohn.[4]

When invited to join a consultancy panel to consider reboxetine, I had mixed feelings, as I didn't yet know what to make of the Halcion story. Stuart Montgomery, who had helped prepare P&U's application for the registration of reboxetine with the Medicines Control Agency (MCA) in Britain, chaired the panel meeting in London. This application had been approved so quickly that it left me wondering whether either sympathy for Upjohn or the company's apparent intention to take legal action against the UK authorities for banning Halcion had played a part in the decision.

What advice could a consultancy panel give Pharmacia about how to sell an NRI in an SSRI marketplace? In some European countries, E. Merck had successfully marketed the norepinephrine reuptake inhibitor, lofepramine, by emphasizing the "tired all the time" patient. Roughly half of the patients who present with "depression" complain about fatigue, and the other half complain of anxiety. It seemed sensible that a drug active on the norepinephrine system might be better for the first group and a drug active on the serotonin system better for the second group. This echoed the ideas that led to the creation of the SSRIs: that drugs active on the norepinephrine system would be drive-enhancing and drugs active on the serotonin system would do something else.

Reboxetine threw up a dilemma for me. In any clinical trial, company monitors check whether all boxes on all rating scales and all tests have been completed satisfactorily. Sometimes they insist side effects be recoded to fit the terminology of side-effect dictionaries. In short, the data are massaged. The question is whether the massaging has been done acceptably or not. Some years previously, a colleague had mentioned reports suggesting potential cardiac abnormalities with reboxetine. Had these been airbrushed out of the picture?

What do you do without firsthand information when a colleague asks this kind of question about a drug and a company? If the drug caused trouble after launch, that was a different matter. I raised the subject with Max Lagnado, Pharmacia's medical adviser on reboxetine. Max seemed trustworthy.[5] Even after he'd left the company, he seemed to know of no hidden cardiac data in the system. Maybe he didn't know, as he had joined only after the merger. How vigorously would anyone chase a doubtful practice if the rumors came from people linked to a competing company? After all the mergers, would it be possible to find anyone in the company who knew? As it turned out, several years after its launch in Europe, there was no evidence of cardiac abnormalities on reboxetine.

These general points are important when it comes to considering what faced people working in Lilly, or as consultants for Lilly, who might know of abnormalities secondhand. Even Ian Oswald conceded that despite all his trouble with the company, Upjohn UK seemed a decent lot.[6]

DIFFERENCES BETWEEN ANTIDEPRESSANTS

When Pharmacia's panel convened, Max Lagnado presented data on a Social Adaptation Self-Evaluation Scale (SASS), a scale company scientists had developed. In addition to the usual Hamilton Depression Scale (HAM-D), the SASS had been used in clinical trials where reboxetine was compared with Prozac. Where both reboxetine and Prozac looked similar on the HAM-D, there was an obvious difference in their SASS scores.[7] In the patients who got well on either Prozac or reboxetine as measured by the HAM-D, fewer than two out of every three taking Prozac returned to "normal" on the SASS, whereas more than three out four taking reboxetine did so.

In 1997, the conventional wisdom said it was impossible to show differences between antidepressant drugs. They might be very different in terms of the brain systems they worked on, but they all got the same number of depressed patients well, and they got them well within roughly the same time frame. There was a suspicion that clomipramine was a "stronger" antidepressant than the others were, but little conclusive clinical trial evidence.[8] A few distinguished voices could be heard crying from the wilderness that the different antidepressant drugs were *so* different in terms of their pharmacology that if they ended up all looking the same, this was because companies engineered it that way.[9] But no one could see an easy way to bring out the differences.

The scene was about to change. After the demise of mianserin (see pages 21–22), Organon marketed a sister compound, mirtazapine, with the trade name of Remeron.[10] In the event, what had been thought impossible could in fact be shown rather simply: Compare your drug with Prozac in a more severely depressed group of patients. The first hints of this appeared at a meeting in Amsterdam in September 1996, when Organon presented clinical trial data showing Remeron got more

depressed patients well than Prozac did. After the resulting press conference, the shares of the holding company, Akzo Nobel, jumped several points.[11] So many other newer agents coming to the market, all acting on the norepinephrine system, went on to pull off the same trick
that it no longer seems remarkable. But no company had managed anything similar in less severely depressed patients. In February 1997, these
SASS data collected in less severely depressed patients were surprising.

But what exactly was the SASS? No consultant in the room had ever
heard of it. It turned out that Adriana Dubini and Marc Bosc, while running an early clinical trials program for reboxetine, developed the SASS
specifically to include in reboxetine trials.[12] They had a strong hunch
that drugs active on norepinephrine would show up well on this scale
compared to SSRIs. Drugs active on the norepinephrine system were
more activating, and this should be good for social functioning. In the
midst of repeated corporate takeovers, no one objected. Then, suddenly,
they produced a result no one knew how to handle.

Myrna Weissman was the guru of social functioning. At Yale in the
early 1970s, she and her husband, Gerald Klerman, along with Eugene
Paykel, looked at the question of social functioning in depressed people. They found that while the older tricyclic antidepressants cleared up
many of the symptoms of depression—improving sleep, appetite, and
energy levels, and enabling patients to leave the hospital—many patients took months or even years to get back to normal social functioning.[13] Weissman decided to look at what could be done to improve the
social functioning of depressed patients. To do this, she needed a scale
to map the area, which became the Social Adaptation Scale (SAS).

Klerman and Weissman then created interpersonal psychotherapy
(IPT).[14] Initially, this was designed to complement antidepressant therapy. The goal was to focus on aspects of the social functioning of the patient, such as conflicts at home or at work, in order to promote social in-
tegration. It turned out that IPT did more than reintegrate people. By
the late 1980s, data from some large studies indicated it was potentially
even more effective than the market leader in depression psychotherapies, cognitive behavior therapy (CBT).[15]

As part of my efforts to chase the history of the field, I had interviewed Myrna Weissman in 1996.[16] On the basis of this contact, I agreed
to bring the SASS data to her attention at the APA meeting at San Diego
a few weeks later. We met the day after I had met the lawyers in the
Forsyth case. Weissman might well have responded by complaining

that her original SAS ideas had been hijacked. Instead, she was interested in the differences between reboxetine and Prozac that showed up on the SASS.[17]

But while most companies only dream about an endorsement from a figure of Weissman's standing, social functioning was not something many people would understand. Marketing departments want to control the message, and the SASS scale and social functioning were unknown quantities. There was a huge potential for prescribers hearing the story about the SASS data to "hear" that reboxetine was a new drug useful for patients with the poorest social functioning to begin with, rather than the message that it was a drug that would produce even better social functioning in the average patient who was depressed.

THE LAUNCH OF A DRUG

The first few months in a drug's life are at least as critical as the first few years of a child's. Market development is at the heart of the industrial process, involving PR and communication agencies and a set of techniques shared with political parties.

PR agencies for a pharmaceutical company like P&U, faced with a subject like reboxetine and social functioning, will feed the words *social functioning* into a computer search engine. This then spills out every article ever produced on the subject. Before reboxetine, however, most articles were produced in connection with personality disorders. PR people with no medical background can easily miss this. Their brief is simple—get speakers to talk on the issue of social functioning generally, and reboxetine sales will follow. This model worked in the cases of "Xanax + panic disorder" and "Paxil + social phobia." But the social functioning of personality disorders is not thought to respond to antidepressants. If the company or agency ends up with speakers whose research is on personality-disordered patients, the take-home message for the audience becomes "Forget drug treatments for social functioning!"

The alternative strategy is to go with the "old hands" in the field, who may know nothing about social functioning but who won't make this kind of mistake—"experts" who give the traditional message and who can be relied upon to stay on script and say the things that fit the company's interests. Better a dull formula than an exciting scientific debate that backfires. This is, after all, business, not science.

Reboxetine was due to be launched in Britain in July 1997 during a satellite symposium at the British Association for Psychopharmacology meeting in Cambridge. Satellite symposia had been big business at APA meetings for a decade but were still relatively rare in Britain. My brief at these and subsequent meetings was to talk about the SASS data. Other speakers focused on more conventional aspects of the physiology of the norepinephrine system, or the efficacy and safety data for the drug.

The Cambridge launch led to my involvement in a European College of Neuropsychopharmacology (ECNP) symposium later that year in Vienna. My talks covered the history of the antidepressants and the new SASS data. Fairly quickly, I raised the question of suicide on fluoxetine. If we were talking about differences in social functioning produced by the two drugs, what better ultimate outcome measure could there be than suicide data? The Jick study showed how much higher rates of suicide were for patients on Prozac than on other antidepressants, and in particular how much higher they were than for patients on lofepramine, an NRI and reboxetine's immediate predecessor in Europe.

Selling this message didn't seem to cause P&U any difficulties. Nor did it seem to be a problem to Stuart Montgomery, who shared the platforms with me, despite his previous attacks on me for my views on Prozac. Invitations came to talk on other P&U platforms in Sweden, Denmark, Finland, Spain, Ireland, France; at an APA meeting in Toronto; and elsewhere. I developed a standard talk, saying it wasn't simply a question of trying to get people well but a matter of having people on the right antidepressant, particularly during the follow-up period.[18] Because of emotional blunting and other effects, the SSRIs might well not be the right antidepressants for some people.[19] At no point did P&U put any pressure on me either to tone down my message or to conform to the conventional, safe script.

My lectures were deliberately provocative, but it was hard to gauge their effect. Some audience members said they'd enjoyed the talk, but who could say whether this was going to lead either to sales for reboxetine or to someone picking up the issue of suicide on the SSRIs? Each time, audiences of several hundred listened to what I was saying about Prozac and suicide without arguing back.

In Britain, I was asked to talk at a range of different meetings. At one such in Newcastle, I was close to where Ian Oswald, Halcion's most prominent critic, lived. Since I was chasing the history of psychopharmacology, and getting into the ambiguities of the field was part of my brief, I arranged to visit him.

My first surprise was that he did not appear bitter and twisted. In fact, he was even pleased that his investment portfolio included shares in the new Pharmacia and Upjohn, which he figured as a good bet for a merger.[20] During our interview, he outlined the legal tactics around the Halcion cases.[21] Shook, Hardy and Bacon, who also acted for the major tobacco companies, were the law firm for Upjohn, and Oswald described a range of things they had been up to. He drew my attention to the recently published *Cigarette Papers*, which outlined the legal maneuvers adopted by lawyers acting for the tobacco companies, particularly how research had been outsourced from companies and, apparently, in some cases either not published or not undertaken in order to reduce legal liabilities.[22] In conversation afterward, he talked about how scared he'd been at times. Millions of dollars were at stake. He had often fantasized how easy it would have been to bump him off while he walked in the dark on the neighboring country roads. Driving away, I had one more thing about Prozac and suicide to think about. The lawyers for Lilly in the Forsyth case were Shook, Hardy and Bacon. How different *were* the tobacco and the psychopharmacology industries?

SHADOW SCIENCE

In the 1990s, I wrote a good deal on how information moves around the psychopharmacology world.[23] A number of things influenced my thinking. In 1993, I published an interview with George Beaumont about the history of clomipramine. This led to inquiries from Ciba-Geigy about the possibility of obtaining up to twenty thousand reprints of this article. Ordinarily, even really good articles in distinguished scientific journals, putting forward novel points of view, would be unlikely to get more than two hundred to three hundred reprint requests if they lacked a clear commercial implication. It doesn't take much thought to realize which set of ideas is going to go further.

Around the same time, a series of articles began appearing in major journals, outlining the fine line between education and marketing; how meetings designed to produce consensus statements may, in fact, present only one point of view;[24] or how journal supplements may deceive readers into thinking they are dealing with peer-reviewed publications.[25]

At this stage, I was speaking for four different companies. This meant dealing with a number of PR and communications agencies as well as patient groups. A picture began to build up of a new world—a world of meetings in which industry could send delegates at up to £1,000 per day to find out how to form or influence patient groups; a world where articles from some of the leading figures in the field were ghostwritten by communications agencies; a world of supposedly scientific meetings having much in common with trade fairs.

PATIENT GROUPS

In October 1996, for instance, I could have attended a meeting, organized by the Institute for International Research in London, on "Creating Targeted Patient Education Campaigns—That Deliver Real Results."[26] This was billed as a must-attend meeting for marketers, product managers, brand managers, and medical information officers in the pharmaceutical industry. "Whilst the promotion of pharmaceutical products direct to the consumer is still strictly off-limits in Europe," the invitation read, "carefully planned patient education campaigns are allowed and becoming more widespread as pharmaceutical companies realize the benefits of added value services. At this two-day conference, you will discover how to successfully create targeted patient education campaigns which will establish your expertise in disease areas and increase company profile." At the meeting I could "*experience* first hand demonstrations of successful campaigns and new educational techniques, *measure* the real business benefits of effective patient education, [and] *profit* from the experience of international disease management and pharmaceutical marketing experts"—among other things.[27]

Patient groups have become a key pressure point in a market worth billions of dollars. They are the perfect conduits for generating views among the "informed" general public, such as the idea that depression is known to be a chemical imbalance in the brain. The promotion of a new antidepressant by the end of the 1990s commonly meant a patient on the speakers' panel, even for a medical audience. At meetings open to the press, patient speakers were almost more important than medical experts. They could offer journalists a simplistic story of how the correction of low brain amines by antidepressants put people right, which by then was a message few psychopharmacologists would have been happy to present. These patients offered living examples of salvation through chemistry.

Patient organizations developed in the United States, as did their subsequent penetration by the pharmaceutical industry. Patient activism has an honorable tradition in America. This led to the formation of the National Association for the Mentally Ill (NAMI), the first and the biggest patient organization in the mental illness field. By the 1990s, its levels of pharmaceutical company support attracted comment because NAMI campaigned aggressively under the slogan "Mind illnesses are brain illnesses" and argued that the way to reduce stigma was for even more people to be diagnosed and treated.[28]

There is nothing intrinsically wrong with a patient group looking for industry support. But it is worth noting exactly what has happened.

In the 1970s, patient groups in North America and Europe were among the most vigorous critics of psychiatry. A coalition formed within the mental illness field between these groups and anti-industry groups, who together managed to have antidepressants removed from the market in Europe. In response, industry began to court rather than oppose such groups, and in some cases to play a part in the establishing of patient groups. A childhood attention deficit disorder (CHADD) group supported by Ciba-Geigy was set up and became a remarkably effective lobbyist for Ritalin. Other groups were formed specifically for OCD sufferers,[29] social phobics, Touretters,[30] and others.

By the 1990s, speakers at meetings attended by patients who argued for the benefits of older (and perhaps cheaper) treatments for depression or schizophrenia were liable to face a hostile audience who, far from wanting to shake off their chemical straitjackets, demanded access to the newest and most costly treatments. In this situation, a patient group like Depressive Alliance (DA) might receive substantial funding from pharmaceutical companies and even share office facilities with PR agencies handling the accounts for antidepressant-producing pharmaceutical companies.[31]

Such arrangements provide badly needed opportunities for the patient group, but the PR agency and pharmaceutical company gain also. A patient group may be "helped" to support awards for best clinical practice in their particular illness. It might be offered funds to produce a piece of self-help literature for patients that would appear under the logo of the patient group, with an expert's name attached. When, as is likely, the original piece is ghostwritten in a PR agency (see below), the patient group risks becoming little more than a conduit for distribution of marketing copy. Such arrangements also typically land the patient group with legal liability for any statements made.[32]

In recent years, patient groups have supported campaigns concentrating on depression in children and young people.[33] These campaigns all begin innocently, geared toward increasing recognition rather than instituting treatment. But recognition is a prelude to medication. Lilly has supported the generation of patient information on depression in pregnancy and postnatal depression, for instance. This will tend to lead to use of SSRIs in women being treated for depression in pregnancy, despite concerns about the effects of SSRIs on the fetus.[34]

GHOSTWRITING AND COMMUNICATION AGENCIES

Another new beast in the psychopharmacology jungle is the communication or medical writing agency, often owned by just one or two people, with a background in medicine or a related science, who work closely with one or two pharmaceutical companies. Essentially, they have become the outsourced communication divisions of the major pharmaceutical companies. One advantage to the companies is that they can shop around among agencies if they think a quality product hasn't been delivered quickly enough at a competitive price. Companies can, for example, put out a contract for twenty-five articles with big-name authors to be placed in good journals, and wait for offers from agencies.

Well-run agencies can turn around material very quickly indeed. In the case of several symposia, I received my proposed talk from a communication agency shortly after agreeing to participate. The understanding in these cases was that I would agree to give the talk sent to me. This would then be put together with the other contributions and sent on to some journal, which had already agreed to publish the resulting supplement. Ghostwritten contributions like this get to the journal on time, unlike those from experts who write their own material. The supplement business is a lucrative one for journals, whose brief is to get the supplement ready for distribution at the company's satellite symposium.

Much to my surprise, a ghostwritten article incorporating elements of my style and references to my published work can seem like a *bona fide* Healy article. Even though the writers may have little or no background in psychiatry, they nonetheless quickly become confident enough to produce an article not immediately detectable as ghostwritten. One obvious conclusion is that in the process, psychiatric language must necessarily have been reduced to the level of a psychiatric *National Enquirer,* and indeed, in most of these journal supplements it is very hard to find anything that is not simply a rehash of material repeatedly presented elsewhere.

What is likely to happen if I decline to go along with an article sent to me? The company might be quite happy for me to produce my own article. I might be told that because certain commercial aspects of the previously produced version were important to the company, they will arrange for it to appear under the name of another senior figure in the field—perhaps someone who didn't actually present anything in the symposium of which these are supposed to be the proceedings. One result might be to have two recognizably "Healy" articles appear in the same supplement under different bylines.[35] Of course, the medical writing slips sometimes, so that articles from big names who are not native English speakers will appear dotted through with regional Americanisms or Anglicisms.[36]

Usually, ghostwritten articles arrive with a covering letter authorizing me to alter the piece in whatever way I see fit. One such letter arrived linked to a meeting aimed at promoting Wyeth's SSRI Efexor.[37] This Laguna Beach meeting came complete with honoraria, expensive travel and accommodation provision, and the opportunity to have one's article ghosted, in this case by CMED, a medical writing agency based in Toronto. The message being promoted was that compared to other SSRIs, which might make your patient well, Efexor got the patient fully better. The centerpiece was an article by Michael Thase, which later appeared in the *British Journal of Psychiatry.*[38] The Thase article led to follow-up correspondence querying how appropriate it was for a journal editor to be publishing articles from a company with whom he had a consultancy.[39] A growing concern led to a *Lancet* editorial asking, "Just How Tainted Has Medicine Become?"[40]

In this case, I left the main article intact but inserted two "viruses." One drew attention to data from trials with one of Efexor's closest competitors, Remeron, at odds with the message Wyeth wanted to convey in this meeting. The second referred to evidence that SSRIs could make some people suicidal. Getting people better than just well was academic if the patient was on the wrong drug.

The first "virus" drew an immediate response: The CMED author questioned the claims made for Remeron. I refused to back down. The article went through further drafts and was already submitted to the *Journal of Psychiatry and Neuroscience* before I got to see it again. Completely rewritten, it was an even more Wyeth-friendly version than the original draft, but what most concerned me were two specific changes. The references to suicidality on SSRIs were gone, and a message had been added at the end, stating evidence suggested venlafaxine was most effective at getting depressed patients completely well.[41] This was completely at odds with everything I believe about venlafaxine. The academic organizer of the symposium for Wyeth had chosen to sign off on the final version of the article—without consulting me.[42]

The usual company line in these instances is that, even when articles are ghostwritten, their notional authors check them closely and sign off on them. As Bert Spilker of the Pharmaceutical Research and Manufacturers of America put it when the issue was raised in the *Washington Post*, "Academic researchers participating in studies 'are given every opportunity to review, make suggestions and sign off on manuscripts [and] except for some very, very rare exceptions . . . [the process] is working very well.'"[43] In practice, as shown in the litigation surrounding Redux, senior figures are prepared to incorporate any changes suggested to them by companies or agencies and to sign off on articles without suggesting a single change of their own.[44]

In some cases, I've had requests from agencies to release to other speakers' slides from a talk that I have given. When the slides weren't prepared by me in the first instance and don't cover research that I've actually done, the fiction that these are "my slides" becomes positively Orwellian. When the name of a senior psychiatrist goes on material like this, whether slides or articles, the potential legal consequences are interesting. It would get even more interesting if it were established that big names had been put on articles produced to order by pharmaceutical companies specifically for legal purposes. As things stand, the process of discovery in legal cases involving the SSRIs and suicide has uncovered correspondence to senior figures in the field enclosing "their" article. Where article bylines include a company author among clinical authors, the company has often drafted the article in the first instance. Even if the clinical authors sign off on the final version, the writer of the first draft has primary control of the message.

A variation on this process is for companies to prepare data for clinicians. By the time the data have been tabulated by the company, the issue of what the data show may have been settled. In SSRI trials, for example, patients who drop out with agitation may be coded under a failure to respond to treatment or as experiencing side effects of treatment. Coding under a failure to respond to treatment immediately does away with data indicating that the drug causes side effects. Unless clinicians inspect the raw data themselves, they won't see this. In clinical trials of psychotropic agents, it is not the norm for senior clinicians to inspect the raw data for themselves. Nevertheless, the reports from studies they participate in end up in the most distinguished journals in the field, including the *Archives of General Psychiatry,* the *American Journal of Psychiatry, JAMA,* and the *New England Journal of Medicine.*

The process becomes complicated when, for instance, such companies as Pharmacia and Upjohn convene an expert panel hoping to provide a consensus statement on social functioning. In this case, invitations will go to key figures in psychopharmacology circles, none of whom may have any background in social functioning. Companies will, regardless, aim to produce a statement on social functioning bearing these names, ideally in as prestigious a journal as possible. The experts will be convened, and a secretariat from the communication agency typically produces draft materials for consideration and a draft statement. Those present are invited to sign off on it. There may be little wrong with what is being said, making argument or noncooperation difficult, particularly given the remuneration involved. But whoever drafts the original document effectively controls the message, and the whole process hands over the authority of distinguished names cheaply.[45]

Many senior figures in clinical psychopharmacology are involved in these processes at one level or another. Some who would not accept a ghostwritten article find it acceptable that their lecture is transcribed and published. But the "uncompromised" participation of these "honorable" figures in symposia enables the participation of others, the content of whose talks is completely dictated by the company. And the presence of these "honorable" figures adds a veneer of respectability to the others.

Companies also have the power to block publication of articles likely to clash with their marketing interests. Two senior figures in the field, Ian Oswald and Isaac Marks, claim this has happened in journals as reputable as the *Archives of General Psychiatry* and the *New England Journal of Medicine*.[46] There would seem little doubt that something of this sort did happen in *The Lancet* in the case of mortality related to asthma treatment.[47] The dynamic in the Marks and Oswald cases is more complex. The issue may not involve direct penetration of editorial offices. Effective censorship may mean it just so happens that articles get sent to the obvious reviewers without editors making much effort to determine whether these reviewers have a conflict of interest. An editor cannot be held to blame for the fact that *all* of her potential reviewers have a conflict of interest. But equally, one criterion of a great editor must surely be a capacity to discern when it is important to accept articles that buck the trend, despite the opinions of reviewers.

CURRENT MEDICAL DIRECTIONS

It has been possible to rationalize ghostwriting by passing it off as something that happens only for satellite symposia and in journal supplements. Given that everyone knows that journal supplements carry a health warning, where's the problem?

For some time now, the Web sites of some of the major writing agencies have indicated that their reach extends far beyond writing for symposium supplements. Take Current Medical Directions (CMD), for instance, a medical information company based in New York, established in 1990 "to deliver scientifically accurate information strategically developed for specific target audiences."[48] This agency writes up studies, review articles, abstracts, journal supplements, product monographs, expert commentaries, and textbook chapters. It conducts meta-analyses and organizes journal supplements, satellite symposia, consensus conferences, and even advisory boards for its clients.

In the course of 1998, CMD, on behalf of Pfizer, coordinated the authorship of approximately eighty-seven articles on Zoloft. Of these, fifty-five were published by early 2001. They targeted the leading journals in the field, including the *New England Journal of Medicine* (*NEJM*),

JAMA, Archives of General Psychiatry, and *American Journal of Psychiatry,* in addition to journals well known for the placement of psychopharmacology articles.[49] Many of these fifty-five articles seem to have originated within communication agencies. A list of articles being managed by CMD indicates three sets of articles. First is a number of publications that CMD's list indicates originated within communications agencies, with the authors' names listed as "TBD" (to be determined). The subsequently published articles in this series have authors' names similar to those in a second series of articles with very similar academic and company authors, which did not apparently originate in a communication agency. A third, small set of articles that do not appear to have been written within a communication agency or to have a Pfizer name on them acknowledges Pfizer funding or support. Some of these are review articles and involve no data. Based on contact with the authors and other sources, my judgment is that in only five cases were the authors likely to have the raw data from the studies they reported on.

Few of these fifty-five articles seem likely to have been authored—in the traditional sense of that word—by the people who appear to have written them. In even fewer of these articles would the distinguished apparent authors have had access to, or have been able to share, the data linked to their names. The importance of this possibility lies in the fact that in science traditionally an author should be able to hand over his or her data for others to analyze. But this new data is proprietary data—something fundamentally at odds with the nature of science.

Aside from these fifty-five articles, there were forty-one therapeutics articles on Zoloft in the world literature in 1998. Of these, three report ambiguous findings for sertraline, twenty report negative findings, and eighteen report positive findings. When the journals in which the CMD and non-CMD articles are compared for impact factor, the CMD articles appear on average in journals with a threefold greater impact factor than the non-CMD articles. When the number of publications of the authors in the CMD series is compared with the number of publications of non-CMD authors, one finds the CMD authors have published, on average, three times more articles than the other authors. When the rate at which CMD papers are later cited is compared to the rate for non-CMD papers, the CMD papers have a three times higher citation rate. Based on this it seems safe to say that by the turn of the century, around 50 percent of the "scientific" literature in pharmacotherapeutics was ghostwritten, originated within companies, or was published in non-peer-reviewed supplements to journals.[50]

The profile of the CMD articles suggests that CMD and Pfizer recruited those whose background increased the possibility of the company's publications appearing in the most prestigious journals. Specific journals seem to have been targeted. CMD "strives to exceed the expectations of our clients and to assist them in achieving their strategic objectives."[51] Whether the combination of distinguished journal, distinguished author, an efficient distribution system, and sponsored platforms achieved results beyond Pfizer's expectations is uncertain, but the impact of this literature on third-party payers and other interested parties seems likely to have been substantial. The question of literature impact seems to be tied closely to the nature of ghostwriting. Authorship lines from perceived opinion leaders, with minimal company representation and nondeclaration of medical-writing agency input, can be expected to increase the likelihood that these articles will be influential with prescribers and purchasers.

The other side of this coin is that many of the most senior figures in the field are becoming "ghost" scientists; an ever-larger part of their work is not theirs in any meaningful sense of the word. These academics become opinion leaders in a therapeutics field because they appear to have their names on a larger proportion of the literature in the most prestigious journals than do others, and because they get asked to international meetings to present the data, with which they may not have firsthand acquaintance. Regardless of whether CMD's authors see the raw data the CMD articles are based on, nontraditional authoring must usually be involved, in the sense that these authors cannot share proprietary raw data with colleagues, as has been traditional in the scientific domain. Allied to the volume of industry-linked authorship, this distance from primary data indicates that scientific authorship is changing. And the culmination of this change could be that the dominant figures in therapeutics will soon have comparatively little firsthand research experience and little raw data that they can share with others.

The key issue in ghostwriting is not whether the true authors are being deprived of recognition or whether academic authors are putting their names to articles they shouldn't get credit for. The key issue is whether there are likely to be discrepancies between these new-style articles and the raw data from the studies they purport to report.

Take one of the studies on CMD's list that seemed most likely to be independent. This was a study undertaken by Ulrik Malt from Norway that compared Zoloft, mianserin, and a placebo in general-practice depression. Malt had received sponsorship from Pfizer and sent a draft of his article to the company. In it, Malt and colleagues stated, "One patient on sertraline committed suicide, and three others reported increasing suicidal ideation which prompted premature stop of the treatment, in contrast to just one case on mianserin and none on placebo. Since the introduction of the tricyclic antidepressants [TCA], it has been known by clinicians that TCA could increase suicidality in the first week. For this reason a close supervision of depressed patients given TCA was recommended."[52] Replying for Pfizer, Roger Lane cautioned against drawing inferences from small numbers (over three hundred patients), especially inferences that had been shown to be without foundation by the Beasley analysis on Prozac.[53] He suggested a rewording: "Close supervision of depressed patients during the first few weeks of TCA therapy has always been recommended as it was recognized that patients remain at risk of suicide in the early stages of treatment." The final draft published in the *British Medical Journal* (*BMJ*) contained no mention of any suicides or any need for warnings.[54] In all likelihood, there was no coercion or corruption here, between Malt and Pfizer, Malt and the *BMJ*, or Pfizer and the *BMJ*. But it is hard to avoid the impression that the "friendships" set up by company sponsorship exert a subtle influence.

It is more difficult to discount the discrepancies in the six published pediatric psychopharmacology articles involving Zoloft from the CMD series, one of which appeared in *JAMA*. These articles mention only one suicidal act on Zoloft, when in fact there were six suicidal acts on Zoloft in the subject group on which these articles are based—a rate approximately six times higher than the published rate in adults.[55]

This demonstrates there is no longer any guarantee that publication even in the most prestigious journals means that the results adequately reflect the data from clinical trials. As the SSRI and suicide story unfolds in succeeding chapters, we will see how a number of the best-known journals have published articles on the SSRI and suicide issue so riddled with gross methodological inadequacies that it becomes difficult to see how they could ever have been published on the basis of scientific merit. We will also see that in some cases, company defenses have depended on articles that are startlingly inconsistent with the raw data.

In contrast, when I approached *British Medical Journal* and *The Lancet* attempting to redress the balance, or at least to open a debate on the issues, initial enthusiastic responses tailed off while third parties called me to tell me the articles would never be published for "political" reasons.

PSYCHOPHARMACOLOGY TRADE FAIRS

Another disturbing aspect of the changing face of psychiatry is the extent to which the psychopharmacology circuit has become a circus. There are now megameetings ranging from the American Psychiatric Association meeting, which may have close to twenty thousand delegates, down to smaller meetings of two thousand or three thousand delegates. Pharmaceutical companies will have brought many of these delegates. At some meetings, almost all delegates have been sponsored in this way, with expenses covered including travel costs, often business-class flights with limousine service to and from airports, accommodation in better hotels, meals in better restaurants, and all registration and associated costs to attend the meeting.

The delegate arrives to be greeted with a bag bearing some sponsor's name. Coaches to and from hotels to the conference center will also be sponsored by one of the companies, as most probably will the president's dinner, a range of committee meetings, social events, the meeting program, and abstracts and associated material. At the meeting, delegates can read a congress newspaper sponsored by one or another of the companies. Within the meeting are ordinary and satellite symposia, both sponsored. At present, the only item *not* likely to be sponsored will be certain plenary lectures, which likely will be balanced by a series of company-sponsored "special" lectures.

Many delegates brought in this manner, when not out visiting the city in which the meeting is held, will spend a great deal of time wandering around the exhibition halls, where pharmaceutical companies locate their glossy stands, handing out trinkets of various sorts.[56] It's hard to believe anyone can be interested in them, but interested they are. For insiders, the gradual development of this scenario has lost all power to shock. Walking an unprepared outsider around one of these exhibition halls can provide a healthy glimpse of the problems—the modern equivalent of selling Manhattan to Europeans for a few baubles.[57]

In defense of delegates, it must be pointed out that the main programs are often so unexciting that wandering around the exhibition hall becomes an attractive alternative. The principles behind the construction of programs for these meetings appear to involve a combination of factors. On a quid pro quo basis, certain senior people appear to invite each other; in the process, all get represented heavily at all major meetings, and get to see the world in the bargain. Another aspect is a virtual bait-and-switch tactic. (A well-known ruse in the secondhand car industry is to bait the buyer with a really good car and then plead unavailability of that particular model.) In psychopharmacology circles, meeting organizers bait themselves into believing they have organized a respectable scientific meeting because of the presence of a handful of really big-name speakers. Delegates meanwhile avoid both quid pro quo and bait-and-switch slots and wander around the exhibition halls because few (if any) of the lectures engage with the real issues of the day. Even in the main program of these meetings, finding a lecture on the merits of older, cheaper drugs, or on the place for nonprescription therapy, or even on subjects such as drug-induced akathisia or suicide, would be like finding snow in the Sahara.

In addition to the obviously commercial company stands in the exhibition halls at meetings, often costing companies tens of thousands of dollars apiece, an ever-greater part of the program for meetings consists of satellite symposia.[58] These were introduced at major meetings such as the American Psychiatric Association meeting during the 1980s. They have so grown in frequency that now major meetings will schedule one or two days worth of satellite symposia before the meeting proper starts. The main meeting will last for three or four days, including, usually in the evenings, further satellite symposia. As of 1999, APA meetings featured up to forty satellite symposia, whose organizers might have paid up to $250,000 apiece.

Delegates brought to meetings by companies are usually expected to attend the satellite symposia. The company will often arrange to wine and dine them at other times, making them less likely to attend the symposia of competitors. Even for those who do attend other satellite symposia, there will usually be free meals before or after. Junketing psychiatrists cannot lose. They can shop during the day and move around from one satellite symposium to the next in the evening, perhaps without ever attending anything on the main meeting.

Speakers at these symposia are drawn from a small handful of figures who rotate from one company symposium to the next. They will frequently say uncritically congratulatory things about the drug produced by the symposium sponsor, making essentially the same statements about all drugs despite their manifest differences. Hard as it is to understand how senior figures can agree to take part in such a charade, it's harder to see how anyone in the audience manages to stay awake, other than in the hope that a speaker might mistakenly mention the name of a competing drug rather than the one he has been asked to talk about. The chance of this happening is not insignificant—those speaking at one symposium often leave the platform to participate immediately in another symposium scheduled at the same time.[59] Sometimes speakers stare at their slides in a manner that makes it obvious they have never laid eyes on them before.

Of course, speakers operating at this pace, and asked to produce articles perhaps for all the different symposia in which they participate, cannot be expected to write all their own articles. Equally clearly, this is a slippery slope that may finally give senior figures an extensive publication record, very little of which they will have produced themselves. Some senior figures now express surprise that anyone still writes their own articles. In the process, control of what is said has passed from clinicians to companies.

There is more than black humor here. A recent analysis of clinical trial results claims the multiple reporting of clinical trial outcomes by senior figures, often in satellite symposium proceedings, makes it very difficult to know just how many trials have actually been performed. This confusion leads to significant overestimates of the efficacy of new drugs—a 23 percent overestimate, by one calculation.[60] This is even before the publication bias from companies not publishing their negative results is taken into account. This is a sobering thought for someone like me, who has presented data from reboxetine studies in a number of different publications.

The extent to which major meetings are "penetrated" by pharmaceutical companies becomes ever harder to establish. In addition to satellite symposia at an increasing number of meetings, most if not all of the symposia or workshops in the body of the main meeting are supported by "unrestricted educational grants." The content of these symposia and their presenters will almost inevitably overlap heavily with the content of satellite symposia.[61] Big names become big names in this field because they are pushed forward by pharmaceutical company support; some of these people may have little scientific achievement to justify their inclusion on the programs of major meetings. In addition to symposia, most meetings also now have educational workshops or "meet the expert" sessions also sponsored by companies.

The returns for the figures at the top of the pyramid, including consultancy fees, fees for being principal investigators in trials, speaker's fees, chairman's fees, and other fees, may be substantial. Some idea can be gleaned from an October 4, 1999, report in the *Boston Globe*, which indicated that some individuals might earn up to $800,000 a year.[62]

Money is one thing, but companies also make these physicians highly visible in a manner that has to be personally gratifying. These players will be seen as the opinion leaders in the field. These individuals, who may be too busy to do hands-on scientific work or even to see patients, and who may never have observed the effects of the drug they are talking about, will be the ones informing others about the drug in some exotic location, perhaps by delivering a message worked out by the pharmaceutical company beforehand. All that is really required of the big name is to remember the brand name of the drug and to stick to the script.

BIG BUSINESS OR SUCCESSFUL SCIENCE?

This control of the scientific media means that certain aspects of the field are selected over others. A premium is put on certain data in a manner that builds up bandwagons and skews the field. This process is not confined to psychiatry. In the cardiovascular field, for instance, in the late 1960s there were competing views as to the important factors in preventing heart attacks. One lead suggested that blood homocysteine levels were important, another that blood lipid levels were the critical factor. The homocysteine hypothesis suggested a range of dietary approaches that might help, such as taking folate or B vitamins. The lipid-lowering approach gave rise to a generation of patented drugs aimed at lowering lipid levels, which became among the most profitable agents ever made. Rival evidence for homocysteine was effectively buried for almost thirty years.[63]

In the field of ulcer treatment, the H-2 antagonists cimetidine and ranitidine, which lowered gastric acid secretion, made Glaxo and SmithKline, respectively, into giants in the pharmaceutical sector in the 1990s. These were ideal drugs, fitting in with the dominant view that ulcers were in some sense a psychosomatic condition in which stress led to excess acid secretion. The H-2 antagonists managed ulcers in a way that made it much less likely that surgery would be needed. But they often needed to be given long-term, as ulcers commonly recurred once treatment was stopped. When evidence emerged from Australia that many ulcers were, in fact, linked to a bacterial infection caused by *helicobacter pylori,* and that a course of antibiotics might clear them up completely, the major companies ridiculed the new ideas. Far from embracing scientific breakthroughs, for many years the programs of international meetings continued to focus on the H-2 antagonists and the proton-pump inhibitors that followed in their wake.

In the case of the SSRIs, this capacity to mold the scientific agenda was the force that made anxiety almost vanish and helped replace it with depression. This is the force that buries talk about drug-induced suicidality. It is the force that overwhelms lithium and electroconvulsive therapy as treatments for depression. It seems reasonable to have psychopharmacology conferences dominated by presentations on the latest drugs, but neglecting ECT and lithium, even though these treatments appear more specific to mood disorders than the SSRIs, does not help psychopharmacology. Nonclinical researchers reading the literature or attending meetings risk being deflected into thinking that changes that occur in their animal models with SSRIs are better leads for further research than studying ECT or lithium.

Research in psychopharmacology, like other areas of medicine, has regularly been compared to the progress of a drunk searching for his keys under a lamppost because that's where the light is.[64] In this case, the drunk seems to be searching under the lamppost with the advertisement for alcohol on it, in preference to the one with the functioning light. Scientific advances may emerge from this process, but they will not do so because the scientific community is behaving rationally.

Control of the message about what psychotropic drugs do has progressively slipped from the hands of clinicians. Around 1980, American federal funding for independent research and educational programs dried up and was replaced by industry funding. The salaries of many academics now depend on money pulled in through grants from industry sources. This dependency may well have contributed to a situation where several of the players in the Prozac story were told by senior figures in the field that it would not be a wise career move for them to raise concerns about Prozac.

The new situation, however, is full of ambiguities. For example, I arrived at the March 1999 meeting of the American Psychopathological Association in New York to find everyone gossiping about the latest media exposure. It turned out the *New York Sunday Post* had run a piece called "Shrinks for Sale" that listed the names of a large number of people at the meeting,[65] together with the amounts of money these clinicians had earned during the course of the previous year running clinical trials and giving talks for drug companies. Someone who knew nothing of the field would react with horror to the portrait painted of researchers who became involved in this kind of exercise in order to put their children through college. The question behind the article was how much the public could trust the kind of information produced by people with such clear conflicts of interest.

One critic cited in the article was Loren Mosher, a social psychiatrist and a senior figure in U.S. psychiatry in an earlier period. He had resigned from the American Psychiatric Association in protest against the corruption he saw visited on the APA by its increasing involvement with the pharmaceutical industry. Mosher's message was that the APA had, in effect, become the American *Psychopharmacological* Association, the change of names conveniently avoiding any change of initials; its meetings were sold out to the interests of drug companies, its offices bankrolled by companies, and its educational and political messages completely subservient to the interests of companies.

From my point of view, the trouble was that the amounts of money being cited were hardly extraordinary for senior figures in the field. Even relatively small amounts of extra earnings could be painted in a very bad light. Someone had to do the talking, and no one was going to do it for nothing. On the one hand, if I wanted to hear an independent message, some of the people cited in the article were the ones I would listen to, even with a company paying for the lecture. On the other hand, some of those listed did not command my respect, and it was common to hear talk of "hired guns"—tough characters who would do a job for the money. At times, it was hard not to think in terms of the Wild West: If there was a marshal in this town, he wasn't hanging out in plain view.

The other obvious comparison is with the packaging of politics, where key figures are given a script to stick to and required to keep on message. A great deal of what happens at some apparently scientific symposia in association meetings is aimed at generating a few bits of information, or sound bites, that get fed into articles in the general media or the specialized medical media. In many respects, the less the experts know about the drugs they are talking about, the better. After presenting the results of research they have not been involved in and talking about the side effects of drugs they have never prescribed, these experts may be seen being chaperoned to press briefings by glamorous PR officers.

Audiences for the most part believe *someone* actually did the work. But even this is now less than certain. Richard Borison—a former professor of psychiatry at the Medical College of Georgia, a big name on the psychopharmacology circuit in the 1990s and a key investigator for many of the antipsychotics and antidepressants now on the market—was jailed in 1997 on convictions rising out of a clinical trials business whose patients did not always exist.[66] Where the patients were real, they were assessed and monitored by junior staff who, instead of being encouraged to detect hazards that a new drug might be causing, were under pressure to get patients successfully through the protocol. Nobody believes the Borison case was an isolated one; the *Wall Street Journal,* the *New York Times,* and *The Guardian* have since reported on others.[67] The extraordinary thing is that the field does not seem to feel any need to account for itself to the public.

Another scientifically indefensible practice is the failure to make any mention of clinical trials that are not published. Many clinicians will have participated in trials that they then discover have been sealed. In some cases, this is because of a suspicion of fraud on the part of the clinical investigator—although, surprisingly, none of the trials involving Borison appears to have been retrospectively "pulled." In other cases, the suspicion has to be that the sealing has happened because the results don't fit what the company expects.[68] Having personally been involved in trials whose results have been sealed (have never seen the light of day), I find it difficult to avoid this conclusion.

A final corruption is the publishing of selected results from trials. In my efforts to come to grips with the meaning of the SASS data, I concluded that this scale functioned more as a quality-of-life indicator than as an actual assessment of social functioning. The next question was, did any other quality-of-life scales show the same differences between SSRIs and norepinephrine reuptake inhibitors as the SASS had shown for reboxetine and Prozac? A search of the literature produced a surprise: As of 1999, there were only seven separate clinical trials in which quality-of-life results were reported.[69] This was odd, as I had personally been involved in seven trials in which these scales had been used. Checking with colleagues produced agreement that these scales had been used, but no one could point to a resulting publication. My estimate is there have to be at least a hundred trials whose results remain unpublished.

BACK TO THE SASS

In the early 1990s, seduced perhaps by their own touting of the benefits of SSRIs over older antidepressants in terms of side effects, Lilly, SmithKline, and Pfizer produced their own quality-of-life scales. This was a between-the-lines acknowledgment that the SSRIs were not as potent as the older antidepressants; companies would instead show that the SSRIs produced a better quality of life. But having gone to the trouble of producing these scales, validating them, and then using them in clinical trials, the companies hadn't published the results.

Getting hold of all these results would be a useful scientific exercise. Stacking them together with the SASS data and analyzing them by age, sex, and other variables would have produced new scientific information. But my industry sources told me I would get nowhere writing to the companies. There were big names in the system who had the power to break a company, and if someone like that were to write, he or she might be able to get the information. Such a figure would be in a position to do considerable good. Maybe many of them were, in fact, doing a great deal of good. It was increasingly difficult to tell the good guys from the bad guys. The stage seemed increasingly populated by players.

In the case of Prozac, there was a more disturbing aspect to this lack of data. In other illnesses, quality-of-life scales show what the person's quality of life is on treatment. In the case of kidney dialysis, for instance, quality of life may be very poor even though the treatment is working.[70] But in depression, quality-of-life scales do double duty by offering the patient's assessment as to whether the treatment is working.

As a series of memos from Lilly Germany to Lilly headquarters, regarding the failed application to have Prozac licensed there, put it: "The BGA[71] stated that there is a disagreement between patients' and doctors' judgment of efficacy . . . in their opinion the patient's impression is more important."[72] Or: "Most self-rating methods, which are decisive for the assessment of efficacy of the preparation, indicate little response [or] no improvement in the clinical picture of the patients during the treatment with the preparation at hand [Prozac]."[73]

The inescapable conclusion from the combination of published and unpublished quality-of-life results is that from the patients' point of view, the SSRIs either don't work or at least haven't been shown to work, or if they work, they are also producing some mental effect, such as emotional blunting, that no one is talking about.[74] All of this is grist to the mill of the critics of psychopharmacotherapy who have never been convinced that the drugs work. For someone like me, who is pretty certain that psychotropic drugs including the SSRIs do work, it means either that randomized controlled trials don't work or else the companies are doing something badly wrong—at least from a scientific point of view.

Much of what I learned about the psychopharmacology world and the interface between academia and industry, between being approached as a consultant for Pharmacia about reboxetine in 1997 and the Forsyth case in March 1999, was implicit in my book *The Antidepressant Era*, published at the end of 1997.[75] While it all remained implicit, a psychiatric audience—such as that at the APPA meeting in New York in March 1999—could respond favorably. Academia can tolerate a certain amount of ambiguity. T. S. Eliot's "Humankind cannot bear very much reality" sounds great—until you ask how much ambiguity we can tolerate.[76] A week later, aboard a plane to Hawaii, I was headed right into the heart of the ambiguities. At that stage, with no experience of legal actions, it hadn't occurred to me that this legal process might relentlessly seek to make explicit what had previously been implicit. I was to learn at first hand that many academics find explicit ambiguity intolerable.

5

A Pacific Fault Line

BEFORE LEAVING BRITAIN for the American Psychopathological Association meeting in New York in March 1999, I gave the lawyers from Baum, Hedlund my time of arrival in Hawaii. Requests for responses to motions from Lilly came through the week in New York. Then silence. Had the case settled at the last minute? No one seemed to be waiting for me in the airport terminal. At last a man dressed in shorts and a Hawaiian shirt, with flowers around his neck, greeted me, and I belatedly recognized Andy Vickery, whom I had last met in San Diego almost two years before.

Headquarters was a nine-bedroom house. There were boxes and boxes of files in the garage. Computers had been installed, as well as fax and phone lines. All the key documents of the case were arranged in one of the living room areas—the operational center of the house. Things got going at 6:00 a.m. and continued past midnight, as the team waiting for me at this base—Cindy Hall; Rhonda Hawkins, a paralegal in Vickery's office; Karen Barth, an attorney from Baum, Hedlund; and Skip Murgatroyd, who apparently had taken time off from surfing to cover for Bill Downey, who had died two months before—sought to answer queries raised by the court.

This was a marriage of two companies. Vickery was a partner in a small Houston company that specialized in medical injury cases.[1] They had prosecuted recovered-memory therapists in one of the first cases in this area, *Abney v. Spring Shadows Glen,* which in 1996 led to a substantial settlement in favor of a parent accused of abuse, and the closing down of the Dissociation Unit in Spring Shadows Glen Hospital. This outcome should have made the company heroes with biological psychiatrists, since most are hostile to recovered-memory therapy.

The others were part of Baum, Hedlund, which had chased airline companies on safety issues and taken on cases involving hemophiliacs infected with contaminated blood. The link that brought the companies together was Barth, who had moved some years previously from Vickery and Waldner to Kannanack, Murgatroyd, Baum, and Hedlund. This California company had brought fifteen Prozac cases, including that of Del Shannon, to the table in 1992, and through Paul Smith had settled fourteen of them. Lilly didn't want to settle the fifteenth—the Forsyth case. Skip Murgatroyd, far from being just a surfer, had retired after several successful cases. The first person the Forsyths contacted, he had helped obtain and review documents during the early stages of the Prozac litigation in 1990 and 1991.

But I knew nothing of this background, and they knew little about me, which seemed extraordinary. Lots of their money might hang in my hands; my very career might hang in theirs. This was my introduction to a world in which, on one side, serried ranks of besuited attorneys worked in large legal offices for corporate clients. These lawyers regarded with disdain the informality of the ambulance chasers on the other side of the fence. It would have been easier to begin on the side of the suits.

The case started almost six years to the day after William Forsyth murdered his wife and killed himself. Two years before, Susan Forsyth had said they might settle if Lilly provided enough money so that they could mail every single clinician in the country material warning them about the hazards of Prozac. A few weeks previously, there had been a final settlement hearing, but no deal was struck.

GOING LEGAL

The judge was Alan Kay. At no point during the week I was there did Kay seem anything other than a thoughtful man. The first step in jury selection had been his. Faced with a panel, he could question and remove anyone who should not serve as a juror. The attorneys for either side then had their opportunity to question jurors, based on their responses to the judge's questions. This could lead to the dismissal of a juror "for cause."

Then both sets of attorneys—Vickery and Barth for the plaintiffs and Andy See and Michelle Mangrum for Lilly—had three opportunities to remove a juror. No reason had to be offered. Vickery was faced with a woman on Prozac, whom Kay had not dismissed for cause, and three insurance claims managers. The latter were considered the kiss of death for a plaintiff's case; but the woman on Prozac also had to go.

There was reason to think See might want to remove one of the claims managers, Julie Ugalde, as she had been involved in a lawsuit against a doctor who failed to warn her mother of potential adverse reactions to a drug. But Lilly never asked her a question. The jury later dropped from twelve to eleven, after one discovered a conflict of interest through ownership of pharmaceutical company shares.

The lawyers spent a great deal of their court time watching how the jury responded to various questions. One man slept a good deal of the way through. Another admitted from the start he had memory problems but took no notes. Two young women just sat back during jury deliberations and let the others argue it out. The one who did most of the arguing in the jury room was Julie Ugalde, the surviving claims manager.

Apart from the jury, there were members of the legal teams, certain witnesses, and lay watchers to feed impressions back to the lawyers. There was the local press. And there was a power-dressed woman whom no one could place. She had appeared the day after Lilly lost a bid to have media coverage banned.

Skip Murgatroyd took me through key documents that might be presented to me on the stand. These included minutes from the Fluoxetine (Prozac) Project Team, dating as early as July 1978, which indicated that Lilly monitors had noticed a large number of reports of patients on the drug developing akathisia and restlessness.[2] One patient had even become psychotic. In response, Lilly's Project Team suggested that in future studies, benzodiazepines could be coadministered in order to minimize the problem.[3] In the mid-1980s, Lilly encountered a problem with the German regulators, the BGA (Bundesgesundheitsamt), who seemed of the opinion that the suicides observed in clinical trials of Prozac were attributable to the drug. When Prozac finally obtained a license in Germany, the drug came with a clear warning that it could cause problems during the first few weeks of treatment and that it might be necessary to coadminister a sedative.[4] Seeing these documents again in this judicial setting, it was hard to imagine they would not stun a jury.

More was to come. A memo by Joe Wernicke, a clinical trial coordinator for Lilly from July 2, 1986, conceded that the suicide factor, item 3 on the Hamilton Rating Scale for Depression, was not a sensitive indicator of suicidality.[5] This was the very point I had made in my letter to the *BMJ* in 1991, which Lilly had been at pains to deny,[6] and the key to the adequacy of the Beasley study. In his response to my letter, Beasley had expressed surprise that I should question this point.[7] Another memo showed that Lilly recognized the same flaws as I had in the Beasley study.[8]

A key memo from 1986 recorded the number of suicide attempts on Prozac in Lilly's clinical trial database at that point as forty-seven on fluoxetine, two on tricyclic antidepressants, and one on mianserin.[9] Correlation of these figures with the numbers who had entered clinical studies at this point revealed that rates of suicide attempts were three to four times higher on Prozac than either on other antidepressants or on placebo.[10]

In a September 1990 memo to Leigh Thompson, the chief scientist at Lilly, John Heiligenstein stated, "We feel caution should be exercised in a statement that 'suicidality and hostile acts in patients taking Prozac reflect the patient's disorder and not a causal relationship to Prozac.' Post-marketing reports are increasingly fuzzy and we have assigned Yes, reasonably related on several reports. . . . You may want to note that trials were not intended to address the issue of suicidality."[11] Here was apparently a frank admission from within Lilly that even the company itself had been forced to conclude that what was being reported to them in some cases was Prozac-induced suicide or suicidality.

Further, this memo established the company had a strategy: to blame the disease, not the drug. This was reinforced by another memo to Leigh Thompson, from E. "Mitch" Daniels in April 1991, regarding a forthcoming TV appearance, where Thompson was encouraged to emphasize the general message "It's in the disease, not the drug."[12] The other messages were that Prozac was the most researched drug in history and, in an echo of the indalpine story, that the real people who were going to suffer because of all this controversy were the people denied access to Prozac. Here was the strategy that appeared to shape everything from the first response to the emerging problem to the Wesbecker tactics and the Rosenbaum article. Alongside memos showing that there had been an explicit strategy to blame the disease and not the drug were reports to Lilly of problems developing in patients who weren't depressed—patients with bulimia, for example.[13] This was just the kind of patient Bob Temple had flagged at the September 1991 FDA hearing on antidepressants and suicide.

Just as surprising was the emergence in the papers of someone I knew, Paul Leber. Early in the documents was an internal FDA memo noting that Tony DeCiccio had stated that Dr. Laughren said, "The firm has a friend in Dr. Temple, who wants an action letter by the end of this year."[14] (This was 1986, when the registration of fluoxetine was proceeding slowly and trickily.) Then, on February 7, 1990, the month the Teicher reports appeared, a memo from Leigh Thompson stated, "I'm concerned about reports I get re UK attitude towards Prozac safety. Leber suggested a few minutes ago we should use CSM database to compare Prozac aggression and suicidal ideation with other antidepressants in UK. Although he is a fan of Prozac and believes a lot of this is garbage, he is clearly a political creature and will have to respond to pressures. I hope Patrick [P. Keohane, CEO, Lilly UK] realizes that Lilly could go down the tubes if we lose Prozac and just one event in the UK can cost us that."[15]

Then there was a letter by Lilly to the FDA regarding a summary of the safety experience with Prozac during its first two years of marketing; a note at the bottom of the page stated, "At the request of Lilly, Mr. A. W. DeCiccio was able to pull and destroy all copies of this submission except Dr. T. P. Laughren's desk copy."[16] Tom Laughren had written a chapter on the assessment of the adverse effects of drugs with none other than Leigh Thompson, which came out in 1994 during the Wesbecker trial.[17] Regulators were supposed to cooperate with companies, but writing a chapter on the issue of drug-induced adverse events with personnel from a company involved in a major controversy such as Prozac-induced suicidality seemed extraordinary.

From July 1990 came a memo: "Paul Leber called yesterday; I contacted him at 6.15 this morning. The call was about suicide. He asked that we FAX nothing to him unless he has agreed beforehand. Paul is taking a position in talking with outside folks today that Lilly and FDA were working together on the suicide issue and following closely the post-marketing events, but that there are no denominators and the best that can be done is to put 'a cap' on the number of events."[18]

Later in the year, on September 12, a memo between Max Talbott of regulatory affairs in Lilly and Leigh Thompson states that "one possible strategy if FDA presses for an additional labeling change vis-à-vis suicide is a class-wide cautionary note; however we should take this position only as a last resort." A reply from Thompson states, "That report MUST move swiftly through approval and to Dr. Leber's hands . . . he is our defender."[19] I respected and indeed liked Paul Leber, but it was clear there were documents here that could paint him in a bad light.

Lilly was also, it seemed, prepared to have warnings put on all other antidepressants from all other companies; it was difficult to see this as other than an effort to avoid putting Lilly itself at a competitive disadvantage.

A further series of documents returned the story to Lilly's difficulties with the BGA. The first involved a memo from Claude Bouchy, the chief executive in Lilly Germany, to Leigh Thompson.[20] It was a memo regarding "Adverse Drug Event Reporting—Suicide, Fluoxetine," which stated, "Hans (Weber) has medical problems with these directions and I have great concerns about it. I do not think I could explain to the BGA, a judge, to a reporter or even to my family why we would do this especially on the sensitive issue of suicide and suicidal ideation." There were then replies from Leigh Thompson explaining the problem that they were having about coding for suicidal ideation, followed by a further response from Claude Bouchy in which he stated, "I personally wonder whether we are really helping the credibility of an excellent ADE system by calling overdose what a physician reports as suicide attempt and by calling depression what a physician is reporting as suicide ideation."[21]

ON THE STAND

The case began with Billy Forsyth in the witness stand, followed by David Capellulo, a friend of William Forsyth, and Bobbi Comstock, a friend of June Forsyth. This went on until 3:00 p.m. on the second day, when the jury was dismissed. I was going to be on the stand that day, but not in the main *Forsyth* case.

Lilly was to be given yet another chance to dislodge me as an expert, in a "Daubert hearing." Daubert hearings were aimed at determining whether an expert's opinions were appropriate. Consulting later with senior colleagues in the United States who had been involved in medico-legal cases, on issues from tardive dyskinesia through to SSRI-induced suicidality, I found none who had heard of this new beast stalking the medico-legal jungle.

It seemed to me that nobody knew what to do. See, whose brief was to show I didn't have the specialized expertise for this case, mixed up arguments about randomized controlled trials with elements of the *Forsyth* case. Vickery looked prepared to fight fires but unsure where they might break out. The hearing continued the following morning. Finally, Judge Kay decided that my credentials as an expert witness had been tested thoroughly enough, and he was satisfied as to my ability to testify on the case.[22]

The jury was reconvened and the case went ahead. The first brief involved being examined by Vickery, who went through my background and reasons for involvement in this case. How would one establish cause and effect following the intake of a drug? What was the basis for saying Prozac made William Forsyth suicidal? It was going well. It looked like it was going to be sensational to be faced with the "documents," with the jury there to listen. See objected that I had not included these documents when deposed, as part of the evidence I had used to come to my opinion, and that therefore they should not be allowed in. Judge Kay agreed.

At the midday recess, a woman from the press approached me. I agreed to meet with her at the end of the day. The unknown power-dresser in the court hovered nearby. At the end of the day, there was no sign of the journalist, and it became clear the stranger in court was handling media relations for Lilly.

Vickery's examination went through the early afternoon. He looked impressively the part compared with the man in shorts and a lei who'd met me at the airport. His rapport with the jury seemed to strike the right combination of cleverness and humanity.[23]

On cross, See opened up with a statement about my 1994 article: "Dr. Healy, in an article you wrote, 'these data from several thousand patients and the evidence that fluoxetine reduces suicidal ideation, must on any scientific scale outweigh the dubious evidence of a handful of case reports.' Have I quoted you correctly?" I said he had. He moved quickly on to his next point. I was surprised. I had expected him to provide me with the opportunity to explain that the point was made ironically and that the follow-up correspondence made this point. When he asked me if he had quoted accurately, I should have said no. In the matter of second-guessing what was going to happen next, I hadn't started well.

He then presented me with a paper by Meredith Warshaw and Marty Keller.[24] This paper had been extracted from a study called the Harvard/Brown Anxiety Disorders Research Program. See emphasized the Harvard connection. He asked me to read the conclusions. Wasn't it correct, he asked me, that this Harvard study had concluded there was no increased risk of suicide from Prozac? I was given some time to look at the study, which I'd never bothered to read before. I pointed out that it was a study in anxious rather than depressed patients, involving so few patients that no conclusions could be drawn. Later that evening, when I got a chance to look at the Warshaw and Keller paper, the problems of this study became glaring. It was a small study involving 654 patients, of whom only 191 ever got Prozac. It did not have the power to support the conclusions that See wanted to draw from it. But it was also a study in anxious patients, in which the only suicide had occurred in a nondepressed anxious patient taking Prozac. As a consequence of earlier legal jousting, there was a ban on me mentioning anything to do with people who were not depressed becoming suicidal on Prozac. But if See had introduced the issue, I was free to pick up the theme and run with it. I had just missed it.

The next day, See introduced a range of documents that I could dismiss as being either Lilly-sponsored or not peer-reviewed publications. We got into a conversation about the work of Stuart Montgomery, who had produced a description of two patients who had become akathisic on Prozac that showed a dose response relationship between their Prozac and their akathisia.[25] I was invited to comment on differences there might be between Montgomery and myself. I found out later that evening that everything I said would be on the Internet the following week.

GOOD GUYS AND BAD GUYS

After an evening meal, Andy Vickery wondered whether I could get involved in a case against Pfizer involving a 13-year-old boy, Matthew Miller, who hanged himself in the bathroom in the middle of the night, next door to his parents' bedroom, after a week on Zoloft. I could point to lots of reasons for not getting involved. Apart from being able to blame a suicide on a drug, there was an issue of being able to persuade the jury that the company had also been in some way negligent. Given that Paxil and Zoloft had come after the Prozac-and-suicide controversy had blown up, surely Pfizer and SmithKline would have managed to avoid leaving as obvious a set of footprints through the data as Lilly had left. Besides, it didn't seem like such a good idea for someone with a career in psychopharmacology to be at war with all the SSRI companies.

Going back to the documents, I questioned whether things were all that they seemed. The documents painted Paul Leber in a pretty bad light, but I was far from being convinced. I knew the man. For my money, he was on the side of the angels. One of the other documents showed that he was advocating a large prospective study, which would have Teicher as a consultant. Just because Thompson from Lilly thought Leber was Lilly's friend and defender, did that make it so?

I had first met Paul Leber at the British Association for Psychopharmacology meeting where I had presented my Prozac cases. He was an imposing man, not one to buddy up to in a hurry. I next saw him featured on a BBC *Panorama* program on the Halcion controversy. There the material had been presented so that it appeared that while nearly everybody else thought Halcion should be withdrawn from the market, Leber was standing firm, in a manner that suggested he must be in the pocket of the industry. Books such as Breggin's *Toxic Psychiatry* had all but claimed that Leber was controlled by the drug bosses. *Talking Back to Prozac* a few years later painted Leber as a supposed defender of the public who in fact was the defender of the pharmaceutical companies.

By this stage, as secretary of the British Association for Psychopharmacology, I sent the invitations for the annual meeting, one of which regularly went to Paul Leber. The man presented his material well. People came to hear what he had to say about things. The drug companies came because, clearly, this was the man who controlled their entry into the marketplace, and every nuance of what he might have to say was going to be analyzed closely. Off the platform, over a drink or a meal, he turned out to be friendly and upright. This man seemed to be a genuine type who in social gatherings didn't migrate toward the people it would look good to be seen with.

During one of these meetings, in 1993, he introduced me to one of his colleagues, and in the course of the conversation he praised a new book on psychiatric drugs I had just published.[26] He was the first person I was aware of who had read this book, which then had just come out. It contained a piece saying clearly that antidepressants, and in particular SSRIs, could trigger suicidality. He didn't say that he liked the book except for the piece on SSRIs and suicide; he just said that he liked the book.

These contacts set up a further meeting. As part of background research on the history of psychopharmacology, which developed into *The Psychopharmacologists*, volumes 1, 2, and 3,[27] it seemed a good idea to try to interview Paul Leber. He had contributed significantly to the use of placebos in clinical trials with antidepressants. The first interview was in Washington, D.C., in June 1994. I got to know a lot about the man—where he had trained, how his career had progressed, why he had ended up in psychiatry (having begun in pathology). I knew why he'd ended up in the FDA. In all this, I heard a forceful but not an arrogant man.

When I mentioned Breggin's *Toxic Psychiatry*, he became defensive. My interviews for the history were intended to seduce people into saying slightly more than they would have wished to say, but I certainly did not want to lose the interview because they felt they had been pushed into things. Nothing much was said; he just looked more uncomfortable than I'd expected. But there were reasons to explain this. I knew that in the Halcion controversy, opponents of the drug had taken extraordinary steps to take an action against Leber himself. In the ordinary course of events, he would have been protected by virtue of being a government employee, but people had found ways, it seemed, to get at him individually. A picture emerged of someone who really was caught between the industry on one side and pressure groups on the other. It seemed a vulnerable and lonely position to be in, and maybe even a physically dangerous one.

That interview was never published. Leber still had several years to go with the FDA, and he thought it would be imprudent. He promised to give me a further interview, and in 1997 we got together again for an interview that was published just before Paul Leber left the FDA.[28]

So, when faced with Andy Vickery seemingly being convinced that Leber was Lilly's friend in the FDA, I had difficulties. From what I knew of the man, putting him on the stand might be a good idea. He more than anyone else might have sunk Lilly. We were debating all this when I launched into the influence of the Scientologists on the whole Prozac controversy. If they hadn't intervened, U.S. psychiatry wouldn't have stood behind Lilly the way it had.

At this point Andy stopped me. Cindy, he said, was a Scientologist. More than one person in Baum, Hedlund was. He wasn't. Karen Barth and Rhonda Hawkins weren't. But Bill Downey had been. I was stunned. It took time to come to grips with this. Was I now working for the Scientologists?

Cindy and Bill Downey had seemed very normal people to me. Then again, I liked a lot of the people whom I knew from Lilly. I had great respect for Paul Leber; but who knew which side of the debate he was on? Could these Scientologists not be reasonable people too? Cindy gave a story of being wild when younger, of having had a life that was spiraling out of control, from which she had been rescued by becoming a Scientologist. Her life had stabilized. She'd gone on to get married and have children. She was now working solidly. How could you complain about something that had done this for someone? Regardless of what Scientologists believed, the process of becoming a Scientologist had done the same thing for Cindy that the process of becoming, say, a Christian or a Muslim had done for others. If this was the case, there had to be decent people within Scientology also.

The line between the good guys and the bad guys was blurring fast. I then blundered into praising Paul Smith based on the depositions I'd read, only to find that in this company, Smith was not one of the good guys. These lawyers were taking an action against Paul Smith for breach of fiduciary trust.

THE SHOW MUST GO ON

The case moved on through Amy Lee, a former local representative for Lilly, to Randolph Neal, the doctor from the Castle Medical Center who'd been in charge of William Forsyth's care while he was there. At one point, Vickery and Barth had hoped he would help their case. He had expressed incredulity when seen first after the event and offered the view that it must have been a double murder done by an intruder. William Forsyth was not a man who could have committed suicide or homicide.[29]

As Neal took the stand, I noticed what I thought was a knowing glance between Julie Ugalde and a man who also had come in with Neal. It turned out Neal had brought an attorney with him. Ugalde worked for an insurance company that had been represented by this legal company, and she played golf regularly with the Hawaiian defense bar.

Examined by Vickery, Neal agreed that William Forsyth had not been suicidal. He agreed, in fact, that Mr. Forsyth had become aware that there was some mention of him being suicidal in the notes, and that he had been very upset about this, as he most definitely was not suicidal. He agreed that Mr. Forsyth and his wife seemed to be getting on very well. The examination was almost genteel. This was strange, because either Neal had made a bad mistake by failing to recognize the potential for extreme violence in William Forsyth, and had discharged him inappropriately, or he had failed to recognize the effects of the drugs. There was no middle ground.

See took over.[30] He set up an easel on which he was to place a series of hugely enlarged copies of the Castle Medical Center notes, for both Neal and the jury to look at. He started into a series of questions. I eventually noticed a pattern when Vickery interrupted to object to the "leading nature of these questions. This man isn't really a hostile witness to Mr. See." He had interrupted after the ninety-fourth question, when eighty-three had essentially been answered yes, no, or correct. The monotony had almost sent me to sleep, but now I was awake. The answers became even more monosyllabic, ending up with 135 answers that were basically yes, no, or correct, with only 16 going beyond that.

See went to take down the notes. Vickery stood up and asked him to leave them there. He asked Neal if it was hard for him to believe that any drug that he gave this man could have caused him to kill his wife and himself. Things were heating up. Vickery moved on to mention that he couldn't help but notice that Dr. Neal had given only three answers—yes, no, or correct. Had he been coached? No.

Q. Do you feel threatened? Has anybody threatened you in any way?
A. No.

You could have heard a pin drop. Vickery moved on to ask, "Why do you have your attorney here?" Neal replied that he had involved one from the beginning. Vickery then went back through the notes See had just worked his way through, dismantling Neal's testimony as he went. Then he went on to the final enlargement, which showed the discharge summary.

Q. The other document that you, as a doctor, dictate with respect to someone is the one when they get out, right?
A. Correct.
Q. And you usually do that right away?
A. Sometimes I don't do it right away.

Q. You didn't in this case, did you?

A. I did not.

Q. You didn't dictate your discharge summary until 20 days after this man was dead, did you?

A. That's correct.

Q. And you didn't dictate your discharge summary until after you already had a lawyer advising you, isn't that true sir?

A. That probably is correct.

Q. And is it not true, sir, that the lawyer that was advising you at the time you dictated the discharge summary was with Mr. Burke's law firm that's representing Lilly in this case?

A. I believe that is correct.

Q. Now you said some things in this discharge summary that really help Eli Lilly, didn't you?

A. I don't know.

Q. Well you said, for example, "At the time of discharge, he was requesting to be discharged because he was in a hurry to get back to Maui to take care of business, and although it was my feeling that he might benefit from a couple more days' stay, he did not request to live."

After noting the Freudian slip about not requesting to live, Vickery confronted Neal with his handwritten notes the day before William Forsyth had left the hospital, which said nothing about believing Forsyth should stay in the hospital and even mentioned stopping the tranquilizer, Xanax, he had been on—not the kind of move that was consistent with feeling this was a man at risk. Vickery closed by asking Neal if he had warned Forsyth that he must continue to take the Inderal[31] that he had been put on. No, he hadn't.

This was marvelous theater. Any jury would have had to be impressed. I'd never seen anything quite like it. It was brief, but Neal had been eviscerated. However, the person most pleased in the courtroom was probably See.

At this stage, I'd been there for an emotional roller coaster of a week. For the rest of the people involved, the ride wasn't over. Ron Shlensky was due to take the stand on Monday, as the next expert for the Forsyths. As an old hand, he was amazed there *was* a trial; no one could or should go through many rides like this. I wondered if See and

Mangrum were hunkered down in their bunker, getting as deeply involved as the Forsyth team was.

I had updates later on Vickery's cross-examination of such people as Gary Tollefson from Lilly. Tollefson had joined Lilly in 1991, after the Prozac story blew up. Vickery had wanted Beasley brought to the court, but Lilly refused to provide him, and to the surprise of Judge Kay, as it had been to Judge Potter in Kentucky before him, they were apparently under no obligation to produce him. Leigh Thompson had left the company after the *Wesbecker* case. Tollefson had not been there when the documents at the heart of the case had been generated. Judge Kay ruled that many of the internal documents could not be admitted. As for the rest, someone who had not been there when they were generated could, with a relatively clear conscience, testify truthfully to not knowing exactly what they meant.

Tollefson was also faced with correspondence he had sent to the *American Journal of Psychiatry,* complaining about the medico-legal precedent the Teicher report might have introduced. The theory was preliminary and potentially counterproductive, he had written. Teicher and Cole had replied with concern at the implication they should not bring things to clinicians' attention.[32] The letter had been written when Tollefson was seemingly an independent academic, but several months later he was a Lilly employee.

The next witness for Lilly was a professor of forensic psychiatry in Hawaii, Daryl Matthews:[33]

> Q. Do you believe that if he [Forsyth] had been kept in the hospital longer, that he would be alive today?
>
> A. I think a lot would have depended on how he was treated and what happened in the course of his depression. He was suffering from a severe depression. He was discharged still severely depressed, and I think if his depression had been in remission, had been gone, that this would not have occurred.

Matthews had earlier in the trial criticized the fact that William Forsyth's Xanax had been halted—"Finally, it is noteworthy that Mr. Forsyth was discharged without Xanax as described above. He disliked the idea of taking Xanax. It may have well been helpful in reducing his symptoms."

Vickery was later to ask:

Q. Do you stand by that report?

A. I do.

Q. Do you stand by your testimony this morning that no more Xanax is one of the substantial factors that contributed to the deaths of Bill and June Forsyth?

A. I think it's probably true, yes.

See, in opening for the defense, made an issue about the package insert for Prozac being enough. One of Lilly's witnesses was Byron Eliashoff, a psychiatrist in private practice in Honolulu. Vickery presented him with a copy of the package insert and a yellow highlighter pen:

Q. Doctor, . . . I have, on page 2, highlighted . . . the warning section. What I'd like for you to do, if you would, is find those warnings that Mr. See was asking you about that deal with akathisia or suicide or any of the kind of things that you think they have given proper warnings about, and highlight them in that document for me.

A. I believe in this earlier version of the drug insert, I don't believe there is a reference to akathisia. I'll have to read this. Do you have a larger copy? I'm having trouble reading this.

Q. I know. That's a problem for the prescribing physicians, too, isn't it, sir?

A. Not if they have time.

Q. Okay. Well, take your time because you've just sworn that this is an adequate warning, so take your time, if you would, and just highlight for us in yellow where the warnings are about this problem.

A. There's no reference in this section to suicide.

Q. Is there a reference to akathisia?

A. No, there is not.

Q. So at least in the warnings section of the package insert, there is nothing about either of those two things at the time this drug was prescribed for Mr. and Mrs. Forsyth; is that true?

A. Yes.

Q. Okay, sir. Now, you have testified, just a few minutes ago, that this package insert contains some warnings somewhere that fully apprise prescribing physicians of the dangers of akathisia or suicide, so all I'm asking you to do is to find the language in there upon which you base your opinion that it's fully apprising them.

A. What I'm about to say is that the package insert is adequate for prescribing. It does not mention suicide because suicide is not a risk of using Prozac.

Judge Kay. Mr. Vickery wants you to read through the rest of the insert.

A. Well, I don't see a place to—where akathisia or suicide is mentioned to highlight.

Q. Let's see if I can help you. I have now highlighted for you the precaution section. Is that different from the warning section?

A. Yes.

Q. And I highlighted for you what Eli Lilly had to say about suicide in the precaution section. Would you just read that for me, the section about suicide or akathisia . . .

A. "Suicide, the possibility of a suicide attempt is inherent in depression and may persist until significant remissions occur. Close supervision of high-risk patients should accompany initial drug therapy. Prescriptions for Prozac should be written for the smallest quantity of capsules consistent with good patient management in order to reduce the risk of overdose."

Q. Now, that doesn't say anything about Prozac causing either akathisia or suicide for some patients, does it?

A. That's correct.

Q. And, in fact, when it talks about overdose or prescriptions written for small numbers, the bells that go off in your head are overdose bells, don't they?

A. Yes. Well, that's part of it. Also, the reminder that suicide is inherent in depression.

Q. Which, of course, you knew as a psychiatrist anyway? . . . Dr. Eliashoff, are you able to point in that document, sir, in the entire document, anywhere in that document to where there's some warning about akathisia?

A. Did you highlight it for me?

Q. No, sir, I didn't do that one for me [sic] because I'm not the one that swore that it was adequate.[34]

These exchanges did much to build the confidence of the Forsyth team, despite their failure to get the documents in. The highlighter pen had stood embarrassingly beside Eliashoff on the witness stand. Viktor Reus, a professor of psychiatry in San Francisco, another witness for Lilly, had been faced with a Pfizer article by Roger Lane stating that akathisia could lead to suicide.[35] Reus conceded that SSRIs could cause akathisia. See later suggested to Vickery that this article was an attempt by Pfizer to skewer Lilly.[36]

But See had his winners. William and June Forsyth had kept diaries. Many of the entries were from a time period well removed from the events of March 1993 and could be mined for dark forebodings of what was to come. These See picked over with Matthews. I had not been worried about the diary contents, but absolutely normal people put all sorts of strange things into diaries, and the Forsyth diaries could certainly be used to portray an unhappy state of mind.

See's summation stressed familiar messages—Prozac was the most studied drug in history.[37] Major depression was a terrible illness that caused terrible things. William Forsyth never had akathisia. Lilly had offered sufficient warnings consistent with the evidence. They had also done tons of epidemiological studies. Throughout, he came back to the testimony of Dr. Healy—it took up over a quarter of his summation. To underline the contrast between Lilly's approach and mine, he threw in a predictable friend: "These data from several thousand patients and the evidence that fluoxetine reduces suicidal ideation must, on any scientific scale, outweigh the dubious evidence of a handful of case reports."

Vickery objected that See had never questioned me on this issue. See said he had. Judge Kay remembered that the issue had come up, but nothing more about it. See was allowed to proceed. "Questioning me" was a fascinating description of our brief exchange on this point.

THE VERDICT

The jury recessed. The stakes were high. As I understood it, Lilly stood to lose up to $20 million. Not only that, but the case would then go into a punitive damages phase, where the court would be invited to consider further penalties for the company if it were agreed this case stemmed from a pattern of poor behavior. At this point, among

Vickery's options was to introduce a videotaped testimony from Judge Potter of the *Wesbecker* case. Potter would recount the story of how Lilly had settled the *Wesbecker* case but had managed to fool him and everyone else into thinking that the case had gone to a verdict. He would describe Lilly's efforts to block him from scrutinizing the outcome, and his final victory in having the verdict reclassified from won to settled. This and other testimony was likely to be extremely damaging to Lilly, which had just paid another company, Sepracor, $90 million for the rights for a derivative of fluoxetine, a drug on which they could take out a new patent and have a genuine "son of Prozac." Vickery would argue that setting a $90 million price tag on a molecule from which Lilly might later earn up to $2 billion per year also set a benchmark for punitive damages in the *Forsyth* case.

The jury went into recess. First indications were not encouraging. According to Skip, they weren't asking for the right documents. If they'd asked for the documents early on, it would have been a good indicator that they had made up their minds that Lilly was guilty. Perhaps they were going to take a long time deliberating and then ask for the documents. But if they took a long time deliberating, the judge had an option to introduce a detonator. He could force them to make up their minds. Finally, they began to ask for the documents. Judge Kay, however, decided that although some documents could be shown in court, the jury couldn't have them.

After two days, late on a Good Friday afternoon, the jury returned. There had been confusion. Apparently, the judge had sent a letter to the jury, requesting they close their deliberations as soon as possible. The jury, it seems, had misinterpreted this. Federal court rules as they applied in this case, unlike in the *Wesbecker* case in Kentucky, required unanimity. It seemed that some members of the jury believed they had to come to an 11–0 verdict. It had become clear they could never come to an 11–0 verdict against Lilly and Prozac. This began to sway others. It was Easter weekend, and they would have to stay there over the weekend.

On Easter Saturday in the United Kingdom, I got a telephone call from Good Friday in Hawaii that the verdict had been in favor of Lilly. Vickery's brief call conveyed a sense of disbelief. Ten thousand miles away, I was insulated. I could only guess what the mood in the bunker was like. What had happened?

I began to hear disjointedly from several members of the Forsyth team. After getting back to headquarters, they received a phone call from one of the jurors, Donna Grain, an older woman, unhappy at the verdict. She talked about pressure on her to vote for the defense. She filed an affidavit. Another juror, Glen Mayeshiro, followed two days later. Both would have voted for the Forsyths. In brief, the story that came out in the affidavits was that the initial jury vote had been nine to two against Lilly and Prozac, with only Julie Ugalde and Daniel Hong voting for Lilly. The affidavits suggested that Ugalde, from close to the start of the trial, had indicated she was going to find it difficult to find against Lilly. Armed with his affidavits, Vickery approached Judge Kay and filed motions for a hearing on juror misconduct. The hearing was held on July 1, 1999.

Julie Ugalde had been involved in a medical practice lawsuit against a doctor who had failed to warn about a possible drug hazard that had left her mother brain-damaged.[38] Donna Grain swore that Ugalde "seemed to base her decision about the doctors in this case being at fault on her own personal experience rather than on the evidence. She said that she did not trust any doctors and, if the Forsyths wanted money, they should sue the doctors, not the drug company." Grain and Mayeshiro swore they had also heard her say she had a family member who had benefited from a new AIDS medication, and for this reason she would never award damages against a pharmaceutical company. Counsel for Lilly argued that snatches of conversation had been misinterpreted by two jurors, but this was hard to reconcile with the fact that during the course of the trial the court reporter, Tina Stuhr, had raised with the plaintiffs' attorneys the possibility of getting one of the jurors removed—Ugalde. Stuhr was concerned that Ugalde was not listening to the witnesses for the plaintiffs; in fact, she would barely look at them. During Billy Forsyth's testimony, she seemed openly hostile.

After hearing the testimonies, Kay ruled that this was just one of the hazards of the jury system. But this hearing had gone to the heart of what had gone on in the jury room. The action taken had been solely against Eli Lilly. The Forsyths did not want either Randolph Neal or Riggs Roberts included in the action. People, it seems, don't want to sue their doctors.

Lilly, however, had implicated Randolph Neal in what had happened, with Matthews, their expert, testifying that had the Xanax not been stopped, and had William Forsyth been monitored properly, there was every chance he would still be alive. But almost the only clear reason why this would have been so was if Xanax was managing a Prozac-induced problem. This was exactly what the Germans had required to be in the labeling for Prozac, when it was finally licensed:

> Contraindications—Risk Patients—Risk of Suicide: "FLUCTIN does not have a general sedative effect on the central nervous system. Therefore, for his/her own safety, the patient must be sufficiently observed, until the antidepressive effect of FLUCTIN sets in. Taking an additional sedative may be necessary.[39]

Faced with Matthews's testimony on warnings in the trial, Vickery had tried yet again to bring the German warning into play, but Kay had overruled him.

Based on this, on April 20, the Forsyth team filed a motion for an appeal on two grounds. One was that Alan Kay had misinterpreted or been unaware of important details of Hawaiian law, which imposed a strict product liability as the cost of doing business. Lilly had tried to water this down to responsibility for "danger that was known or knowable in light of the best scientific and medical knowledge available at the time of manufacture and distribution."[40] Vickery had argued that this was a mistake, and that under Hawaiian law, the focus was not on what Lilly knew but rather on what the doctors did not know; that under Hawaiian law, a "product is defective if it contains substances that are dangerous to the user and does not contain directions or warnings regarding dangers in its use [that] were known or by the use of reasonabl[y] developed human foresight could have been known."

The other ground for appeal lay in Kay's exclusion of key documents, such as the German warning insert or the memorandum by David Graham of the FDA, which offered the views that Lilly's trials were not intended to address the question of suicidality, that the Fava and Rosenbaum study supported an association between Prozac and suicidality, and that there were flaws in the Beasley paper in the *BMJ*. Even though I had used some of the documents in replying to Lilly motions to have me disbarred, I wasn't allowed to testify to any of them in trial. Of 150 exhibits, Judge Kay had excluded forty outright and made seventeen available for cross-examination only. Not only did I not get a chance to comment on them, but when jurors, faced with Ugalde asking them to show her the documentary evidence that there was any problem with Prozac, asked for fifteen documents, they found they could only be shown one. Documents such as the memos on Lilly's strategy to blame the disease, not the drug, were denied to them.

As it turned out, there were even stronger grounds on which to appeal. Vickery had, in the course of the trial, registered but not appreciated the significance of another player in the courtroom—Doug Norman, a patent lawyer working for Lilly. What was he doing at this trial?

6

Kafka's Castle

WHEN THE PROZAC CONTROVERSY first took shape, Lilly responded by meta-analyzing its clinical trials database—or so it seemed. Lilly brought this evidence to the FDA hearing that "cleared" Prozac in 1991, and the company confronted Martin Teicher with it at an ACNP meeting in December 1991. Finally, this was the evidence published in the *British Medical Journal*, with Charles Beasley as first author, in September 1991, just as the FDA hearing on Prozac took place.[1] Perhaps more than anything else, this article influenced the events that followed. For many, the science was on Lilly's side.

Lilly had consulted widely with senior figures in psychopharmacology in the United States and Europe; so when the article was published, it would have influential support. It was first submitted to the *New England Journal of Medicine*, which sent it back stating that its readers would not be interested.[2] The *BMJ* then agonized over publication, since the document had an entirely company authorship line.

The Beasley article represented itself as a meta-analysis of randomized controlled trials undertaken by the company. It claimed, "Data from these trials do not show that fluoxetine is associated with an increased risk of suicidal acts or emergence of substantial suicidal thoughts among depressed patients." Reading between the lines, the message was that this was *science*, compared with the anecdotes produced by Teicher and others. Which was a scientist to believe—the meta-analysis or the Teicher anecdotes? Which was a journalist going to believe?

I wrote to the *BMJ* to point out that the Beasley article's dependence on item 3 of the Hamilton Scale was unjustified, and that these trials had not been designed to investigate the emergence of suicidality. What I missed at the time, obvious in retrospect, is that the analysis omitted patients who dropped out because of anxiety and agitation,[3] which amounted for up to 5 percent of all subjects in the trials analyzed—

about 85 of the approximately 1,700 patients who went on Prozac out of the 3,067 total. These patients, at the heart of the debate, were eliminated at the stroke of a pen.

What I didn't know at the time was that the Lilly studies involved patients coadministered benzodiazepines in order to suppress manifestations of akathisia and suicidal ideation.[4] Further, of seventeen sets of patients contained in the meta-analysis, a Dr. Cohn had enrolled six sets; others involved Louis Fabre. When Lilly filed to register Prozac in 1985, the FDA suggested work by Dr. Cohn be left out of the frame.[5]

Still more pertinent, John Heiligenstein and Charles Beasley, both physicians with Lilly, had reanalyzed the trial data. Their brief was to investigate suicide attempts or suicidal ideation reported in trials and to categorize events as completed suicides, suicide attempts, or "suicide gestures." The last category was effectively invented for the purpose; the paper reported on suicides and suicide attempts but not suicidal gestures. Catherine Mesner testified that similar data had been forwarded from clinical trials in Europe to Beasley and Heiligenstein to assess and categorize, and that those analyzing the trials managed to reclassify nine out of ten suicide-related events as nonsignificant.[6]

While Beasley and Heiligenstein's reclassifications may have been correct in some cases, their approach was entirely inappropriate scientifically. The correct approach is to leave the matter to the statistics to sort out. If suicidal events were happening on Prozac but not caused by it, similar events should be happening on placebo or other antidepressants. The assessment process was therefore neither independent nor conducted with any clinical sophistication. Indeed, Charles Beasley had never practiced clinically, and Heiligenstein had prescribed Prozac once in his life—to a child. Heiligenstein's testimony in his *Wesbecker* deposition was as follows:

A. Suicidal ideation is not an adverse event.
Q. Why not?
A. It's a component of the illness.
Q. Doctor, is it your testimony that nobody has ever become suicidal because of the use of fluoxetine?
A. In my estimation, to the best of my knowledge, no.[7]

Beasley's testimony in the same trial was:

> *Q.* Have you seen an instance where you in your medical judg-
> ment have believed that ideation was caused by ingestion of
> Prozac?
>
> *A.* No.[8]

This was not an analysis that might show Prozac to be less likely to be associated with suicidality than other antidepressants or placebo, but one in which Prozac could not *in principle* be associated with a single case of suicidality. You couldn't go on Prozac in these studies if you weren't depressed. If you became suicidal, it couldn't be because of Prozac, because only depression causes suicidality. You could have insomnia, a feature of depression, caused by Prozac; or sexual dysfunction, another feature of depression, caused by Prozac; or fatigue, also a feature of depression, caused by Prozac—but never suicidality.

At his deposition in the *Wesbecker* case, Leigh Thompson faced a December 7 memo from Richard Huddleston to Hans Weber, inquiring about a German patient who committed suicide. This patient had been on no other medications, and his physician had explicitly connected the suicide to a surge in serotonin. The Indianapolis monitor "judged the report to be not related."[9]

A similar mindset is demonstrated in the *Miller* case several years later, in the deposition of Wilma Harrison of Pfizer by Andy Vickery:

> *Q.* An eight-year-old boy who was on Zoloft for 36 days and
> here's what it says about him. "Patient was hospitalized for
> a suicide gesture, and dropped from the study. The patient
> mutilated himself by cutting his feet with a razor blade and
> tying a tie around his neck. There was no previous history of
> self-mutilation or suicidality, although family history was
> significant for affective disorder (mother, maternal uncle)
> and suicide (maternal uncle). The event was attributed to
> study drug by the investigator.
>
>   What does that last sentence mean to you?
>
> *A.* I would like to see the report.
>
> *Q.* The question is: What does the last sentence mean to you?
>
> *A.* I can only answer that in context. This is a patient who was
> in a study because the patient had major depression, and the
> patient has a strong family history of both depression and

suicide, so this is a patient that's at very high risk for developing suicidal ideation or behavior.

The patient was in the study, and the time in the study was probably not sufficient to completely treat the symptoms of depression, so the fact that this patient made a suicide gesture while being treated says that the patient probably was still depressed and feeling suicidal at the time that the patient committed the suicidal gesture.

Now, in order to attribute it to the study drug, I don't see how anybody could attribute it to the study drug. While it's a possibility that you could say that it could be attributed to the study drug, the illness itself is associated with suicidal ideation and behavior, so it is more likely that this patient had made a suicidal gesture because of the underlying depression that was not yet treated.

Q. That's not what your investigator concluded, is it?

A. I'm a psychiatrist, and I have to assess each case on the basis of facts given to me.

Q. You're not going to tell me that you know the eight-year-old boy, are you?

A. I know about treating patients with depression, and, in my clinical judgment, I would not have attributed this to the drug under study. I would have attributed it to the illness under study.

Q. Do you know anything about this eight-year-old boy?

A. It is not necessary for me to know about this specific eight-year-old boy. You have given me the history of a family history of affective disorder, a child only eight years old who has a serious enough depression to warrant treatment, and a family history of suicidality. That's very strong risk factors for suicidal behavior.

Q. What did Pfizer's clinical investigator conclude with respect to the cause of this boy's suicidal attempt?

A. The investigator attributed it to the study drug.[10]

Part of the fascination of this deposition is that Vickery had already inquired as to whether Pfizer had confidence in their clinical investigators and had been told the company did. Put aside the fact that this study was conducted when some American clinical investigators' practices were about to lead to jail terms; this eight-year-old boy, far from being in a study for the treatment of severe depression, was listed as having an obsessional rather than a depressive disorder and was in a tolerability study that meant pushing his dose of Zoloft to 200 mg.

Lilly had conducted a similar analysis of its depression database to review aggressive events, and this, too, not surprisingly, cleared Prozac. Beasley and Heiligenstein managed to reduce 1,115 adverse events to just 11 that called for further analysis.[11] Let's examine Heiligenstein's deposition in the *Wesbecker* case again:

> Q. And is it fair to say that some of these adverse events listed in and of themselves would indicate risk factors for somebody becoming more violent, aggressive?
> A. They may.
> Q. And that wasn't taken into consideration . . . ?
> A. Depression itself is a risk factor and that was taken into consideration, yes.[12]

There were further grounds for concern. Reading the Beasley paper in 1991, I had the impression that Lilly had analyzed all the relevant clinical trials from their database, even though the article clearly stated that the company had analyzed only American studies. But, in fact, not even all American studies were analyzed. A sample of 3,067 patients had been analyzed out of a total of more than 26,000 patients enrolled in trials. About 23,000 patients simply vanished.[13]

After all this, the figures presented in the Beasley paper point to "an excess risk with fluoxetine."[14] This led one reviewer to recommend a change of title from the original "Fluoxetine and Suicidality: Absence of an Association in Controlled Depression trials"[15] to the more neutral "Fluoxetine and Suicide: A Meta-Analysis of Controlled Trials of Treatment for Depression." Far from setting the matter to rest, then, the Beasley article makes it less possible to write off the whole episode as just incompetence, given the steps taken by Lilly. This raised further the issue of the failure of the field to notice what had transpired.

The Beasley article was only one element in the equation. In the course of the *Forsyth* trial, Andy See raised a Daubert challenge against Ron Shlensky, claiming Shlensky had no data to satisfy the standard that he himself ought to apply what is generally accepted in the scientific community. . . . In this case to the contrary we have many epidemiology studies, all going the same way. . . . The Fava, if you read what the authors did . . . shows nothing adverse about Prozac. The Jick study, if you hold to looking at statistically significant conclusions . . . supports the conclusion that there's no difference between Prozac and other antidepressants. The Leon study that I talked to Dr. Healy about, the Wirshing study, that I talked to Dr. Healy about, as well as the Beasley study . . . all of those come to exactly the same conclusion. The Beasley study is . . . a very big group of controlled clinical trials but the rest of them are in the nature of epidemiology studies. There were how many lawsuits regarding Bendectin and, in fact, there was no evidence that it caused birth defects, it is almost like that. Every one of these epidemiology studies came to the same conclusion.[16]

Lilly tried hard to persuade Judge Kay that the epidemiology was on their side. Why? Because we were in an era when epidemiology and clinical trials talked in the courts. This stab at winning by default should shock any reader, academic or lay. Where the Fava and Rosenbaum study was concerned, See was correct if, as he suggested, one only "read what the authors did." If you read what anyone else made of the same figures, you saw they concluded these figures suggested that suicidality was three times more likely on Prozac than on other antidepressants. Besides, this was not an epidemiological study, it was a postmarketing surveillance study.[17]

The Wirshing study, which See had raised with me in the *Forsyth* trial, was the study by Warshaw and Keller involving 654 patients, of whom 191 had been on Prozac.[18] This study appeared to demonstrate the opposite to what Lilly claimed it proved. More to the point, it could not even remotely be described as an epidemiological study.

Warshaw and Keller, along with personnel from Lilly, were authors of another study put forward by Lilly—the Leon study, conceived almost twenty years before Prozac was launched and begun ten years before Prozac's launch.[19] This involved 643 patients, of whom 185 had gone on Prozac at some point. To imply this study was in any way designed to test for the possibility that Prozac might be associated with suicidality was ridiculous. Besides this, the numbers of patients involved would almost certainly have made any characterization of this as an epidemiological study a breach of any trade description act, if there were such a thing for epidemiological studies. The puzzling aspect was why the *American Journal of Psychiatry* published the Leon study.

Following the litigation on breast implants, epidemiology had become one of the weapons in the "tort wars." Lilly was trying to portray Fava, Warshaw and Keller, and Leon as epidemiological studies. But an epidemiological study by definition requires a study of populations. It is rare to get good epidemiological studies with fewer than tens of thousands of subjects in their sample, and even then, these studies specify steps taken to make these huge samples representative of the population at large—all but apologizing for the fact that the entire population has not been studied. These Lilly papers, in contrast, were dealing with studies where only between one hundred and two hundred were taking Prozac, and no effort was made to show what steps had been taken to produce a sample representative of the larger population. To call this epidemiology was at best misleading, if not an effort by force of money to commandeer the current legal high ground. Randomized controlled trials (RCTs) and epidemiological studies had become accepted in court as appropriately scientific methods. However, it takes a great deal of money to run RCTs or epidemiological studies of the kind being proposed. It also requires the cooperation of the psychiatric profession. This is not something that could be undertaken by plaintiffs or their lawyers.

AN ISSUE FIT FOR THE *BRITISH MEDICAL JOURNAL*

There was an issue here any decent scientist could support, even if she thought that Prozac did more good than harm. I drafted an article on the power of the pharmaceutical industry to "buy" the scientific agenda, questioning how it had become possible to claim that randomized trials and epidemiology were the *only* way to prove cause and effect in cases of drug-induced injury, and how the industry had ended up in a position where companies were the only ones able to conduct such studies. Wealth and power often win in legal cases, but it was getting to the point where companies could ensure that cases didn't even get to court.

Graham Dukes, editor of *International Journal of Risk and Safety in Medicine* and author of the standard textbook on drug-induced injury,[20] had responded to my first attempt in this area, before the *Forsyth* case:

> It seems to me your approach is original and fair. . . . I had not seen the issues of litigation, regulation and patents juxtaposed in this way before but . . . I agree entirely from my own experience with many of your comments; there are some striking examples of companies tenaciously hanging onto a profitable and patented drug despite the evidence that it is doing more harm than good. Their motives are a mixture of opportunism and genuine belief that the product is being wrongly accused. I also agree with your remarks about the failure of the present overall research approach to elicit a reliable picture of adverse effects and the sometimes unrealistic defenses put up by industry when their products are the subject of injury litigation.[21]

This article got put on the back burner during the months leading up to the *Forsyth* trial, but I revisited it while awaiting the outcome. The verdict in favor of Lilly had implications for prescribers. In any future action, the prescriber might well be put in the dock along with the company. If it seemed possible a jury might acquit Lilly on the basis that the prescriber should shoulder some of the blame, one legal option for plaintiffs would be to adopt a "Cutthroat." This involves putting prescribers in the dock as well, forcing them to sink with the company or swim by testifying they had never been at any educational meeting of any sort that raised the issue of Prozac-induced agitation and suicidality. These options, it seemed, had been in Lilly's mind when the controversy blew up, because the company offered to indemnify any American doctors who ended up in a legal action because of Prozac.[22]

There was another, flesh-and-blood reason for doing something. After returning from Hawaii, I met Dave Wilkinson, then secretary of the child psychiatry section of the Royal College of Psychiatrists, who told me that he and colleagues had been using many more SSRIs in the past year than before and were noticing problems. He described the case of a 15-year-old boy who experienced a personality change on Prozac. A normally quiet lad, within days of going on Prozac he became involved in fights. This moved on to burglary and risked escalating further. Dave stopped the drug. A few days later, the lad said he was back to normal. Dave asked the boy, would he do any of those things now?

Definitely not. He'd be too scared. While on the drug, it was as if his adrenaline had been turned off.[23] The realization that I had authored a consensus statement that might be used to promote increased prescribing to teenagers worried me.

I decided to call in to the offices of the *British Medical Journal* to explain the situation to the editor, Richard Smith. Since the *BMJ* had carried the Beasley article, he might be interested to learn about the background to this article. Smith could hardly be faced with a better offer, in the sense of a newsworthy issue from someone who had been the secretary for a national association.

Medical journals are essentially journalism, even if of a rarefied kind. What determines entry into the *BMJ* or the *American Journal of Psychiatry* is the same as what determines entry into the *Boston Globe* or the *Wall Street Journal*. Knowing the editor or the editor's friends helps. Toeing the party line helps. Defensibility of the story line helps. Something that might hit advertising revenues will be a consideration for most journals. Quality of research is further down on the list of priorities.

When I called the *BMJ* offices, Richard Smith wasn't there, but I filled in the deputy editor, Jane Smith, on the story. We agreed that I would follow up the visit with a formal submission. I sent in the article with a four-page letter explaining the background and acknowledging the issues as tricky and complex. I stated that I would be happy to discuss matters further if the *BMJ* felt the piece was of interest and to modify my submission in the light of any editorial suggestions on how the issues might better be handled.

Richard Smith wrote back:

> I think a version of your paper could well be suitable for publication in the *BMJ* if you can shorten it to not more than 2000 words. . . . I think the Prozac story is especially interesting, and it clearly would make sense for something to be published in the *BMJ* when we have played such a crucial part in the story. I remember clearly the meta-analysis that we published, and I remember something about the debate around the paper at the time. Some people said we shouldn't publish the paper because it would inevitably be biased, making the point, I remember, that if the study had proved the link between Prozac and suicide then they undoubtedly wouldn't have sent the paper to us. Others said that we couldn't reject a paper simply because it came from a

pharmaceutical company and that we didn't see many major scientific problems with the study. In retrospect, there is clearly a problem with the fact that the study suffers heavily from publication bias,[24] but I think it's true to say that we were all much less conscious of publication bias in 1990 than we are in 1999. . . . I hope you will have a go at revising the papers, but if you decide to publish them elsewhere then perhaps you could send us copies. We would then pick up on them in the *BMJ*.[25]

The *BMJ*'s "Education and Debate Section," toward which I was led to believe this piece was being steered, took two-thousand-word pieces. I spent a weekend reducing everything to this length. By Monday, I had an article called "A Failure to Warn," which I put in the mail with a further letter emphasizing that should the *BMJ* take the piece, I would be open to revising and rephrasing in line with any constructive editorial comments.

The piece was sent to John Geddes, a senior lecturer in Oxford, to review. I have no idea what the covering letter said. At this stage, as I saw it, given the statements and internal documents from Lilly that the company had assigned "probably related" to a number of the case reports of suicidality and suicides on Prozac, it was difficult to see how any further evidence was needed. There was a particularly interesting situation in the light of the fact that Lilly had chosen not to publish conventional clinical trial evidence that confirmed that Prozac could induce suicidality. Smith had been campaigning on the issue of company failures to publish data during the previous year, one more reason to think he might be interested.[26] I left synopses of the Lilly documents in the *BMJ* offices.

Geddes, of course, didn't have this evidence. The next letter from Richard Smith stated: "I'm afraid we don't think it suitable for publication in the *BMJ* in its present form." The Geddes review was the review of a person considering whether this piece proved Prozac did or did not cause suicidality. As it stood, the greatly abbreviated piece focused on the bioethical issues and wasn't intended to prove this. Geddes raised the issue of how certain we need to be that a risk exists, and how great that risk must be, before we must warn patients and doctors. But this was not a matter for Smith or Geddes to agonize about. FDA statutes *require* companies to warn if there is an association, even if cause has not been proven.

I wrote back immediately, spelling out that the issues we were dealing with were comparable to the issue of informed consent, first raised by Henry Beecher in 1966. Beecher's article detailed twenty-two pieces of research where explicit informed consent had not been sought from the research subjects. Beecher criticized no one and called no one guilty, but no reader could fail to recognize that at least some of the patients in some of these studies had to have entered the research not knowing what was being done to them, and might have suffered an injury they would not have chosen to risk. It seemed to me that we were in a similar position. Even if the *BMJ* or its readers thought Lilly was not guilty, if clinical studies were generally happening in this way, then it was certain that at some point in the proceedings, wrong was being done.

Two letters were exchanged, then Richard Smith phoned me.[27] When I protested that data hadn't been provided because he had asked for an "Education and Debate" article, he brushed me aside. When I assured him that data could be provided, he replied to the effect that no matter what I wrote, the article would not be accepted. Things had evolved rapidly and surprisingly.

The *BMJ* in 1991 faced a dilemma. As far as I can make out, the Beasley paper was the first major article to appear in a major journal with a company-only authorship line. Its acceptance by the *BMJ* probably facilitated the appearance of a great number of other articles with predominantly company authorship lines in major journals—the Leon paper may be a good example. At a 1998 meeting on new antipsychotic drugs at the American College of Neuropsychopharmacology conference, delegates bewailed the fact that published clinical trials now invariably supported the sponsor's compound. They complained that some of these company-only authored articles on new drugs contained data that simply didn't add up; efforts to reanalyze the data independently indicated the data had been massaged beyond acceptable limits.

BEYOND THE *BMJ*

What could happen next? I'd made contact with Sarah Boseley from *The Guardian,* the leading liberal broadsheet newspaper in Britain.[28] I gave her a draft of the "Failure to Warn" piece, letting her know there was a good chance it would appear in the *BMJ.* She was geared to picking up on it when it did and running with the story from there. John Geddes later offered the view that a *Guardian* article would have much greater impact than anything in the *BMJ*. Would it?

Following the rebuff from Richard Smith, I met with Sarah. After she left, the phone rang in my office. It was the *Sunday Times* and another Sarah. I ended up spending nearly two hours on the phone with Sarah Tonge, who had gotten hold of the *Forsyth* documents and details of the case through the Internet and then made contact with Baum, Hedlund. She wanted to know more.

I wanted the story done thoroughly. Boseley seemed to be offering a four-thousand-word piece in the review section of the *Guardian*. Tonge was offering a much shorter piece in the *Sunday Times*. I contacted Boseley, who was alarmed and began work on a shorter first piece, which the *Guardian* published on the Saturday before the proposed *Sunday Times* piece. This outlined in brief the details of the *Forsyth* case and the fact that not all the relevant information had come out. Nothing appeared in the *Sunday Times* the next day. Some months later, a pro-Prozac story ran in the *Times*,[29] mentioning "the booming anti-Prozac lobby, with its strident pieces in the middle-market tabloids, its raucous sites on the World Wide Web, its best-selling books."

The main *Guardian* piece came out October 30, Halloween weekend. The review section sported a lurid black, Halloweenish cover with the title "Prozac: Can It Make You Kill?" Inside was a five-page article detailing the *Forsyth* case.[30] It went through the documents indicating that Lilly knew there were hazards from early in the development of the drug—gripping stuff. But after this there was not a peep from Lilly.

Four days later, the *Daily Telegraph* carried an article detailing the death of Robert Woods.[31] The coroner in Carmarthen in South Wales, a Mr. Owen, had noted the fact that Mr. Woods, a farmer who shot himself through the forehead, had been on Prozac for the previous two weeks. Mr. Owen apparently wondered whether Prozac should carry warnings. How many cases like this were coroners seeing?

After the first *Guardian* article, two people approached me: Jane, described in the preface to this book, and Jenny Clark. Neither wished to take legal action. But Jenny did want to know more about Prozac. Shortly after Christmas two years earlier, her 23-year-old son Craig had been put on Prozac by his GP, unbeknownst to his family. Craig did not appear depressed or different to them. But his GP had noted that he had been flat and apathetic since the breakup of a relationship, that he seemed to be moving from job to job, and that he was drinking more than was good for him.

Over the New Year period, Craig did seem different to his family: more agitated and less able to settle, doing things out of character, getting involved in fights. None of the family members had any idea why he was behaving this way. Craig returned to his GP after a week to ask for counseling. This was fixed for the following week. But the day before he was due for his first counseling session, and two weeks after he had gone on Prozac, Craig Clark hanged himself in his apartment. At the inquest a few months later, Jenny raised the possibility that the Prozac her son had been on—which at the time she had not known he'd been on—might have played a role in his suicide. The coroner dismissed her concerns. The inquest lasted a matter of minutes. She felt that Craig had been written off as unimportant. Jenny thought her GP was excellent; she didn't blame him. Maybe one of the reasons there were so few legal actions against primary-care physicians was that people didn't want to take action against doctors they saw as good.[32]

In addition to the two women who approached me after the *Guardian* piece ran, a man named John Marshall was referred to me with a request from his lawyers for a report on whether an action could be taken against the psychiatrist who had prescribed the Prozac that had made him suicidal. His story did indeed point to a Prozac-induced agitation. Communication had broken down between him and his psychiatrist, who hadn't fingered Prozac in a deteriorating relationship. A psychiatric pharmacist had written a report saying the entire world knew that Prozac could cause difficulties like this and therefore there was a case against the doctor. But was there? It still seemed to me that the coin wouldn't have dropped for many clinicians, given the constant reassurances from Lilly and the appeals to science. In this era of evidence-biased medicine, who was going to be unscientific and blame Prozac? While I was pretty sure about John Marshall's Prozac, I found it difficult to support this action against his psychiatrist. How many other patients had cases that went nowhere because experts like me felt that even if the drug did cause suicidality, it was difficult to hold the clinician responsible?

Jenny Clark's case suggested coroners might be a way forward. I wrote to all 146 coroners in England and Wales; 30 replied. Some said they hadn't noticed anything but would keep an eye out in future. Others said they had noticed something and would keep a closer eye out in the future. Reginald Browning, Craig Clark's coroner, didn't reply. I wrote to him several times without reply. I then wrote and specifically asked him about Craig Clark. Mr. Browning finally replied, stating that he had known nothing about Prozac, and that even if he had, it was not his place to do anything other than record a verdict.

I wrote to the British Secretary of State for Health, Alan Milburn, and got back a reply that would have brought a smile to the face of Franz Kafka. It seemed that, writing from Wales, I should address the Welsh National Assembly. I wrote back and apologized for not doing so, but I suggested this was not simply a Welsh issue but of significance to the rest of the United Kingdom. Nevertheless, I was informed by phone that if I had written from France, the Department of Health would have considered the issue, but because I was writing from Wales, they couldn't. This had to go through Cardiff. Cardiff referred me back to Whitehall—to the Medicines Control Agency (MCA).

I had already written to the Medicines Control Agency. Several months later, I got a bland rehash of old statements in reply. They'd considered things in 1990 and decided nothing had been proven. Lilly did include a warning on Prozac, I was told—that there was a suicide risk inherent in all cases of depression, and prescribers should therefore take care. I had also asked the MCA to consider the possibility that, because of the way side effects were not being recorded, all patients participating in clinical trials in Britain and elsewhere were putting themselves and others in legal jeopardy. The MCA gave no answer. I wrote to them again mentioning this. Their subsequent reply made it clear they didn't understand the point.

There were other people to write to. I got a friendly letter back from John Cox, the president of the Royal College of Psychiatrists, who noted my concerns and said that he'd hand my letter on to the Psychopharmacology Committee. A year later, even after a follow-up letter, I was still waiting. Two years after that I was still waiting, despite my further overtures. I also wrote to Denis Pereira Gray, from the Royal College of General Practitioners, who noted my concerns and said that he would liaise with Cox on this issue.

Several TV companies made contact, interested by the possibilities the story offered. However, when they submitted program proposals to the Central Authorities, the reply tended to be that the Prozac story was an old one. Unless something new turned up, all any program could do was repeat what had already appeared in the *Guardian*, and this wasn't sufficient. A later *Guardian* editorial suggested the British media had turned against exposing corporations.[33] It was hard to know where things were going at this stage. On the basis that there is no such thing as bad publicity, maybe all I'd done was increase sales of Prozac.

In hopes of getting ideas about how to move things forward, I sent documents to friends within companies. Longtime friends replied asking me not to send anything else like this to them again, especially to a company address. Others have not been in touch since. Several senior contacts drew my attention to the pharmaceutical industry Code of Conduct, according to which companies are not supposed to denigrate another company. This prohibited them from even discussing things with me. Others listened at greater length. They agreed, as many senior clinicians have, that Prozac could trigger a suicide, but that it was probably a rare event. One executive told me he was horrified and had put the documents in the company safe to make sure no one else saw them. He had no suggestions about what I might do. It was so messy when these things got into the media.

To try to get a take on whether I was seeing this right or not, I took the documents and the case to key company people who had been through the messiness of drug stories in the media. The view that came back was that marketing was marketing and had to be vigorous, but there was a line and it seemed from the documents that Lilly might have crossed it. What should I do about it? "Write an article to the *BMJ*" was the suggestion. Offers to talk on the issue on company platforms were not taken up. I wrote to the Association of the British Pharmaceutical Industry. The letter wasn't acknowledged.

I presented the material in a series of UK and Irish settings, including Bristol, London, Oxford, Leicester, and Cardiff. The response from audiences was almost completely supportive. None of the points made here were contested. But my employer, the University of Wales College of Medicine, insisted I make it explicit that I was speaking in my own capacity. Everyone, it seems, was scared of being sued by Lilly. At the Institute of Psychiatry at London, I gave the talk at a "Suicide Club" whose program was ordinarily sponsored by Lilly. Lilly withdrew the funding for my talk.

I wrote an article for the special March 2000 Prozac issue of the *Hastings Center Reports* to accompany pieces written by Carl Elliott, a professor of bioethics in the University of Minnesota, and Peter Kramer.

Lilly, which had been the biggest private sponsor of the Hastings Center, withdrew its support.[34] Bob Michels, the dean of medicine at Cornell and a member of the editorial board of the *Hastings Center Reports,* persuaded the center to have my article re-reviewed, on the basis of which they would either apologize to Lilly or make it clear, if called upon, that they stood behind the piece. It was sent out to three reviewers, one of whom was Max Fink from New York. Fink's review made it clear that the only shortcoming with my piece was that it didn't go far enough.

But while Max Fink and others stood publicly behind me, I was introduced to a new definition of friendship—your friends are the ones who will tell you they can't be seen talking to you. A string of colleagues from Japan through Europe to the United States called or e-mailed to tell me that they had been told to have no contact with me—that I was trouble, and about to be *in* trouble.

There was also some good news. After the difficulties with the *BMJ,* I sent "A Failure to Warn" back to Graham Dukes at the *International Journal of Risk and Safety in Medicine,* who accepted it. "We were unforgivably slow in dealing with your excellent paper. . . . It was approved by our reviewers . . . no modifications were proposed. I am wondering whether you would agree to our printing it as a guest editorial. I prefer that papers which we are anxious to emphasize get this status."[35]

BACK TO THE *BMJ*

It was time to try a second piece in the *BMJ,* an editorial on the question I had raised with the MCA about clinical trials and legal jeopardy. This seemed an even bigger issue than the issue of whether Prozac causes suicidality.

Both the *Wesbecker* and *Forsyth* trials, as well as the *Guardian* article and every talk I gave on the issue, included the stunning memo from the chief executive in the German branch of Lilly, Claude Bouchy, in which he stated, "Hans had medical problems with these directions and I have great concerns about it. I do not think I could explain to the BGA, to a judge, to a reporter or even to my family why we do this especially on the sensitive issue of suicide and suicidal ideation."[36] Another memo followed, stating, "I personally wonder whether we are really helping the credibility of an excellent ADE system by calling overdose what a physician reports as suicide attempt and by calling depression what a physician is reporting as suicide ideation."[37]

Lilly countered this in the *Forsyth* trial by reading the reply to Bouchy from Leigh Thompson, who noted this "good and important point. . . . I would like very much to emphasize again that we never diminish information content in a report by DELETING any words of the reporter—NEVER EVER."[38]

Reading the whole correspondence made it clear this was not a matter of a drug company fiddling results to get itself out of tight situation, but rather a systematic bias affecting all companies and trials. When new things went wrong on a drug, there might be no box in which to code the problem. You didn't have to delete any reporter's words if the boxes the FDA would analyze didn't mention suicidal ideation. All the events might be present, but if they were coded depression, where was the problem?

The real issue was not what this said about Lilly and Prozac but what it said about all companies and all drugs. The FDA would never analyze side effects happening to patients in clinical trials if a box corresponding to the side effect didn't exist. This might be tolerable if the data from these clinical trials were just used for marketing purposes. But if companies were using the lack of data to argue that clinical trials had proven these side effects didn't happen, then patient participation in trials was putting everyone else in legal jeopardy. This held whether one believed that Prozac induced suicidality or not. I knew a number of companies unhappy with the situation.

Surely, this was the sort of point even Richard Smith couldn't argue with. A 580-word editorial maybe was something he could commit to. Shorn of references, it went as follows:

> In the clinical studies, prior to its launch in 1988, Prozac had been associated with akathisia and agitation, occurring with sufficient frequency and intensity to lead to recommendations that benzodiazepines be co-prescribed with it in clinical trials. A post-launch randomized trial recorded a 25% akathisia rate on Prozac. Leading textbooks on the clinical profile of psychotropic agents mention Prozac's well-known propensity to cause akathisia. Akathisia has been implicated as a mechanism whereby Prozac may in certain circumstances lead to violence and suicide. The physiological mechanisms by

which this happens are relatively well understood. Yet Lilly's presentation of the side effects of Prozac from their clinical trials database contains no mention of akathisia.

Emotional flatness or blunting is a not infrequent side effect of treatment reported by patients on Prozac. Arguably this effect is all but intrinsic to the mode of action of the drug, which generally reduces emotional reactivity. It has been reported in observational studies, where it has been linked to other potentially harmful behaviors. But nothing resembling emotional blunting appears in the clinical trials side-effect database for Prozac.

There is published and unpublished randomized controlled trial evidence that SSRI use is associated with a higher rate of suicidal ideation early in the course of treatment than other antidepressants, strongly suggesting that treatment may induce suicidality in some. Whether or not the reader believes that an antidepressant could induce suicidal ideation, as a matter of fact treatment-emergent suicidal ideation is not recognized by any code in current clinical trial systems. It is not recorded as a side effect of Prozac in the Lilly database.

There are a number of problems with the side-effect data from clinical trials. One is the failure of systems to cope with "new" problems. Another is a current dependence on self-reporting methods for side-effect collection. In the case of the SSRIs it would seem that these methods only detect one in six of the side effects detected by systematic checklist methods.

If the side-effect profile of a drug drawn from clinical trials were used just for marketing purposes, there might be little problem with this state of affairs. These profiles have, however, also been used in academic debate and for legal purposes to deny that claimed adverse effects are happening. Against this background, it would seem that patients entering clinical trials where side-effect data is collected by spontaneous reporting methods are putting anyone who may suffer a drug induced adverse event into a state of potential legal jeopardy. The consequences for prescriber liability are also uncertain.

This is a problem that could be readily remedied. If UK ethical committees were to insist that consent forms for trials include a statement that side effects collected by current methods could be used for marketing but for no other purposes, the present poor arrangements could continue without posing a threat of legal jeopardy to all of us. Alternatively ethical committees could request better side-effect collection

methods, which would both enhance the scientific information provided by clinical trials and minimize the risks of jeopardy. As many
important trials are now multinational and must adhere to the same
protocols, these simple maneuvers would have an immediate international effect.

Ethical committees came into existence because the process of recruitment of patients to clinical studies was not transparent. Beecher's
review of practices in 1966 indicated a situation where it was likely
that some abuses were happening or could happen. The same situation applies today to the use of data emerging from clinical trials.[39]

Following the reception of the earlier article, it was no surprise this
editorial was rejected. Rather, the reasons were surprising:

> The main reason for this is that we find the editorial very far from
> clear. We think few BMJ readers would make it to the end, and those
> that did would, we think, be very unclear about the exact message. I
> can understand that you must be worrying that we keep rejecting your
> paper because we are covering up a mistake. Perhaps unconsciously
> we are, but I obviously don't think that is the case. I think that we are
> rejecting your papers because they are too long, too unfocussed and
> insufficiently clear.[40]

It was impossible not to reply, "It's difficult to see how this could be too
long." I suggested we could get blind raters to rate for focus. I told
Richard Smith I was due to lecture on the issues at the Institute of Psychiatry, not far from the BMJ offices, two weeks later, and he would be
welcome to attend there or in Oxford some weeks later. In the meantime, he might be interested to know we had completed a new study in
which healthy volunteers had, astonishingly, become suicidal on SSRIs.

> I'm sure you will agree that very few people in my position with
> another article on these issues would approach the BMJ but believing
> that the playing field is indeed level I would be happy to do so. I ac-
> cept that any paper will need to be peer reviewed and your response
> will depend on the reply from your reviewers but I also know that
> publication in any journal is not a simple matter of scientific merit. . . .
> Would you advise me to send the manuscript to you or would you ad-
> vise me to go elsewhere?[41]

I had a quick reply from Richard Smith: "To be honest I cannot see how a study like that you propose would help answer the very important question of whether fluoxetine increases the risk of suicide. It seems to me that this is a question that can only be answered by the methods of clinical epidemiology."[42] So the playing field *wasn't* level.

I went elsewhere. In the United Kingdom at least, if all ethics committees (institutional review boards, or IRBs) were to act together, companies would have little option but to play ball. But the omens for IRBs weren't promising. I presented my talk at an enhancement technologies workshop attended by a group of North American ethicists. Their reaction was that ethicists on one committee blocking an industry protocol would simply find industry going down the road to another committee at another university. There was no North American forum through which ethicists could act in concert. To my further astonishment, I learned that review boards were being rapidly privatized and run by the organizations that run clinical trials for the pharmaceutical companies.[43]

The situation might be easier in the United Kingdom, which had a much smaller number of ethics committees. Richard Nicholson, editor of the *Bulletin of Medical Ethics,* said he was prepared to take an article on this issue. Several months later, while waiting for this article on "Clinical Trials and Legal Jeopardy" to appear,[44] I had a surprise. Max Fink, a New York contact, e-mailed to say he had just been given a copy of my article and that he agreed with what I was saying. He said Jonathan Cole had given him a copy. I had sent nothing to either of them.

HOW MANY DEATHS?

By the time my relationship with Richard Smith went into decline, it had become evident that there were even more data of the kind that he would like than I had suspected. In 1986, a document had been sent to Lilly headquarters in Indianapolis from Hans Weber, Lilly's medical director in Germany, and Barbara von Keitz; this gave figures from clinical trials to that date which seemed to indicate a greatly increased frequency of suicide attempts among patients on Prozac, compared with other antidepressants.[45]

On Prozac, there appeared to be 54 or 56 suicide attempts in 5,427 patients, a rate of roughly 10 per 1,000 patients. In the patients randomized to imipramine, amitriptyline, doxepin, or mianserin, there were 3 suicide attempts in 1,981 patients, a rate of 1.5 to 1,000 patients. On placebo, there were 7, 5, or 1, depending on how one read the data, from 1,169 patients; this could give rates of 6, 4.3, or 1 per 1,000 patients.

Why the variability in the placebo rate? Lilly had included at least several patients who made a suicide attempt in the placebo washout period of clinical trials in their placebo group. This was highly inappropriate. There were two ways to respond. One was to count only 5 suicide attempts in the placebo group, giving a 4.3 per thousand suicide attempt rate. The other was to count all patients who went into clinical trials as placebo cases also, giving a one per thousand suicide attempt rate. Overall Prozac was three times more likely to lead to a suicide attempt than all other treatments combined, and the figure might yet be four or five times as high.

In September 1999, I spoke for the French pharmaceutical company Pierre Fabre at a European College of Neuropsychopharmacology meeting in London, in a symposium on their dual serotonergic and norepinephrine reuptake-inhibiting antidepressant, milnacipran. Stuart Montgomery, one of the other speakers, presented the results of a meta-analysis of the company's clinical trial database looking at suicide attempts on SSRIs, on tricyclic antidepressants, and on milnacipran. The data had been published two years previously in a review article.[46] This again showed an approximately threefold greater rate of suicide attempts on SSRIs than on milnacipran or tricyclics.

At the same meeting, David Baldwin, a colleague of Montgomery, spoke on a study done by Montgomery on recurrent brief depression being treated with either Paxil or placebo. In midpresentation he flashed up data that showed suicide attempts were three times higher on Paxil. The data had not been published, but this presentation put it in the public domain.[47]

Ross Baldessarini from Harvard was also working on suicide attempts in clinical trials on both old and new antidepressants. Data from early analyses gave higher figures for suicide attempts on SSRIs than on placebo, and up to five times higher than on older antidepressants.[48] Shortly afterward, in April 2000, an article appeared in the *Archives of Psychiatry*,[49] looking at rates of suicide attempts on newer antidepressants compared to placebo. Again, the rates for SSRIs were higher than for placebo.

These clinical trial figures made it possible to estimate how many people had made suicide attempts because of Prozac. If ten per thousand make an attempt on Prozac and five per thousand or fewer do so on placebo or other antidepressants, and if (as is conventionally estimated) forty million people worldwide have had Prozac, then there will have been two hundred thousand more suicide attempts on Prozac than had Prozac not been used. Conventional wisdom is that there is one suicide for every ten attempts. These would give twenty thousand suicides over and above the number who would have committed suicide if they had been left untreated or been treated with older agents.

At this point, I had accessed the FDA's Adverse Events Database to look at suicides reported on Prozac.[50] As of October 1999, there were over two thousand. The FDA estimated their database picked up only between 1 and 10 percent of serious adverse events. This gives a spread between twenty thousand and two hundred thousand suicides on Prozac. Over a quarter of the accompanying descriptions of the patients' mental state prior to suicide gave clear indicators of akathisia. There was one extraordinary feature to the figures. Ordinarily, the ratio of male to female suicides is four to one; in the Prozac database, the sex ratios were equal. Either there was a strange reporting bias here, or some abnormal factor was cutting across natural responses.

Then there were the figures from the Jick study of primary-care depression: 189 suicides per hundred thousand patient years on Prozac. These needed to be set against the only available figures for suicides in primary-care depression—approximately thirty suicides per hundred thousand patient years (see Chapter 3). This would give a total number of forty thousand or more suicides for the forty million people who have gone on Prozac since its launch.

These figures from three different sources converge on a similar number of suicides. While extrapolations are involved, we must remember the FDA database records several thousand actually dead people. Applying these figures to countries such as Canada or the United Kingdom, where there have been up to twenty million prescriptions for Prozac during the 1990s,[51] would give a minimum of one million people put on Prozac, and as a result at least five hundred deaths per country over the decade—one for every week of the 1990s, and ten attempted suicides per week. Applying the figures to the United States leads to estimates of one suicide per day.

Could something like this be missed? As I now knew, British coroners could easily miss something happening at this rate. There were 150 coroners, and this suicide rate would give them, on average, less than one suicide per year each.

But what about Britain's postmarketing surveillance systems, supposedly superior to the FDA's Adverse Events system? Here another surprise waited. Inquiring in emergency departments, I found that a standard exchange went as follows:

Q. Do you guys recognize that among the suicide attempts you get, there is a group of people who come in after a first overdose or suicide attempt, who simply aren't chronic parasuicides?

A. Yes.

Q. Do you have any sense that these patients are much more likely to have recently been put on an SSRI than any other kind of antidepressant?

A. Yes.

Q. What do you do about their antidepressant?

A. We send them home and tell them that this shows the drug is working. It's kicking in.[52]

This disastrous advice explained why surveillance schemes weren't picking up a warning signal. There wasn't much point in reporting that the drug was working. Lilly played some part in this. It had been telling primary-care practitioners for some time about something called serotonin pickup syndrome[53]—a new term to me. But the point behind telling primary-care physicians about this was that if they didn't warn the patient, the patient might stop treatment. Lilly was warning people not in order to minimize hazards but in order to keep patients from going off Prozac.

In the case of the South Wales farmer Richard Wood, the coroner had publicly wondered about warnings: "Perhaps Eli Lilly should reexamine the literature they supply to doctors as well as their patients." Contacted by the press, Lilly's response was that the care of patients was the responsibility of doctors: "We provide a patient information leaflet with Prozac and provide clinicians with the best advice."

They did provide a patient information booklet in the United Kingdom, called *Day by Day*. The advice included:

Day 5

Keep going! No matter how bad you are feeling now, you should feel better in a few weeks.

Day 6

Keep going! The success of treatment is up to you—don't give up on your treatment now.

Day 11

Did you know? Anxiety and nervousness are often troublesome in depression but they usually respond well to treatment in a few weeks.

Day 12

Keep going! Don't give up now—it may take a little longer to feel better but it's well worth it in the end.

Day 13

Keep going! Don't worry if you are still feeling bad, you remain on the road to recovery as long as you carry on with your medicine.

Day 17

Did you know? The more severe the illness, the more likely that antidepressants will help.

Day 20

About your treatment. Any side-effects of treatment are usually nothing to worry about and go away after the first few weeks.[54]

It was hard to know whether the pills or the "advice" was more poisonous.

7

Experiment at the End of the Millennium

FROM THE DEPOSITION of John Heiligenstein, taken for *Fentress vs. Eli Lilly*:

Q. Can you conceive as a clinical research physician and scientist, anything that would change your opinion on whether or not Prozac has a causal relationship between it and suicidality?

A. I doubt if there is any study that could be done that could possibly demonstrate a relationship between fluoxetine and suicidality.[1]

Before I became an expert witness, in the course of lectures for Pharmacia and Upjohn following the launch of reboxetine, I had wondered why the quality-of-life scale they used (the SASS) showed better results for reboxetine than for Prozac (see Chapter 4).[2] One possibility was that the emotional indifference caused by Prozac and other SSRIs might be associated with some people improving but not returning to normal; a pervasive indifference might lead people to rate down their quality of life. Reboxetine had no actions on the serotonin system. As early as 1997, I suggested that a study in which healthy volunteers took reboxetine or an SSRI might lead to a lowering of quality of life as represented by SASS scores.

Rudolph Hoehn-Saric and colleagues from Johns Hopkins University had examined emotional indifference as early as 1990.[3] Hoehn-Saric described four people on either Luvox or Prozac who had become indifferent or disinhibited. One woman changed personality completely, presenting herself almost naked at parties. Hoehn-Saric speculated on serotonin connections to the frontal lobes and wondered whether in some patients the effects of an SSRI might not amount to a "mild" lobotomy. Other articles making similar arguments have followed.[4]

Clinicians occasionally see extreme disinhibition in patients taking SSRIs, but milder forms were, in my experience, relatively common. One man on Zoloft I treated memorably described a loss of concern for others. Normally he would help older women having trouble crossing the road, but on Zoloft he found himself much more likely to walk past them. Since I was prescribing Zoloft frequently, similar cases often came my way. In one, a sophisticated professional described a split within himself, part of him consciously watching the more instinctive side. He found he was having to intervene much more deliberately than usual to stop himself doing socially unacceptable things—such as bludgeoning to death kids he caught trying to break into his car. This seemed to lie midway between disinhibition and blunting.

There might be a good side to this. One wonderful woman found that where normally she was too conscientious at work and wouldn't relax until every last "t" was crossed and "i" dotted, on Prozac she could leave work at 5:00 p.m. without anxiety and handle bosses' comments on her work without taking them to heart. Prozac had produced a certain beneficial nonchalance or mellowness in her case. Was this woman being chemically "lobotomized" to fit into a stressful work situation? Should she instead have protested bad working conditions or sexism from her boss? The medical students who saw her argued she should have protested and perhaps resigned. I suggested they were being young and romantic, and that life would teach them otherwise. Was it our decision whether she should protest or take pills? Who gave medical people that authority? This is the country that Lauren Slater explores in *Prozac Diary*.[5]

The possibility of emotional blunting occurred to me when the April 1999 killings in Littleton, Colorado, hit the news. One of the students, Eric Harris, was reported to have been on Luvox. Within hours of this news, the APA Web site posted a message saying, "Despite a decade of research, there is little valid evidence to prove a causal relationship between the use of antidepressant medications and destructive behavior. On the other hand, there is ample evidence that undiagnosed and untreated mental illness exacts a heavy toll on those who suffer from these disorders as well as those around them."[6] Here came the "blame the disease, not the drug" message again.

Against this background, I suggested to my contacts in Pharmacia that it would be valuable to see what happened to SASS scores in a group of healthy volunteers taking an SSRI or reboxetine in a design that had them taking one drug for two weeks, halting for two weeks, and then crossing over to the other drug. Would SASS scores end up, on average, lower in people taking the SSRI than in people taking reboxetine? If the figures panned out, they might allow P&U to make some statements about the levels of well-being that depressed people who remained on treatment were likely to experience on reboxetine, compared, for instance, to an SSRI.

Submitting such ideas to pharmaceutical companies is a hit-and-miss affair. They shuffle through bureaucratic scrutiny at local, national, and finally international levels. Companies tend to be very risk averse. Even when a company is broadly speaking in favor of the idea, should someone spot a potential snag—however minor and improbable—it will likely stall the project. You wouldn't want to base a scientific program on support from the industry. Pharmacia didn't bite.

Most university departments have "slush funds" built up in endowment accounts from work done on clinical trials or legal work, or where companies or others have offered general support to a department. The department in which I was working luckily had a small fund, to which SmithKline Beecham had been the biggest contributors.

GETTING ORGANIZED

There were a few key things to be sorted out before pursuing the comparative study. First, with which SSRI should reboxetine be compared? Prozac was a nonstarter because of its long half-life. Even after two weeks' washout, most subjects would still retain it in their bodies and feel its effects. Luvox was too likely to cause nausea. Paxil had become too associated with withdrawal problems. I had treated withdrawal problems of a number of nursing colleagues put on Paxil, some still suffering three months later despite short durations of treatment. No one would have volunteered.

That left either Zoloft or Celexa. Zoloft was the natural choice for two reasons. Even though I had first noticed the phenomenon of emotional blunting in patients taking Zoloft, I was nevertheless well disposed to this pill, so that when it came out I was among its main prescribers in North Wales. As the psychiatric representative on our hospital's Formulary Committee two years before, I had argued for the removal of Prozac from the formulary and its replacement with Zoloft and Celexa. There were good reasons for this, quite apart from any suicidal ideation that Prozac might trigger. Prozac's long half-life and risk of interacting with other pills made it unsuitable for use in a general hospital setting where, by definition, people would be on other pills.

My second reason for picking Zoloft was that it came in 50 mg and 100 mg forms. There was consensus that 100 mg of Zoloft was the equivalent of 20 mg of Prozac. The 50 mg tablet was generally perceived as being a weaker dose. This made it possible for us to draw up a protocol that involved a step up from either 4 mg of reboxetine, which our volunteers would take for the first five days, or 50 mg of Zoloft, to 8 mg of reboxetine or 100 mg of Zoloft for the subsequent ten days of that arm of the study. Nobody was going to accuse us of exceeding the normal clinical doses and bringing about the results by poisoning our volunteers.

I considered the demands of the study on its subjects, who would take pills for four weeks, ingesting chemicals that affected their brain function, and fill out rating scales for eight weeks. How much should we pay the volunteers? Institutional Review Boards (European ethical committees) have struggled with this policy question for some time. IRBs came into being in response to public perceptions that medical students, patients, or other subjects such as company personnel—because in some way dependent on the goodwill of the person running the experiment—might feel coerced into participating. Deciding whether subjects are being unfairly influenced by the prospect of financial gain is an easier issue to resolve than whether other, subtler forms of pressure are involved. An ideal arrangement is where subjects are so persuaded by the merits of the study that they volunteer without payment of any sort. However, this ideal is neither expected nor demanded. Instead, some inconvenience money is usually paid.

After taking this through our IRB, a figure of £400 to be paid to our subjects at the end of the study was recommended, £50 for each week.[7] By the end, everyone thought the amount of money compensated for the inconvenience research subjects were put through.

Our group was made up of eleven women and nine men, aged between 27 and 52.[8] Some were consultant or trainee psychiatrists. There were senior and junior nursing staff but no nursing trainees. Some were senior administrative staff. Most knew the others. One woman dropped out as coincidental developments in her personal life made it difficult to know whether any assessments of her mood, emotional state, and sense of well-being would reflect the actions of the drugs or her circumstances. This left us with nineteen subjects.

Why were they doing this? The primary motivation appeared to be simple curiosity. Some wanted to know what these pills they regularly handed out to their patients were like. For others, it was curiosity about themselves. We told them we would be assessing their personalities and would feed them back the results of assessments. We also told them the study was of the "better than well" phenomenon described for Prozac. For yet others, it may simply have been something novel to do. These various motivations can skew a sample: For instance, risk takers might be more inclined to participate in this study than others who were more conservative.

I was influenced by a study done by Peter Joyce and Roger Mulder in New Zealand with depressed patients.[9] They had shown that certain personality profiles were more likely to respond to drugs active on the serotonin system, while others responded to drugs active on the norepinephrine system. The world had paid no heed to this study; the findings were not good for business. The results suggested that SSRIs should be used for certain people who were depressed, and not others; a drug like reboxetine for example, instead of being a general antidepressant, would have its own, smaller niche. To test whether the personalities of our volunteers might influence their response to Zoloft and reboxetine, we asked them to complete a number of personality scales, including the ones Joyce and Mulder used.

First baseline assessments of personality and completion of other rating scales were done a week before the trial proper began. We organized all drugs to look identical. Everyone involved in the study was blind as to who was getting what. All drugs were handed out the same day to all subjects.

Conventional wisdom holds that antidepressants do not work for the better part of two or three weeks. Keeping our volunteers on each of these drugs for four weeks would have been optimal, but two blocks of four weeks' exposure to each of the two drugs seemed far too long for healthy volunteers. So we compromised on two weeks' exposure to each drug. This left me worried that we might expose these colleagues to risks without learning anything, but it was the best we could manage.

FIRST IMPRESSIONS—"BETTER THAN WELL"

From the very first day it was obvious something was happening. One of my closest colleagues, Tony Roberts, was so changed by whichever drug he had first that even his patients noticed. Everyone agreed he was mellower than usual. Tony himself was aware of this and provided a number of examples of situations that would previously have bothered or irritated him. This was emotional blunting in its good form.

One woman in the group, Joanna, experienced a similar effect from the first day. She was much more relaxed and commented that this "chill pill" she'd just been put on was something that she might be able to get used to.

Pretty soon, however, we realized that things weren't going to fit easily into our original ideas about trying to map emotional indifference onto the SASS. For a start, it was surprisingly difficult to decide who was on which drug. We had assumed the known side effects of the two drugs would enable us to guess. But both drugs seemed to be causing nausea, although only Zoloft had been supposed to do so. Both were causing sleeplessness, where reboxetine was supposedly much more likely to do so. Both interfered with sexual functioning, especially in men—something we had expected only on Zoloft.

We encountered strange results not on the side effects list for either drug. Subjects complained of feeling cold, with chilblains and patches of cold perspiration. This strange side effect seemed more likely to be caused by reboxetine, but nothing on the company's data sheet prepared me for this. Some volunteers complained from the second day of stiffness or pain in their jaws, pain in their throats, or forced yawning. This was not something they could have picked up by suggestion or read in the data sheets of either drug. But I knew what it was. Several years before, a colleague and I had written about six cases of patients with precisely these problems on SSRIs—then the largest series of cases reported of this potentially ominous problem.[10] It later turned out that half our volunteers suffered from this side effect in some form. I would never have expected this to appear at all in the course of a two-week study on this kind of dose. To have it happening in half the group was extraordinary.[11]

I had expected reboxetine to make people more aware of their emotions and feelings, maybe making them *too* emotional. Zoloft, in contrast, should blunt them somewhat, for good or bad. Things were more complicated. Was reboxetine having a paradoxical calming effect, just as Ritalin did? The crucial question was whether subjects could tell the drugs apart when they went on to the second drug. If they couldn't, the study would be pointless. Within a day or two of starting the second drug, it was clear that they could distinguish between the two and knew almost immediately which they preferred.

But a significant number of people were doing very well on Zoloft. Tony Roberts had assumed he was taking Zoloft the first time around because he had diarrhea and changes in sexual functioning that pointed strongly toward Zoloft. Now on what he was convinced was reboxetine, he was having trouble passing water, constipation, and a range of other problems. If so, he had clearly had a much better two weeks on Zoloft, and surely his SASS scores would reflect that.

The plan was to finish the study with a focus group before the blind was broken. Participants had been asked to keep a diary throughout. They had been encouraged to check for any effects of the drugs with their partners, parents, or others living with them. The question now was, could our volunteers put into words the differences between the two drugs? This was the heart of the experiment. Did the SSRIs produce some kind of emotional blunting compared with reboxetine? If so, how did this affect daily life? What everyday words expressed what was going on?

BREAKING THE BLIND

Our focus group met two weeks after the study ended. We already knew that almost everyone had preferred one of the two drugs. But two-thirds rated themselves as having done "better than well" on one or other of the drugs. Although this was a study of well-being, antidepressants weren't supposed to make people who were normal feel "better than well." Not even Peter Kramer had said this. The argument of his famous *Listening to Prozac* was that people who were mildly depressed on Prozac became better than well. Here, people who had never been depressed were claiming to be in some way better than normal.

Just as striking, two-thirds of the group felt significantly worse on one of the two drugs—not simply by virtue of inconvenient side effects, such as difficulties in passing water, but in terms of being depressed or disturbed or in some other way realizing this was not a drug for them.

The implication was that there was a very high chance, perhaps approaching fifty-fifty, that primary-care physicians could put their patients on a pill unsuitable for them.

This explained at a stroke why people generally don't take antidepressants for long. It is rare for any survey to find more than 40 percent of people continuing to take their antidepressant after four weeks. The SSRIs had been sold on the basis that they didn't affect transmitters such as norepinephrine or acetylcholine. They were therefore supposedly cleaner and should have fewer side effects. This should translate into better compliance, but it never has.[12]

It turned out that Joyce and Mulder's findings of personality differences between people responding to drugs like reboxetine or Zoloft mapped exactly onto the findings in our group.[13] There was a right drug and wrong drug for people. Simply making a drug cleaner was not going to help if the cleaned-up molecule kept the wrong bit for a large number of patients. Indeed, a cleaned-up and stronger "wrong bit" might be far more dangerous than a messy, older drug.

This had great implications. Pharmaceutical industry trials showed each of the SSRIs appeared marginally, if any, better than placebo. This left companies open to critics' charges that the drugs didn't work. But had industry selected populations along personality profile lines, it now seemed they would have produced results showing much bigger differences between SSRIs and placebo. However, they would then have been able to market the drugs only to a smaller group of people. Our results for Zoloft were, in fact, much more convincing in the group of healthy volunteers who preferred it than the clinical trials Pfizer had submitted to the FDA in pursuit of a license.

When we broke the blind, Tony Roberts found out he had done well on Zoloft and poorly on reboxetine. This led him to expect that everyone else who had done really well had had Zoloft, but this was not the way it went. The proportions of people doing well on one drug and poorly on the other were split almost evenly between the two drugs. Where one person had done well on Zoloft and poorly on reboxetine, the next person at the table had experienced just the reverse.[14]

Despite many people doing well on Zoloft, when we analyzed the overall results, the original hypothesis was upheld—volunteers' quality-of-life or social functioning scores as a group fell on Zoloft but remained unaltered by reboxetine. This seemed to explain why no one had published the quality-of-life results on SSRIs.

Chasing the question of whether Zoloft caused emotional blunting, half the group said it had given them a "nothing bothers me" feeling. Reactions were split about this: Some liked the effect; others found it made them emotionally dead. Reboxetine, in contrast, didn't seem to make anyone feel indifferent—calm, perhaps, but not indifferent. Its effects were better described as energizing—again, good for some but not for others.

One small event in the focus group went unnoticed except by two people there. When I asked whether anyone had noticed any other side effects, one volunteer mentioned vivid and disturbing dreams of killing herself. I skated over this, helped by two other volunteers claiming they had many more dreams than usual. I broadened out the question to whether anyone had become depressed on either of the two drugs. Yes, two had—on reboxetine. Both were women and described the experience as like the "baby blues." Neither, however, was remotely suicidal.

BECOMING SUICIDAL[15]

I now knew two people in our study had become suicidal. The roots of what had happened lay at the start of the study. When Tony Roberts had done obviously well from the outset, Joanna had done equally well. When we switched drugs, Tony became visibly uncomfortable with urinary retention and genito-urinary pain. It seemed highly likely that this was caused by reboxetine. He was the one person who we thought knew what he was taking. But where Tony had physical problems, Joanna had a far more dramatic and worrying change. Within days of going on the second drug, it was evident that, for her, this was no chill pill. The bloom was gone from her normally extraverted and confident self. She now looked almost shrunken, worried, and nervous. She withdrew from interactions with others. She began demanding support from Dinah Cattell, one of the study monitors. Dinah alerted me that Joanna was doing things she would later regret, such as impulsively spending more money than she would normally do. Worse, she was doing other things she was reluctant to tell.

This had worrying implications for healthy volunteer studies. I had not envisaged anything this problematic when I had presented the study to the IRB. I had told them that the scale of any problems should be no worse than what might happen to someone taking an antihistamine. By the end of the first week of her second drug, the effects on Joanna could not be described as minor. She was in turmoil. I was convinced she was on reboxetine; Dinah thought she was on Zoloft.

In the second week, things got even worse. Over the weekend, Joanna had dreams of slitting her throat open and bleeding to death in the bed beside her partner. These dreams woke her at 3 a.m. and left her frightened and unable to get back to sleep. The same dream recurred on three successive nights.

Toward the middle of that week, we decided Joanna couldn't be allowed to continue whatever she was taking. She was told to stop on more than one occasion. We weren't to know she wasn't registering anything we told her. This may not be unusual. When Joseph Wesbecker was advised by his physician Dr. Coleman to stop his Prozac, he had argued that he still felt it was doing something for him.[16]

By this time, the change in Joanna was startling. She might begin to cry for no obvious reason. If anyone asked how she was, she brushed it off, telling him or her that any moment now she would be better again. Her mood was swinging from gloom to doom in a matter of minutes, so much so that a number of people described her as almost manic. She was bothered by how irritable and snappy with others she had become. She described an increasing sense of disinhibition. Her diary entries record a feeling that she had become two selves, an adult and a child, and it seemed her adult could only watch while the child responded to things impulsively and emotionally.

She took a pill that night. When this was discovered the following day, the pills were removed from her. That night alone in her house was one of the worst of her life. She felt things were watching her. She checked behind doors in case there was anything there. She began to write her diary but couldn't concentrate on it; her diary entry records a hope that she would make it through the night. She suddenly decided she should go out and throw herself in front of a car or a train. It was as if there was nothing out there apart from the vehicle she was going to throw herself under. She didn't think of her partner or her child. This lack of feeling for them ate away at her later. When our biology changes, we change, but even in the midst of a high fever, when everything was unreal, she still knew she loved her daughter. Now she felt nothing.

All her anxiety vanished once the thought of death crystallized in her mind. Putting an end to herself, even in this violent way, seemed a way to solve her anguish and pain. She was, in fact, on her way out the door to kill herself when the phone rang. It was as though a hypnotic trance was broken. Joanna had the wit to seek out the company of others, tell them she was having a bad night, and ask them to keep an eye on her. They laughed, wondering what had gotten into her. She looked normal. No one guessed her state, and although having company helped, no one looked after her. The following morning, deeply distressed, she called Dinah, who spent most of the day with her. Joanna had become a fragile, vulnerable woman, still at serious risk of suicide. On my instructions, she said nothing about all this in the focus group.

Then Max spoke. I had known nothing about Max's problems. She also had done well on whatever the first drug was, feeling both more energetic and more calm. But from the start of the second drug, she found herself irritable and snappy. A lot of her colleagues remarked on the change—more assertive, some said. But Max didn't see it that way. She saw herself become impulsive and disinhibited. Where others saw her speaking out assertively, she saw herself doing things without regard for consequences. Her mood, like Joanna's, veered from high to low. Both could swing from tears to mania within an hour.

Max became disinhibited in a more serious sense. Driving home one day from shopping with her mother, she came to a point where the road narrowed and traffic had to slow. A group of 18-year-old boys began making obscene gestures and shouting derogatory remarks. Max stopped her car in the middle of the traffic and climbed out. She went over to the youths and manhandled one, warning him that if he continued she would "deck him."

She should have been alarmed at taking on a group of young men this way. How did she know they wouldn't take down her car registration and follow her home? What then—slash her tires, steal her car, or throw a brick through the window of her house? Her mother, who knew that in the ordinary course of events her daughter would have realized this, was frightened at what was happening. Where others had seen her as merely assertive at work, Max knew she had gone past mere assertiveness. But it was not her new aggression but her ideas about suicide that led her to the brink of quitting the study. She is a woman prone to lucid dreaming—someone who can rise and talk in her sleep and appear wide-awake while doing so. This makes it difficult to be fully sure of what happened. But in the middle of the second week, she had episodes on two successive nights during which she found herself thinking of the beam in the ceiling of her bedroom, planning to hang herself from it. She was drawn to it, controlled by it, and knew she did-n't care that finding her body the next day would disturb the rest of the family.

She later thought things might have been different had she not been a volunteer. Had she been on this drug for weeks and felt trapped be-cause her doctor had told her she needed it, she might well have gone on to suicide. Things were eased because after the first night, she low-ered her dose from two pills to one, knowing she only had three more days of the study to get through. But she would never knowingly go on these pills again.

AFTEREFFECTS

No one had warned these women they might ever feel the way they had done on either of these pills. Our study had been about how well peo-ple could be and whether anyone could be made "better than well." We never thought to warn anyone about suicidal ideation. Even with my background, I saw the possibility of making totally normal people sui-cidal in this way as a merely theoretical risk. Had we set out to design a study to do this, I would have figured on recruiting a hundred volun-teers. Nothing in the published figures suggested we would be likely to pick up an effect like this in so small a group.

Unprepared for what was going on, Max committed nothing to paper. Worried about being diagnosed as crazy, she told no one what was going on until she learned someone else had been through some-thing similar.

Neither woman drew the conclusion that it was "just" the pill. Finding each other reduced the isolation but didn't solve the problem. One of the consequences of this study was to bring home, as nothing else had done, the potential long-term injury we can do to people by making them suicidal. Even I, watching from the outside and firmly committed to the idea that when this happened on drugs it was caused *by* the drugs, found myself pulled by a strange attractor. Surely, some-one in whom this had happened must have had something wrong with her to begin with, some disorder in her personality. It was worse for the two women, who were difficult to reassure on this point.

Nothing on the personality tests we had done beforehand, nothing on the variety of tests of well-being or social functioning that were conducted, indicated any abnormality in either of these two subjects. Nothing on the tests would have enabled anyone from Eli Lilly or Pfizer to predict that these two out of the twenty subjects would suffer this problem. If anything, Joanna and Max showed lower-than-average traces of any kind of depressive thinking. Furthermore, in line with the early reports from Prozac, the effect had been manifest in women rather than men. Maybe this explained why the FDA database on Prozac-associated suicides contained an equal ratio of females to males, rather than the expected four men for every one woman.

While we may have accidentally demonstrated conclusively that the drugs could cause the problem, even looking the beast straight in the face, we didn't know what we were dealing with. Two volunteers on reboxetine became "depressed," but neither became suicidal. Neither Max nor Joanna became depressed on Zoloft. It didn't seem to be akathisia either; two other subjects on Zoloft became akathisic, but not suicidal. There did seem to be some link with disinhibition. Zoloft had caused disinhibition, and perhaps in these two more markedly than in others. This was not something we were geared up to explore. Clinical trials suggest this may be happening with considerable frequency, but as of yet it has been left unscrutinized by the entire psychiatric field.

Max's case highlighted the theme of hanging, so common to SSRI suicides. At close hand, our impressions were that someone who did finally hang herself would do so in an almost calm frame of mind. This fit with what I've heard from people about children or partners who had hanged themselves in bedrooms next door to their children or to their siblings. If they had wanted to commit suicide, why didn't they go elsewhere? People who kill themselves by hanging ordinarily don't do it in the middle of the night in a bedroom next door to the rest of their family. Nor do they throw themselves out fourth-floor windows to land on concrete where their children likely will find them. The common theme seemed to be of lack of concern for those left behind.

This was the experiment in which Richard Smith said he could see no value. Doubtless, an archskeptic would have required us to reexpose Max and Joanna double-blind to see if the problem recurred. Obviously, we could not reexpose these two women in circumstances where we could not guarantee their safety. Quite apart from the impossibility of ethical committee approval for such an experiment, someone who didn't believe the original study would find a means of dismissing the results of a subsequent reexposure. We might have been told, "Second time around, they could have told the drugs apart by their side effects, and this time around both women would have had so much invested they would have 'put on' suicidality."

The injury we had done both women was greater than these escapes suggested. Both remained disturbed several months later; both seriously questioned the stability of their personalities. At first this struck me as ludicrous. But we had great difficult persuading them that it had been the drug—and only the drug. Their view of themselves had been shaken. We had had at least a medium-term impact on both women's self-esteem.

This connected a number of facts. A case in point was John Marshall, whom I had seen a few weeks before (Chapter 6). His medical notes indicated that those seeing him interpreted his drug-induced nerves and later suicide attempt as evidence of a personality disorder. Another woman was referred to my clinic after an overdose. She had received news her father was dying; her partner had left her in financial straits just as she returned to university as a mature student; her eldest son, who was ill, had suddenly decided to return home to live. Stressed, she consulted her primary-care physician, who had put her on Prozac. She carried out a number of concealed suicide attempts over the following few weeks, until one brought her to the local accident department. Clinical impressions were of a possible personality disorder. There were no more suicide attempts once the Prozac was stopped. But how long would the label "personality disorder" remain in her medical notes? Then there was a 61-year-old woman assessed after a suicide attempt. She had been on a benzodiazepine, which her primary-care physician had been reducing for months. At the last step, when she was on 0.5 mg of benzodiazepine per day, he switched her to Prozac. Within a week she became suicidal for the first time in her life.

These were typical cases. How many similar stress reactions were being labeled as personality problems? This connected all the way back to Tony L., the first person I'd seen have problems on Prozac, for whom the long-term effects were disastrous.

To the outside world, the suicide attempts caused by Prozac and other SSRIs were near misses, lucky escapes. But everything known from research into suicide indicated that one of the factors that made successful suicide most likely was a previous attempt. If Prozac and Zoloft induced suicide attempts or marked suicidal ideation, might this in some way lower the threshold for a future suicide attempt?

Perhaps the best analogy is with precancerous cells of the cervix. If, in the course of a trial of an experimental drug, a subject developed precancerous cells in the cervix, which cleared up when the drug was halted, the manufacturers would almost certainly claim their drug had caused nothing. But it seems a distinct possibility that such an event would make future development of cancer of the cervix more likely.

Even forearmed with theoretical knowledge, it was difficult not to feel the power of the idea sucking Max and Joanna in: "Something must have been wrong with me to begin with for me to end up this way." "Why didn't it happen to anyone else, then?"

Critics of the pharmaceutical industry sometimes have real problems when they meet the people behind drugs like Prozac or Zoloft. They seem to expect to meet the devil incarnate, rather than some very decent and likeable human beings.[17] It's easy to demonize people after the event, but in real life, it's rare for the good guys and the bad guys to be clearly distinguishable. In this case, however, we had just met a much more medieval devil, something mindless and alien and capable of sucking any good there was out of someone.[18]

A TWIST TO THE TALE

Our obvious next step was to check whether anyone who gave drugs to healthy volunteers as part of their research, or in phase 1 studies for pharmaceutical companies, had encountered anything like this. They had. In fact, our high incidence of serious problems could be topped by other studies.

Prior to reboxetine's European launch, I took part in a March 1998 consultancy panel meeting for Pharmacia with a number of panelists, including Ian Hindmarch, a professor of psychopharmacology at the University of Surrey and an expert on healthy volunteer studies. He was an enthusiastic supporter of the SSRIs, which looked much better than some of the older tricyclic antidepressants on driving simulation tests and other cognitive function tests.

I mentioned an article by Andrew Solomon, just published in the *New Yorker*,[19] in which he compared the effects of Zoloft to taking fifty-five cups of black coffee and Paxil to taking eleven cups. To my surprise, all the others present demanded copies of this piece. No one was keener than Ian. As he explained to me afterward, he'd had a similar experience years before. As part of a set of studies carried out for many companies, he'd run one study, which as he remembered it involved ten to twelve subjects, where all those randomized to Zoloft dropped out because of marked agitation or anxiety. He'd never seen anything like it. At the time, possible suicidality on SSRIs had not been an issue, and no one had inquired about this in particular. But the reactions, if anything, seemed even more marked than in our study.

"Of course we've always known that these drugs could do funny things to healthy volunteers," I was told by Mervyn Whitford, a colleague who had worked extensively in the pharmaceutical industry. Had we? It turns out we had—so much so that workers in this area in the 1980s, such as Berndt Saletu in Vienna[20] and Steven Warrington in England,[21] specifically documented the adverse effects of SSRIs (including Zoloft) on healthy volunteers and remarked on the discrepancy between how bad these drugs could make healthy volunteers feel and how they seemed to have quite the opposite effects in depression. They rationalized this by arguing that the brains of depressives were obviously very different from those of healthy people.

This made sense in the 1960s and 1970s, when people diagnosed with depression were older and their condition didn't respond to Valium but did to ECT. The trouble with the SSRIs was that nobody had envisaged a situation where the majority of people most likely to get these drugs would be much closer to healthy volunteers than to endogenous depressives—13-year-olds stressed out at school, like Matthew Miller, for instance, or Caitlin Hurcombe, or Craig Clark. No one realized cases of Valium were about to become cases of Prozac. Against this background, the fact that companies not only knew about SSRIs' deleterious effects on healthy volunteers but also had commissioned and conducted studies demonstrating exactly this was nothing short of stunning.

This healthy volunteer study also gave us an opportunity to put figures on the extent to which drugs like Zoloft might increase the risk of suicide for someone like Matthew Miller, using the United Kingdom as the backdrop to our study. First, the combined population of England and Wales is slightly over fifty million. Second, there are just over five thousand suicides on average per year in England and Wales. Extrapolating from the second point, we get approximately two hundred suicides per fortnight in England and Wales.

Certain assumptions can then be made. The first concerns how many of these two hundred suicides per fortnight will be in entirely normal individuals with no mental illness and without significant interpersonal legal or financial problems—the biggest predictors of suicide. None of our healthy volunteers had either factor. Many experts would insist there are probably no suicides in totally normal individuals lacking any of those factors. Nevertheless, let us assume that ten of the two hundred suicides involve totally normal, unstressed individuals.

It is generally accepted that for every successful suicide there are ten suicide attempts. This would give one hundred suicide attempts in totally normal unstressed individuals in England and Wales in the course of a fortnight. One more assumption has to be made. How many people become actively suicidal for every suicide attempt? If we assume there are ten people actively suicidal for every suicide attempt, this would lead to one thousand instances of actively suicidality in totally normal individuals with no current interpersonal legal or financial problems over any fortnight period in England and Wales.

How many people are at risk for active suicidality? In a population of slightly over fifty million, we could exclude thirty million as juveniles or individuals with mental illness or significant interpersonal legal or financial problems. This leaves twenty million people at risk.[22]

Calculating the probability for two healthy volunteers without mental illness and no current interpersonal legal or financial problems becoming suicidal during a two-week period on Zoloft gives a probability of $p = 0.0000005$.[23] Put another way, if one thousand out of twenty million totally normal individuals are likely to be actively suicidal compared with one out of ten taking Zoloft, it follows that Zoloft makes you two thousand times more likely to be suicidal than normal.

Critics might argue this involves piling assumption on assumption, but there is considerable scope to modify these assumptions unrealistically in favor of Lilly and Pfizer without changing the significance of the findings. In fact, the more reasonable question would be: How could our finding of suicidality be explained in any way other than being caused by Zoloft?

Far from rising to this challenge, the response of senior figures in the field was to contact the editors of *Primary Care Psychiatry*, in which the first reports appeared, to castigate them for publishing these anecdotes in an era of evidence-based medicine.

A NEW PROBLEM

In the late 1980s, as companies outsourced drug and market development, university medicine departments might witness severe patient agitation on an SSRI and not know what to do. No one had warned them this could happen. In the mid- to late 1980s, the suicide story had not yet begun to roll. There was no overwhelming reason for reporting the findings in a journal or other public forum. Reporting ran the risk of alienating the sponsoring company. Even reporting it to the company might lose business. Why report it if they were all but certain to know it anyway? University people were not to know that it was quite possible that no hands-on work with the drug actually took place anywhere within these vast corporations.

The only group of people who might know something were the regulators. I wrote to the MCA in Britain and the FDA, giving details of our study. Did they have other data on file remotely like ours? My contacts suggested they *must* have—in which case it seemed the regulators were in a bind if they had the data on file, and in just as big a bind if they didn't.

We had now blundered into a situation where, once the chairman of an IRB committee knew about the results of our study and others, they would find it very difficult to permit any study with healthy volunteers to go ahead, even one involving only medical and nursing staff, without clear warnings and close monitoring. Even with these in place, university studies in healthy volunteers must be insured. Would any insurance agency underwrite such a study? And yet these drugs were available without warnings or monitoring, being prescribed in ever-increasing amounts to people for stress reactions rather than depression, and—still more worrying—prescribed ever more frequently for children and teenagers. On the face of it, this was an extraordinary situation.

Let us return to the deposition of Leigh Thompson in the *Wesbecker* trial:

A. Now in terms of whether we specifically designed a study to address the issue of suicidality separate from all of the other issues of efficacy and safety, the answer is no.

Q. You didn't then, did you, haven't now either, have you?

A. We've worked extremely hard on trying to figure out how to address that issue; yes indeed we've spent an awfully [sic] lot of time and money on trying to figure out how to do.

Q. How much time?

A. Of my time or total people at Lilly?

Q. Whatever the time we're speaking of when you say we spent an awfully [sic] lot of time and money.

A. Well I can say that I personally have spent hundreds of hours on this specific issue, talking to experts, reading the literature and trying to decide how we could possibly do these kind of studies. I can only speak for myself, but I know that many other people spent far more time than I did at Lilly working on this.

Q. Has anybody figured it out yet?

A. Not to my knowledge.

Q. How much money has been spent?

A. I don't know what the total amount of spending would be . . .

There followed a series of thrusts and parries until:

Q. You said it's been very expensive.

A. Yes, sir.

Q. I would assume that you had some facts; you're not just pulling that out of the top of your head, are you, Doctor Thompson?

A. No, sir.

Q. All right, how expensive has it been?

A. Millions of dollars.[24]

What a healthy volunteer study does is to take depression out of the equation. If suicidality happens on Prozac or Zoloft or Paxil in these circumstances, it is difficult to see how it cannot have been caused at least in part by the drug. Our study cost only $15,000 to run. Similar studies with even more clear-cut results were sitting in company archives, apparently inaccessible to national regulators such as the MCA in Britain—who, almost a year after I began to correspond with them, apparently ended up with a *four-page summary* of Ian Hindmarch's study.[25]

Few of the many healthy volunteer studies done by SSRI companies as part of their development work on these drugs have been published.

In the case of Prozac, twelve out of fifty-three have been reported on. In the case of Paxil, approximately fourteen out of thirty-five healthy volunteer prelaunch studies have appeared. In the case of Zoloft, as few as seven of approximately thirty-five prelaunch studies are available. It is difficult to have much confidence in the published work when the data reported commonly exclude material concerning behavioral toxicity, even failing to mention suicide when it has occurred.

This material had been lying around for years before the first public concerns were raised about Prozac. Why had it played no part in the debate hitherto? Why did regulators not know what these studies had found? Why were no academic voices raised demanding access to this material? The combination of our healthy volunteer study and my involvement in ongoing legal actions led me to access the healthy volunteer archives of Pfizer and SmithKline. Was it merely coincidence that pretty much as soon as I walked through the door of Pfizer's archives to look for these data, I got the sack?

8

The Plots Thicken

SHORTLY AFTER I WROTE up the healthy volunteer study, the cases of Matthew Miller, Viktor Motus, and Donald Schell triggered access to Pfizer and SmithKline's healthy volunteer studies. Working through Pfizer's internal documents in the *Miller* case, Andy Vickery came across the study Ian Hindmarch had done in the early 1980s, which Hindmarch himself had outlined for me some years before. His results were even more startling than our study:

> [O]f 12 . . . healthy volunteers entered into this study, five in the first week of the study were randomized to Zoloft, and seven to placebo. And of the five randomized to Zoloft, all dropped out in the course of the first week for what appears to have been fairly severe anxiety or agitation.[1]

When I was deposed in the *Miller* case at the end of March 2000, Pfizer's lawyers stated that details of this study had been sent to the FDA.[2] I had just sent the details of our study to both the FDA[3] and the MCA in Britain. The regulators now had more convincing evidence that Zoloft produced agitation than they possessed when they licensed Zoloft for the treatment of depression. My covering letter to both sets of regulators asked whether they had anything comparable on file. I never got a reply from the FDA. But a fascinating correspondence began with the MCA, which showed they simply did not know the contents of the healthy volunteer studies on these drugs.[4]

For example, the regulators did not know that in the 1980s both Zoloft and Paxil were shown to produce dose-dependent agitation and apprehension in healthy volunteers. These studies were often conducted on company personnel and supervised by clinicians specialized in ear, nose, and throat or gastrointestinal medicine rather than psychiatry. Nonetheless, rates of agitation in up to a quarter of volunteers were noted. Many subjects dropped out on the SSRI, and there was even one suicide. In one study on Paxil, after only a few weeks on the drug, a significant dependence syndrome was visible in up to 85 percent of healthy volunteers upon withdrawal.[5]

SUICIDE IN CHILDREN—THE *MILLER* CASE

In the early 1990s, the striking manic-depressive illness of someone like Kay Jamison, which had begun in her teenage years, and the real risk of suicide such an illness poses had stimulated various campaigns, such as DART and Defeat Depression, which hoped to increase recognition of such conditions. This was a legitimate, even a noble cause. Manic-depressive illness and some forms of severe depression may begin in childhood or adolescence. But at that age, these disorders are so rare that no clinical trial has ever been conducted on any antidepressant in these patient groups—there simply aren't enough patients around. Children and adolescents nevertheless experience much unhappiness and distress. Until the 1990s, the received wisdom was that for the most part, childhood or adolescent distress was not the same thing as manic-depression or endogenous depression.

That view began to change in the 1990s. In America and elsewhere, children and adolescents were given psychotropic drugs with increasing frequency. In some cases this might be entirely sensible. For example, classic obsessive-compulsive disorder (OCD) can begin as early as the age of three. SSRIs can make a difference in many cases of OCD in adults; there was no reason to believe OCD in children wouldn't respond to SSRIs, even though the drugs had not been tested in these age groups. Faced with a convulsing child, few clinicians would hesitate to give anticonvulsants, although most anticonvulsants have not been tested in children.[6] A prescription for lithium or even ECT can similarly be justified for a teenager with manic-depressive illness.

Serious depression is extremely rare in childhood, but there are enough distressed and unhappy children to conduct trials of antidepressants in childhood and adolescent age groups. These began in the 1980s and early 1990s. Results uniformly failed to provide any evidence the drugs worked. Some pharmacotherapists argued that these age groups didn't respond to tricyclic antidepressants but the new SSRIs might offer an answer. In fact, the SSRIs fared little better, prompting Seymour and Rhonda Fisher to ask in a 1996 review whether the usual rules of science were somehow being suspended. The trial results were uniformly negative, they pointed out, yet clinicians were prescribing increasing amounts of antidepressants to children.[7]

Clinicians, however, saw children and adolescents respond to Prozac and other SSRIs. The confounding factor here is that clinical trials of antidepressants in distressed children show extremely high placebo response rates. These responses might simply have been because someone was paying attention to these children. High placebo response rates mean it is very difficult for *any* other treatment to do better. When I convened the British Association for Psychopharmacology consensus meeting on prescribing for children and adolescents in early 1997, however, I was assured that a new trial in press, conducted by Graham Emslie, would show Prozac really did work.[8]

In brief, Emslie and colleagues first excluded subjects showing a placebo response. This left them with a group of subjects randomized to Prozac or placebo. In that pool of subjects, Prozac did marginally better than placebo. Critics of pharmacotherapy argue placebo washouts produce an extremely artificial situation. But this design does demonstrate that Prozac does something. An effect suspected by many was in fact demonstrated in some patients, thus providing some legitimacy for prescribing an SSRI to children or adolescents. But the finding does not legitimate widespread prescribing in this age group. Indeed, this trial demonstrated that many children—perhaps a majority—did no better on Prozac than they would have done simply seeing a sympathetic clinician.

Prescriptions boomed nonetheless. *Newsweek* and other periodicals featured the rising tide of Ritalin prescriptions in the mid-1990s. Whatever the rights and wrongs of giving drugs to children, there was a large body of evidence that stimulants could improve many children's lives. By the end of the decade, *U.S. News and World Report* and other periodicals had moved on from Ritalin to question what was going on in the case of Prozac and the SSRIs.[9] The *U.S. News and World Report* article featured Matthew Miller.

Thirteen-year-old Matthew was a restless kid experiencing difficulties after moving to a new school. Concerned about his behavior, teachers administered a set of tests on which his scores fell marginally outside the normal range. His parents agreed to take Matthew to a psychiatrist. In June 1997 he saw Douglas Geenens,[10] who was also a consultant and speaker for Pfizer. Geenens considered either a possible depressive disorder or ADHD. Matthew's depression, if it was present, was mild and nonspecific in nature. There was no indication that this was the onset of a manic-depressive disorder. Hospitalization was not considered. Had the Millers' HMO coverage provided for psychotherapy, this would probably have been the next step. Instead, after a second consultation in July, a prescription for Zoloft was arranged. The initial pills came from a sample left with Dr. Geenens by his local Pfizer representative. He warned the Millers that Matthew might experience some nausea and insomnia.

During the next week, Matthew looked normal to his parents. His grandmother noted at one point over a meal that he was fidgety, "jumping out of his skin."[11] A questionnaire filled out by Dr. Geenens had noted that Matthew had ideas he might kill himself but would not do so. This changed. He met two girls to whom he confided he was thinking of burning down his parents' house.[12] In the early hours of the morning, a week after going on Zoloft, Matthew Miller hanged himself in the closet next door to his parents' bedroom.

Rather than settle, as it had done in the case of Bryn Hartmann, who killed her husband and then herself after ten days on Zoloft,[13] Pfizer fought the *Miller* case. It argued that suicide is the second most common cause of death in 13-year-old males. It is—but only because 13-year-olds don't often die. There had been only 61 suicides among 155,000 13-year-old males in 1997. One expert, Parke Dietz, argued that because Mathew Miller had not hanged himself from a height, this might be a case of autoerotic asphyxiation gone wrong.[14]

During the pretrial process, I was able to examine Pfizer's clinical trial database, involving over eight thousand patients as of December 1991, just before Zoloft's launch in America. My analysis suggested patients on Zoloft were almost twice as likely as patients on placebo to go on to suicidal acts.[15] Pfizer, in contrast, found the relative risk for suicidality on Zoloft to be almost identical to placebo.

Another document reported that six children and adolescents had become suicidal on Zoloft in the course of studies for depression and OCD. There were four suicidal acts in forty-four depressed children—a rate ten times higher than that found in adults. In the case of one 8-year-old boy, the investigator blamed Zoloft.[16] It was in this case that Wilma Harrison of Pfizer had sworn that the drug was not to blame (see Chapter 6), even though Pfizer monitors had agreed that the activating effects of Zoloft had likely led to the child's suicidality.[17] Despite this report filed by the company, and evidence of a high rate of suicidality on other SSRIs in this age group, the FDA did nothing.[18]

I was deposed in the *Miller* case in Boston in March 2000. This led Pfizer to scrutinize our healthy volunteer study comparing reboxetine and Zoloft in details, and in the following weeks to portray it in the media in a manner completely at odds with all the material given to Pfizer's lawyers. It was claimed that all subjects were my employees.[19] Only one of the nineteen had been on my staff—unless you argued that being paid inconvenience money made them my employees. It was claimed I had not examined any of the volunteers medically or psychiatrically. This was true—because it would have been inappropriate for me to do the examinations. Other medical staff examined them. Finally, it was claimed that Max had a significant alcohol disorder, when in fact she took two glasses of wine per week on average. But how could I rebut any of these assertions? This was the start of increasingly personal attacks on me; briefs for court actions and feedback from journalists characterized me as a zealot who said one thing for money, in court or to the media, and quite different things in scientific forums.

THE PROZAC PATENT

The *Miller* case fed directly into the Prozac story. On February 25, 2000, a court in Milford, Connecticut, acquitted Christopher DeAngelo of robbing a bank because he was on Prozac at the time.[20] Another court in Britain acquitted a man who had been on Prozac on an assault charge.[21] The *Forsyth* appeal was also pending.

These interconnected stories led the *Indianapolis Star* to ask how Lilly had managed the legal time bomb of Prozac in the mid-1990s. The paper ran a story on how the MDL cases involving Paul Smith's alleged breach of fiduciary obligations to his colleagues had been held up in Indiana for several years. Mitch Daniels, a spokesman for Lilly, commented that it was an illuminating spectacle to see sharks turn on each other. Daniels, a former top aide to Ronald Reagan and president of the Hudson Institute, and later a member of George W. Bush's cabinet, characterized the over $50 million in known Lilly settlement payments in Prozac cases as "relatively insignificant."[22] Had Lilly been forced to withdraw the drug or substantially alter the labeling, the company might have faced $2 to $3 billion in settlement claims. Lilly's main loss, if any, came from whatever dip in sales the controversy might have caused.

Meanwhile, after the publication in April 2000 of Joseph Glenmullen's *Prozac Backlash*,[23] ABC's *20/20* approached Martin Teicher but were puzzled by his apparent lack of commitment either pro- or anti-Prozac. They found Teicher was now engaged in what seemed to be a study for Lilly of a "new" Prozac.

Celexa and Prozac have structures that mean the parent molecule can come in an original and a mirror-image form (called isomers). It is often difficult to separate the two isomers in early industrial production, and companies therefore develop a "mixture" of the two. The side effects of these mirror images can be quite different. This enables a company to apply for a patent on the more effective or better tolerated of the two mirror images—if they can separate them.

In 1991 the Massachusetts-based company Sepracor isolated the isomers of Prozac—called S-fluoxetine and R-fluoxetine, or dexfluoxetine. Sepracor needed someone to help determine their potential. Who better than Martin Teicher? After describing the hazards of Prozac in 1990, Teicher had turned to animal research in an effort to model Prozac-induced akathisia.[24] This made him the obvious person to establish the behavioral profile of Sepracor's new drugs. His work suggested R-fluoxetine lacked the activating profile of S-fluoxetine. Sepracor took out a patent for R-fluoxetine in 1995,[25] which bound them, Teicher, and McLean Hospital together. In 1998, Lilly bought the marketing rights to the patent in a deal that potentially offered Sepracor up to $100 million per year.[26]

After early hype, *Prozac Backlash* might have died a quiet death. ABC stalled on broadcasting their program. But then the *Boston Globe*, *Newsday* in New York, and other media outlets received a number of unsolicited critiques of the book. These included a commentary from John Greist of the University of Wisconsin, a witness for Lilly in the *Wesbecker* case. Another was by Graham Emslie, whose study of Prozac in children we noted earlier in this chapter. A third came from David Dunner, a clinical trialist for Lilly and member of the 1991 FDA panel on Prozac. A fourth came from Harvey Ruben of Yale. All followed a standard line about the devastating disease that was depression, the weight of research behind Prozac, and the patients who would commit suicide because they had been scared off treatment.

In one commentary, Tony Rothschild claimed to be

disheartened that Dr. Glenmullen bolsters many of his arguments and proves his hypotheses by borrowing liberally from others' work including my own. . . . [A]t no point did Dr. Glenmullen consult me directly to question my studies, two of which he conveniently uses to prove his argument.[27]

I had tried unsuccessfully to contact Rothschild to talk about just this. It was well known that Carol Locke, the senior author on the Rothschild and Locke publication, stood by her view that the study pointed toward a causal relationship between Prozac and suicidality. Jerrold Rosenbaum from Massachusetts General, who apparently owned up to not having read the entire book, was also quoted in the material sent to the *Globe*. When approached by the *Globe* and asked about his consultancy with Lilly, he claimed that nearly every senior figure in psychopharmacology had consultancies with a range of different companies—that, in fact, it was impossible to function in this world without these links.[28]

The commentaries sent to *Newsday* in New York included a delicious covering letter from Robert Schwadron of Chamberlain Communications Group:[29]

> The book preys on the fear of people with clinical depression, and may prompt some people to abandon their medication and seek medically unproven alternatives for a debilitating disease with potentially life-threatening consequences. If we can offer you any information, or some balance to a story you may be planning, we would be more than happy to oblige. We can arrange for interviews with spokespeople from Eli Lilly and Company, as well as with independent researchers from the medical community.[30]

The *Globe* materials came from Rasky Baerlein, another PR group working for Lilly. This prompted Leah Garnett to investigate. Garnett was an assistant health editor who had come to the *Globe* a few months before from the *Harvard Health Letter*. She was on her way to a freelance career and was clearing her desk as the story came to a head. She wanted something new on Prozac that Lilly would find difficult to portray as selected documents stemming from plaintiffs' attorneys. The answer came to her in the middle of the night: She could just go to a government Web site and use the search terms *Teicher* and *Sepracor* to look at the patent for the new form of Prozac. What she found led to a headline feature on the front page of the *Globe* days after she left the newspaper.[31] The new patent stated, "Furthermore, fluoxetine produces a state of inner restlessness (akathisia), which is one of its more significant side effects."[32] "The adverse affects which are decreased by administering the R(-) isomer of fluoxetine include but are not limited to headaches, nervousness, anxiety, insomnia, inner restlessness (akathisia), suicidal thoughts and self mutilation."[33]

If the new "Prozac" ever reached the market, it would presumably carry warnings that it could cause suicidal thoughts—even though it might be less likely to do so than the parent compound. Replying for Lilly in the *Boston Globe*, Gary Tollefson took a familiar tack, arguing that sufferers from the debilitating disease that was depression were being unwarrantedly stigmatized, and the result of this would be that they would fail to seek treatment and lives would be lost. He claimed that the weight of scientific research made it abundantly clear that Prozac didn't cause any of the problems claimed for it.[34]

This opened up the possibility that groups like the Church of Scientology might use Lilly's own clinical trials and interpretations of their meaning to squash the new patent, on the basis that it did not contain a valid new development. Could Lilly deny the basis for patenting and still hold onto the patent?

The discovery of the patent on R-fluoxetine impacted on the outstanding legal cases. One of these was in the hands of Nancy Zettler. This was one of the original cases, dating back to the August 1991 suicide of "Corky" Berman, a Chicago businessman. Berman leapt from the thirty-seventh floor of the Carbon and Carbide Building, a striking art deco skyscraper on North Michigan Avenue in which Berman's psychologist kept his office.[35] Berman had ended up in a style of therapy that became common with managed care—he was seeing a psychologist for "therapy" and a pharmacologist (a psychiatrist)[36] for his prescriptions. On a 10 mg dose of Prozac, he had a range of side effects for which he was prescribed antidotes, including trazodone. Not unlike some of our healthy volunteers, he also underwent a change of personality, which was noted frequently by his psychologist, who had no knowledge about the possibility that Prozac might cause this. Two weeks after his dose of Prozac was bumped up dramatically, and a few hours after visiting his psychologist—who saw him as apparently normal and definitely not suicidal—Berman jumped to his death.[37]

Shortly after Berman's widow took legal action, the prescribing psychiatrist, David McNeil, was persuaded to switch insurers and avail himself of an indemnification package then offered by Lilly to American psychiatrists.[38] The *Berman* case brings out the hazards in this arrangement, under which McNeil had little option but to take the advice of his new lawyers, who were also involved in Lilly's defense. What if the best company defense were to hang McNeil out to dry? He had prescribed the sedative trazodone to counteract Prozac side effects. How would he justify what he had done? *Where is the evidence that you should do this, Doctor? Did Eli Lilly ever tell you this would be a good idea?*

While I was being deposed in the *Berman* case, Andy Vickery was invited to Indianapolis to discuss settlements in his outstanding cases. Meanwhile, Baum, Hedlund and Vickery had filed an action on June 8, 2000, to supplement their appeal against the *Forsyth* verdict, claiming Lilly had perpetrated a fraud upon the court.[39] The final deal between Lilly and Sepracor had been struck in December 1998. Three months later, in the course of the *Forsyth* trial, Lilly's patent lawyer Doug Norman had been present in the court. The plaintiff's appeal was based on a precedent set in a case against the Thompson Tool Company, a gun manufacturer, who had a video on file showing their gun firing accidentally when dropped. The relatives of a Mr. Pumphrey, who had been killed in just this manner, had appealed a "not guilty" verdict. The U.S. Court of Appeals found Thompson had committed a fraud upon the court by failing to disclose the video. The new *Forsyth* action argued that failing to disclose the details of the patent amounted to a comparable fraud, compounded by the presence of Lilly's patent attorney in the courtroom.[40]

Vickery brought the R-fluoxetine patent into play in this and three outstanding cases. One involved Hugh Blowers, a 17-year-old Hawaiian who had hanged himself after a week on Prozac. Blowers had described symptoms of akathisia in an e-mail to a friend just before he killed himself, and his friends described a marked change in character. On his bedroom wall was a poster for Prozac and what normalizing your serotonin system can do for you—part of the reason Blowers pushed for a change of antidepressant. This case would take the doctor (McNeil in this case) out of the equation. But then Vickery was asked to Indianapolis, where he settled the *Blowers* case.

Lilly believed the original Prozac patent held in the United States until December 2003. But in the week ending August 12, 2000, an appellate court ruled competitors could begin to produce generic versions of fluoxetine from February 2001. Lilly's stock fell from a capitalization of $123 billion to $85 billion, making it vulnerable to takeover. Suddenly, it had considerable incentive to settle all cases and to prepare to trash Prozac and the generic fluoxetines that would appear in 2001, making way for the new, improved R-fluoxetine it hoped to launch in 2003. Zettler and Vickery applied between them to depose Teicher, Beasley, and a series of Lilly lawyers, including Doug Norman. Teicher, extraordinarily, would be deposed effectively as a Lilly scientist, and Beasley was to be quizzed about what steps were being taken to determine the suicide potential of this new compound.

Then, in October 2000, Lilly shelved its development plans for R-fluoxetine (Zalutria). The investigation of the cardiac profile of dextra-fluoxetine suggested that the company might not get the new drug to market in time to forestall the competition.[41] Sepracor's stock plummeted by 25 percent.[42] Lilly was left with only duloxetine, a 1980s serotonin and norepinephrine reuptake inhibitor, in its antidepressant pipeline.[43]

I had first been approached about participating in a clinical trial of duloxetine in the early 1990s, before the company shelved the compound, as far as I knew because of bladder side effects. U.S. psychopharmacologists dutifully praised the development that duloxetine constituted, unaware perhaps that duloxetine was on the market as a bladder stabilizer in Europe. Rebranding it as an antidepressant may yet raise interesting questions about duloxetine, among both bladder specialists and the general public, who might well be mystified as to how a drug could be marketed for one condition in one country and an entirely different condition in others.

CONFLICTING INTERESTS

While working on the appeal in the *Forsyth* case, Cindy Hall came across two memos that had gathered dust since 1994. In the first, a memo to the "I Saved Prozac" team on August 1, 1990, Leigh Thompson wrote:

Today at PSC was LRL/Medical's finest hour. Dave Thompson and Gene Stap told me that it suddenly gave them a glimpse of how far medical has come and the vision that they knew (about global data-bases, super handling of ADE, proactive excellent relations with FDA, complex analyses and presentations made simple, DEN, GPT etc) but had never really had burned into their brains the elegance and mastery of the complexity!

So many of us were not here for the Oraflex, Moxam, etc crises, that it is very hard to measure the progress over the last few months on so very very many fronts.

When you battle the media and politicians, the ONLY thing that counts is the first word. The rebuttals are always on the last page and forgotten. You have to get out front and enlist your allies. The rapid flights to Boston to visit Teicher, the trips to FDA, the consultants coming in, the huge complex database, having so many large trials, the ability to quickly perform elegant analyses, DENs mastery of ADEs, have all come together in a significant effort.

I'll try to give a global overview of our past (Oraflex and Moxam especially) and our present and our future (with Mobius, Scientology etc after us) tomorrow at DEN. Please pass on my congratulations and profound thanks to your spouses/friends for tolerating your extra work/pressure and to those colleagues whom I have left off the list of addressees in my rush to get out this note.

I'd like to have some buttons or mementos of other kinds made with a logo along the lines of: "I saved Prozac." Suggestions please for design, memento and words—.[44]

The "I Saved Prozac" effort in 1990 gave rise to the first version of the Beasley article. Laura Fludzinski was then head of the clinical research department in Lilly Europe. By the time she was deposed in the *Wesbecker* case, Smith and Zettler had focused on events in Germany, leaving the British story, and the twenty-eighth and final exhibit in Fludzinski's deposition, to languish. This exhibit included a memo dealing with a trip by Lilly's David Wheadon to Britain and Europe in August 1990, to gauge opinions on the Teicher issues, as well as a set of reports from consultants for Lilly in response to an early draft of what later became the Beasley article.

Wheadon's memorandum mentioned that he hoped Allan Weinstein would be in good form when he saw the expense account. It also noted how some of those he had met were sure they could help Lilly with the problem—"Of course, he had several ideas on how he could assist us with this!" The exclamation mark suggests bids for funding.

After this came a covering letter and a set of reports. The first report up came from Brian Leonard, confirming my hunch that the reason he had asked me about the Teicher paper was because Lilly had asked him for his views. What he wrote was much what I would have written at the time—skepticism that this was anything more than a periodic scare. He pointed to the lack of a neurobiological rationale for what was happening and the evidence from the fluvoxamine story that SSRIs might in fact be useful in suicidal patients.

The mianserin story had shown how a company needs a network of "friends" when a crisis blows up. Roger Pinder put together such a network for mianserin and Organon. Responses from many of those involved in the mianserin story were in exhibit 28, along with input from George Ashcroft, who had put forward the first serotonin hypothesis of depression.

The revelation in Fludzinski's deposition exhibit came in another report. The covering letter noted that the key report came from someone whose views were likely to be particularly influential with regulators; the name was blacked out. It began:

> It comes as no surprise that the issue of suicidality and fluoxetine has surfaced as a problem for Lilly since I predicted it would some four or five years ago. . . . As you know there were questions about the agitation and stimulating properties attributed to fluoxetine and there were fears that this might increase suicidality. . . . I covered this issue in my expert report for the English and later in greater detail for the Dutch and German authorities.
>
> It was for this reason that I felt that Lilly would be wise to undertake a formal prospective study in this area. As you know I promised to examine the effects of fluoxetine or placebo in a group of multiple suicide attempters. At the time you will remember Lilly did not think this study had a high priority, which was reflected in the level of funding. . . . I nevertheless regarded this as a sufficiently important issue to carry out the study using my own resources in my own time.[45]

Stuart Montgomery had begun a Prozac study in multiple suicide attempters around this time. Lilly personnel were quizzed about this in

1994 depositions, but there was nothing in print. Later that year an article appeared titled "Lack of Efficacy of Fluoxetine in Recurrent Brief Depression and Suicidal Attempts."[46] Despite the headline, the text claimed there was no evidence of an increased rate of suicidality and that this lack of evidence disproved Teicher's hypothesis. But the figures in the text belied the claim. The original study had been scaled back so that only 107 subjects from a planned sample of 150 had been recruited.[47] Of those recruited, fewer than half completed the study with its randomization to Prozac or placebo. Of those completing, rates of suicide attempts were reported as the same in both the Prozac and placebo groups. But the fact that almost half the subjects dropped out made it impossible for the study to "disprove" Teicher's claim—almost by definition, all the Teicher cases would have dropped out early. Furthermore, although the paper didn't report the information, internal Lilly memos showed that on other measures placebo had done dramatically better than Prozac (p = 0.006).[48]

Montgomery subsequently undertook a similar study with Paxil in recurrent brief depression. As with Prozac, this study also terminated early. It showed no benefit for Paxil, but some critical details remained unpublished. At a psychopharmacology meeting in London in September 1999, David Baldwin, a former colleague of Montgomery, reported that there had been a threefold higher rate of suicide attempts in those taking Paxil compared with those taking placebo[49]—with a projected rate of forty-five suicide attempts per year in the Paxil group and twelve per year in the placebo group.[50] SmithKline Beecham later defended this study by claiming the results were not statistically significant. But the main reason the results failed to reach statistical significance was that the study terminated early, after only thirty-six patients had been recruited. The most serious suicide attempt involved a woman on Paxil who ended up with spinal injuries and later took an action against St. Mary's Hospital.[51]

These studies can be seen as a worthwhile effort to examine the benefits a then-new group of drugs, the SSRIs, might offer to a particularly difficult patient group—those who are highly suicidal. There turned out to be none. Even had SSRIs reduced suicidality in this high-risk group, this would not mean they couldn't at the same time induce suicidality in other individuals not at any risk of suicide. Indeed, a cynical argument would be that if one wanted to hide or manage an SSRI-induced suicidality problem, the very best group to pick was a high-risk group, where there was less scope for existing high rates of suicidal acts to increase further.[52]

When Lilly's expert went on to characterize the first draft of the Beasley report as "disappointing," it became clearer why Lilly might want the name in this exhibit report blacked out. Lilly had failed to follow the approach taken by Jenny Wakelin, he said, which was to analyze the data from the more suicidal patients to see if they showed more benefit than other patients. "Since these data [Wakelin's] are published it is reasonable to expect Lilly to have performed the same analysis and if it is not reported the assumption may be that fluoxetine has a less favorable effect."

He noted Lilly had reported on a smaller number of trials than it had undertaken: "The decision to report on a smaller number of trials than the full data base may appear as evasive. In any event selective reporting on your data requires adequate explanation, which is missing. . . . Any suggestion that the full data base is not being examined will raise the thought in some minds that the data are potentially misleading."

In passing, he noted that in clinical trials suicidal ideation is not "systematically asked for and therefore is erratically collected and unreliable." He noted how poor item 3 on the Hamilton Scale was (the suicide item), and how much better the suicide item in the Montgomery Asberg Depression Rating Scale was. He concluded:

> [T]he analysis is patchy and apparently not done on the full pool of blinded placebo and reference controlled data, which is available to the company. It is therefore suspect particularly since it contradicts already published data.
>
> The report refers in an offhand manner to the recent change in product labeling, to warn of suicidal ideation associated with fluoxetine. This conveys to me, and, I believe, most clinicians, that Lilly is convinced the data support the presence of a relationship between fluoxetine and the provocation of suicidal ideas. It is difficult to understand why this report provides no evidence to support this, and increases the feeling that other data not presented here must have helped persuade Lilly of the existence of a causal relationship.
>
> Overall the report is disappointing. The review is patchy and inadequate, the analyses undertaken are not in line with published data

and do not give the numbers involved and provide limited data on the main question. The conclusions of the report contradict the recent change in product labeling and this adds to the impression that the question of whether fluoxetine provokes suicidal thoughts or not has not been properly considered.[53]

Lilly had voluntarily inserted a reference to suicidal ideation and violent behaviors into a section on the labeling for postintroduction reports on May 29, 1990. This section reports on claims made after launch. But it is neither a warning nor a precaution nor an acknowledgment of possible causation.[54] Looked at cynically, it allowed Lilly to claim that the wording was there for physicians to see. Jurors might, as a consequence, blame the physician rather than the company.

Despite this comprehensive critique of Lilly's position, a few years later, in the case of Paxil, a very similar analysis to the Beasley analysis appears in publications from Stuart Montgomery,[55] a former consultant to the British MCA. A similar analysis under the name of Juan Lopez-Ibor appeared in 1993,[56] in a two-page symposium supplement. These two articles were the significant planks for SmithKline's medico-legal defense in the first case that came their way—the *Tobin* case. But, as we shall see, there were major mismatches between the data reported in these articles and the underlying raw data from SmithKline's clinical trials.

Nine years after the expert report for Lilly, at an ECNP meeting in London, Stuart Montgomery presented data from Pierre Fabre's meta-analysis showing that SSRIs were much more likely than milnacipran or tricyclic antidepressants to be associated with suicidality. At exactly the same time, Sarah Boseley was writing her *Guardian* article "Prozac: Can It Make You Kill?" When she contacted the company for comments, Lilly offered Montgomery as someone who might offer an "independent" comment. Some experts, it seemed, walked a very fine line.

When the difficulties posed by the patent of R-fluoxetine entered the public domain in May 2000, Lilly's response included the continued assertion that "Teicher's article was a series of anecdotal reports, and his suggestions of a 'possibility' of a causal relationship have been refuted by multiple large placebo controlled prospective and retrospective clinical studies that have demonstrated no increased risk of suicide associated with Prozac use."[57] However, when deposed as a Pfizer expert in the Miller case in 2000, Daniel Casey, who had chaired the FDA hearings in 1991, agreed that he was not aware of any prospective studies designed to test whether Prozac might induce suicidality.[58] John Mann, another Pfizer expert in the same case, agreed,[59] as did Roger Lane of Pfizer, David Wheadon—once of Lilly but then of SmithKline—and Charles Beasley of Lilly, all during the course of 1999–2000.[60]

BOSS OF BOSSES

Charles Nemeroff, professor of psychiatry at Emory University in Atlanta and a senior figure in American psychopharmacology, gave the Annual Guest Lecture at the July 2000 British Association for Psychopharmacology meeting in Cambridge. At this meeting, I presented the results from our healthy volunteer study in poster form. I did not attend the guest lecture, during which Nemeroff apparently criticized drug studies in healthy volunteers.[61] Others present at the lecture brought this to my attention, so I expected Nemeroff to visit me at the poster session. He did.

As I recall it, Nemeroff's opening gambit was that I was doing myself harm publishing such material.[62] Why? It was good clear-cut science, and other, unpublished studies backed up our findings. Nevertheless, I was warned, it would ruin my career to get involved in this. He said he had been approached on several occasions to participate in legal actions against me. This was a frightening prospect—as he phrased it.

Nemeroff claimed he had looked through the Lilly database at the time of the FDA hearings in 1991, and that in his opinion there was nothing there. He had, in fact, presented data on the company's behalf at the FDA hearings. I countered that I had also looked through Lilly's database and those of other companies, and in my opinion there *was* something there. I pointed out that the clinical trials submitted to the FDA for new antidepressants showed an excess of suicidal acts on SSRIs compared to placebo. If the drugs reduced suicidality for some people, as both he and I believed, they must be causing it in others to account for the number of suicidal acts. This was brushed aside.

With the Hindmarch study in mind, I mentioned that our study was consistent with other healthy volunteer studies. Nemeroff immediately said that this other study involved a dose effect. This appeared to be a clear admission of a causal connection between the SSRI and emergent suicidality. Also, his reply, if I understood it correctly, would seem to suggest that he and probably other experts knew of the existence of either this or other studies.[63]

He went on to say that these were big companies in an $8 billion business, and that he himself had had problems with Pfizer some years back, when the company managed to make life very difficult for him, for his research staff, and for others associated with him.

Did I want the consequences of creating a fuss about drugs like the SSRIs? he asked. American primary-care practitioners would simply hear a message that there was a problem with these drugs and would stop prescribing them, and as a result, more people would commit suicide. There would be a public health cost. Could I cope with this on my conscience? Could I cope with the string of flaky individuals who would bring cases my way, individuals who, both he and I knew, had difficulties that were not caused by the drugs?

What about our duty, I asked, as prescribers of drugs available on prescription only, to warn other prescribers and patients of any hazards in order to make therapy as effective and safe as possible? He wouldn't engage on this point. Some would say it was immaterial what people like the two of us did—that these companies were so big they would simply roll over those who got in the way, as tobacco companies had done. They were answerable to their shareholders only, and profit was the bottom line.

But in addition to being a prescriber, under conflict-of-interest guidelines at other meetings, Nemeroff listed himself as a major equity shareholder in Lilly, Pfizer, SmithKline Beecham, Pharmacia, and Forrest—all the SSRI-producing companies.[64] Some weeks later, I stumbled on a copy of a glossy new journal, filled with advertisements for pharmaceutical products, called *T.E.N.: The Economics of Neuroscience*. The front cover was a portrait of Nemeroff captioned "Boss of Bosses: Is the Brash and Controversial Charles Nemeroff the Most Powerful Man in Psychiatry?"[65] There was no hint that the headline or the profile inside was written ironically, or that the authors were aware of what the title and the text implied.[66]

The possible great influence of a small group of people is apparent in Alan Schatzberg and Nemeroff's 1998 American Psychiatric Press *Textbook of Psychopharmacology*. In this, the chapter on SSRIs was written by Lilly's Tollefson and Rosenbaum from Massachusetts General Hospital. The chapter cites the Warshaw and Keller study as the only piece of evidence on the issue of Prozac and suicide.[67] This chapter was later used by Pfizer in the *Motus* case as part of its basis for a statement of undisputed facts claiming that serotonin was low in depression, that SSRIs promote serotonergic function, and that the selectivity of SSRIs meant they were less prone to side effects than other antidepressants.[68]

We have moved into a new world in which the dean of Harvard Medical School publicly agonizes about the issue of conflict of interest. (Harvard had until recently set a ceiling of $10,000 support from outside interests but, alarmed that they might be losing senior figures to other universities, had decided to review their policy.) In this new world, what duty of care or responsibility to the community do academics have? With duties as shareholders come opportunities to have an input into company policy in a manner not available to the ivory-towered academics of yesteryear. As shareholders, individuals have access to the right connections to do great good. George Bush Sr. previously sat on the board of Lilly. Clearly, therefore, board members had considerable influence, but to do the right thing, Bush or others like him need a proper assessment of the situation. If the experts conclude there is no problem, there is little Bush or anyone else can do.

The Prozac story involved the senior figures in American psychopharmacology in a calculus. As shareholders, they were perfectly placed to force a debate on major issues in public and academic forums. Teicher claims that some of these figures had attempted to block his first efforts to raise the issue, offering arguments essentially similar to those with which I was being confronted in 1999 and subsequently.[69] The "advice" in my case could be construed as concern for my welfare, yet, if followed, it could shut down debate. But whatever was going on, who gave either Lilly shareholders or me the right to settle the matters of public importance involved in the Prozac case?

The Fludzinski exhibit indicates that the role of certain players goes beyond their duties as shareholders. Some of these experts are also advisers to regulatory bodies. Given the information that was published, and which MCA knew about, it is hard to understand how Prozac could have remained on the British market without warnings.

The extent to which there are conflicts of interest in FDA hearings was explored in a lengthy article that opened with a front-page headline piece in *USA Today* on September 25, 2000.[70] The article maintains that it has become almost standard practice for advisers to the FDA to have a direct financial interest in the drug or topic they are asked to evaluate. The process of waiving conflicts of interest has become a mere formality. The FDA response to questions on this point is that the best experts for the FDA are often the best experts to consult with industry. But this is not always the case. It is not difficult to find others without the same ties to industry.

Since the controversies surrounding the Prozac and breast implant cases, the FDA "has stopped releasing details on conflicts because of concerns about violating the privacy rights of committee members."[71] This concern is difficult to understand. Exactly what privacy rights are involved here? Similar controversies were being voiced in Britain at almost exactly the same time, in connection with a new vaccine for meningitis C.[72]

REGULATORS AND FRIENDS

After the healthy volunteer study outlined in the last chapter, I wrote to the MCA, drawing their attention to three studies that showed Zoloft could trigger serious agitation.[73] The MCA responded that a series of epidemiological studies indicated there was no problem. When pushed to name these epidemiological studies, they offered six names—essentially the studies Andy See had offered in *Forsyth*.[74] One was the Jick study, which all but proved that Prozac caused suicide. Another was the Fava and Rosenbaum study, but many analyses of these data indicated that Prozac did induce suicidality. The third and fourth were the Leon and the Warshaw and Keller studies, but as we have seen, whatever these are, they are not epidemiological studies. The fifth, a British post-marketing surveillance study, compared SSRIs to each other using the reports of primary-care physicians.[75] If extrapolated to the population at large, the rates cited would have trebled British national suicide rates. The final "study," by Ashleigh and Fesler, was a one-column letter in the *American Journal of Psychiatry* looking retrospectively at 206 patients who had been put on Prozac.[76] The MCA failed to acknowledge two other genuine epidemiological studies that had by this stage been published. One showed increased rates of suicidal acts on SSRIs,[77] and the other increased rates of suicide on SSRIs.[78]

This regulatory response is deeply problematic. It seems to me that there are only a few ways to interpret this specific MCA response. One would seem to be that they are incompetent. A second is that they are under pressure or rushed. A third is that they have taken the word of some advisers that these are epidemiological studies that do not indicate a problem. In a world where advisers did not have conflicts of interest, this might have been reasonable; this is no longer the case. A fourth option is that they have taken the direct word of pharmaceutical companies that these are epidemiological studies. A common factor to all these interpretations is that no one wants to cause trouble.

When I first wrote to the MCA asking for any other studies on file with results similar to our healthy volunteer study, they responded that it would take some time to get back to me with an answer. They wrote to the SSRI companies and asked them for details of the results from their healthy volunteer studies. Four months later, I got my reply—a set of company assessments of what their data revealed. None of these company assessments mentioned any difficulties or hazards; not even Pfizer's, where I knew there had been several disturbing healthy volunteer studies. Specifically challenged on the Hindmarch study, the MCA later revealed that they had acquired a copy of this study with a "pattern of severe adverse side effects and drop outs."[79] But had they received it only in response to my pressure? Everything about their response indicated that this was probably the case; regulators in Australia, for instance, did not appear to have a copy of this study.[80] It later transpired that the MCA possessed a four-page *summary* of the Hindmarch study. Company healthy volunteer studies from this period typically contained well over a hundred pages.

The e-mails within the FDA and between the FDA and Lilly on Prozac in the early 1990s had referred to a number of FDA personnel, including Martin Brecher and Paul Leber. Brecher had gone on to work with Janssen and, later, Astra-Zeneca. And in 1998, Paul Leber left the FDA and set up his own consulting firm. His first customer, and for a period his only one, was Pfizer.

The migration of FDA officials into industry will worry some. In Britain, the trend was just the opposite, although the United States now seems to copying the United Kingdom. When writing to the MCA, I was writing to Keith Jones, who had formerly been in Merck. In early 2001, Ian Hudson, the former head of international safety for SmithKline, became head of the licensing division of the MCA. A few weeks beforehand, Hudson, still at SmithKline, had been deposed in the *Tobin* case, in which all the issues in this book came to a head.

TOBIN VS. SMITHKLINE

In February 1998, Donald Schell, a 60-year-old living in Gillette, Wyoming, became withdrawn and began to complain to his wife, Rita, of difficulty in sleeping. Schell first suffered from his nerves in the mid-1980s, with approximately five subsequent nervous episodes centered on work stressors or bereavements. Don and Rita appeared to those who knew them to be a close couple. They were married for thirty-seven years. They had two children, Michael and Deborah. Deborah married Tim Tobin in 1992, and in 1997 she gave birth to the Schell's first grandchild, Alyssa. Deborah and Alyssa, now nine months old, came down from Billings, Montana, to stay for a few days with Don and Rita in February 1998.

Don's means of handling his nerves was to take time off work, as he could easily get someone to deputize for him. He went for walks with his wife, took care with his diet, and spent time talking with friends or with Tim, if he was around. He had got on well with a Dr. Suhany in 1990, so if he remained low after a week or two, he would go to see the doctor. Suhany had first put Schell on Prozac and noted that it made him tense, anxious, and jittery, despite the fact that he was on several "antidotes" such as Inderal, Ativan, and Desyrel. Suhany stopped Prozac and put Schell on imipramine, to which he responded rapidly.[81] What Suhany didn't know was that Schell might have even been hallucinating while on Prozac. Since Schell had responded to imipramine in 1990, in two further brief episodes in the 1990s he was put on tricyclic antidepressants and again responded rapidly.

In February 1998, when Schell began to complain about his sleep, he and Rita went to see a primary-care physician, Dr. Patel. Dr. Patel did a thorough examination, which included rating scales that indicated Schell's main difficulty was poor sleep and that he felt hopeful about the future and thought well of himself. Patel diagnosed an anxiety state and, unaware of a prior adverse response to Prozac, put Schell on Paxil, without any covering antidotes. Forty-eight hours later, Don Schell put three bullets from two different guns through Rita's head, then through Deborah and Alyssa's heads, before shooting himself.

After more than a year in a mental wilderness, Tim Tobin sought out Andy Vickery and took an action for wrongful death against SmithKline Beecham, then in the process of becoming Glaxo-SmithKline, the world's largest pharmaceutical company. I was retained in the case, just around the time I agreed to move to Toronto.

THE TORONTO AFFAIR[82]

At the end of November 2000, the University of Toronto Department of Psychiatry invited me to speak at a seventy-fifth anniversary meeting on the theme "Looking Back: Looking Ahead." Charles Nemeroff was also on the program.

A year before, I had been appointed to the University of Toronto as a professor of psychiatry in the Mood and Anxiety Disorders Program at the Center for Addiction and Mental Health (CAMH).[83] I was waiting for my visa. A week after the Toronto meeting, I was due to give an annual guest lecture and seminar on the history of psychiatry at Cornell University Medical School, New York. I arranged to give the same talk in both places, visiting Pfizer's New York Zoloft archive in between.

The day before the Toronto meeting, I interviewed a psychologist for a position on the program I would be running, considered decor for my new office, and discussed the practicalities of moving from Britain to Canada with David Goldbloom, the physician in chief at CAMH, whose budget would cover part of my salary. I discussed the SSRI medico-legal cases I was involved in, and he seemed to have no concerns. Some members of the university department on the day of the anniversary meeting were in Indianapolis discussing "work product" with Lilly, which had funded research in the department. In the previous year, the Mood Disorders Program had received over 50 percent of its research funding from pharmaceutical companies.

The talk I gave to Toronto and Cornell had first been worked up for a meeting for Astra-Zeneca. My lecture outlined my forthcoming Harvard University Press book *The Creation of Psychopharmacology*.[84] I reviewed developments over fifty years of psychopharmacology, the key drugs, the development of clinical trials, and the subsequent development of conflicts of interest. I touched peripherally on the central claims of this book—that SSRIs can make people suicidal, and that since the problem arose there had been no research to map its dimensions and decide how best to minimize the risks posed by these drugs.[85] The postmeeting feedback forms I received from Toronto some weeks later showed that my talk had rated the highest for content. After the same lecture in New York a few days later, Jack Barchas, head of the Psychiatric Department in Cornell and editor of the *Archives of General Psychiatry,* told me that this work on the history of psychiatry would be remembered.

Bob Michels, the dean of Cornell, attended a meal after my talk there. He immediately asked me what had happened in Toronto. Surprised, I said I had delivered the same talk he had just heard. I outlined to Michels and others my encounter earlier in the year with Nemeroff, and how after the lecture in Toronto Goldbloom told me he took exception to my claim that SSRIs could make someone suicidal and the implication—as he put it—that Lilly had known about it. The day of the talk in Toronto, according to Nemeroff's lawyer Nina Gussack, Nemeroff had talked to some people in the university about "Healy" and was under the impression that decisions had been taken.[86] In a subsequent letter, Goldbloom indicated Nemeroff had been only one of the people who talked to him. He believed that these people had independently spoken to him. Had they? Or had they all, in one form or another, encountered Nemeroff?[87]

Michels made it clear that I had been fired. I flew home from New York the following day to find an e-mail from Goldbloom:

> Essentially, we believe that it is not a good fit between you and the role as leader of an academic program in mood and anxiety disorders at the Centre. While you are held in high regard as a scholar of the history of modern psychiatry, we do not feel your approach is compatible with the goals for development of the academic and clinical resource that we have. This view was solidified by your recent appearance at the Centre in the context of an academic lecture.

What could explain what had happened? The University of Toronto was still embroiled in the affair of Nancy Olivieri, a researcher dismissed for publishing data on adverse events from a clinical trial.[88] An international outcry forced her reinstatement, and a new dean pledged to uphold the core values of a university.[89] Another Olivieri case would be a disaster for the university. It might be an even bigger disaster for Lilly, Pfizer, and SmithKline, because it was just the kind of story a jury could understand only too well.

The day after my talk in Toronto, just as I entered Pfizer's archive to seek out their healthy volunteer studies, Nemeroff had spoken at length on "Healy and his views" before a group of psychiatrists in New York at a council meeting of the American Foundation for Suicide Prevention. Sometime between Friday and Tuesday, when I lectured in Cornell, a senior figure in U.S. psychopharmacology called senior figures in Cornell telling them, my informant suggested, that "Healy was manic-depressive, violent and a peddler of junk science," intimating that my lecture should be canceled.

I learned most of this through phone calls from colleagues within days of receiving the Goldbloom e-mail message. When overtures to senior CAMH and university figures brought no constructive response, I wrote to CAMH and the university, suggesting that the picture might be a more complex one than they initially appreciated. Given that Lilly withdrew their funding from the Hastings Center after an article I had written covering the same ground, the likely press interpretation would be that the institution had been worried about the threat to funding of its Psychiatric Department.[90] Had the university been complicit even inadvertently in compromising a witness in a legal case?

What would companies do to an awkward witness? Before he bowed out of the Prozac debate in the mid-1990s, Martin Teicher had appeared in one case, the *Greer* case.[91] At his deposition, Nina Gussack, the attorney for Lilly, went through his six cases in detail.

Teicher, as it turned out, had sent his second case to Rosenbaum for another opinion. Rosenbaum claimed the patient said, "I never thought I was any more suicidal on Prozac than I was before or after, but I suppose Dr. Teicher is more sensitive to this issue." Alarmed at the implications, Teicher saw the patient again after receiving a letter from Rosenbaum. Faced with his medical records, the man apparently did remember just how bad it had been on Prozac. Teicher's notes included details of phone calls from the man's mother, confirming that he had been worse on Prozac.

In a letter to Teicher, Rosenbaum "recognized" that a patient is not always an accurate historian. As far as he could gather, the patient had gone on Prozac again without becoming suicidal. Teicher's medical notes revealed a different picture. Faced with a man who did not connect his suicidality to his Prozac intake, Teicher had, in fact, tested him out on Prozac again a year later, and he had again become suicidal. So either the case was strengthening with this rechallenge or Teicher had been fooled. I recognized this failure to remember as one of the difficulties my patient Tony L. had after becoming suicidal on Prozac. It was as though Prozac, like childbirth, produced state-dependent changes, so that afterward the individual sometimes just didn't remember what it was like. But how did Gussack come to have confidential clinical correspondence?

On the second day of the deposition, Teicher and Gussack worked their way from case 2 through to case 6. Teicher stated that he had been instructed by his attorney to discuss only those details of this sixth case that had appeared in print. Gussack nevertheless asked about the malpractice suit that, she asserted, the patient had filed. She inquired about an ongoing legal matter regarding his registration with the Board of Registration in Medicine in Massachusetts.

Gussack asked, "Would you agree, doctor, that she complained you were negligent in your prescribing of multiple medications for her at the same time?" "Did she also allege in her deposition that you had engaged in multiple acts of sexual relations with her?" "Is it accurate to state that . . . you described this [patient] as a grand hysteric . . . who would make up all sorts of things for attention . . . that [she] had serious problems with reality testing, distinguishing fantasy from reality in all areas?" "You said that Jane Doe would call you at home . . . throughout the course of the time you were treating her?" "She had a great deal of difficulty at night . . . she was 'very lonely, very frightened, often very suicidal after her husband had gone to sleep.'"

"Doctor, it is true, isn't it, that in the course of the malpractice suit . . . patient number 6 alleges that you had sexual relations with her starting in the fall of 1984 . . . that you had sexual relations with her at the Battle Green Hotel . . . Have you denied in your testimony . . . that you had any inappropriate touching or kissing with patient number 6 . . . that on three or four occasions she had sexual relations with you at your home . . . , that you engaged in oral sex, intercourse and anal intercourse with you [sic] on a number of occasions . . . that you had sexual relations with her in your office countless times . . . that you have given her gifts . . . an artificial plant . . . a foldout fan . . . a pair of earrings . . . birthday cards, signed 'Love Marty' . . . cassette tapes of recordings of you playing the guitar?"

This was late on the second day of questioning. Even the court stenographer was getting worked up and misplacing pronouns. Teicher refused to answer anything against a backdrop of Andy Greenwald, counsel for Greer, saying, "I don't know why I keep saying objection. I have a continuing objection."

Most clinicians reviewing the bare details of this kind of case, unaware of the context, would assume a considerable possibility that few of the things being aimed at Teicher were in fact true. This woman had been described as a borderline patient in the 1990 paper, and "boundary problems," as they are called, are a feature of managing just this kind of patient. The difficulty for Teicher was that even if nothing was true, he couldn't win on a witness stand, even though the Massachusetts Board of Registration had decided there was no malpractice.[92]

A few weeks before this deposition, he received further news. Divorced, Teicher lived close to his former wife and helped out with the children. But then his wife moved—to a post in oncology in Indianapolis with Lilly.

There was a good chance the first question I would face on cross-examination in the *Tobin* case would be "Dr. Healy, isn't it true that you were recently sacked from the University of Toronto?" Journalists were already asking questions of the University of Toronto, CAMH, and Nina Gussack. Faced with an almost complete lack of response from the University of Toronto or CAMH, I had little option but to raise the affair preemptively in my deposition in the *Tobin* case at the end of March and then to answer media questions on the issue. A few weeks later, in response to an application from SmithKline, Judge William Beaman issued a gag order that prohibited the lawyers from talking to the media and from raising the issue of my employment status in any legal proceedings.

SHOWDOWN IN CHEYENNE

The *Tobin* case was heard in Cheyenne, Wyoming, from May 21 to June 6, 2001. Just before the case started, a Supreme Court judge in New South Wales, Australia, delivered a verdict making it clear that in his opinion, David Hawkins, a 73-year-old man who had murdered his wife the day after going on Zoloft, having had a prior history of an adverse response to Zoloft, would not have committed the act had he not been put on Zoloft. But it was too late to factor this into the *Tobin* case.

The jury of five women and three men heard first from Vickery and Fitzgerald for the plaintiffs. The surviving members of the Tobin and Schell families testified. There was expert input from Don Marks, who had previously worked as a safety officer for Roche Pharmaceuticals; Terry Maltsberger from Harvard; and me. They heard the physician Dr. Patel say that if he had been warned, he would have taken even more care than he had originally taken.

SmithKline put forward a series of experts: John Mann from Columbia, Alan Fraser from San Antonio, Philip Wang from Harvard, and Kenneth Tardiff from Cornell, as well as David Wheadon, Ian Hudson, and others from the company.

The defense rested on a number of claims. One was that Don Schell was chronically depressed and ideally should have been maintained on antidepressants for the rest of his life, from the time he had first become depressed. Part of the basis for this claim lay in a study by Montgomery in which patients who had responded to Paxil were, after several months, re-randomized to either Paxil or placebo. Those who went onto placebo became unwell, leading Montgomery and SmithKline to claim that Paxil not only treated but prevented further episodes of depression.[93] On the basis of this study, the FDA and MCA had licensed SmithKline to make these claims. But in the light of 85 percent rates of physical dependence reported in SmithKline's studies with healthy volunteers, this claim was extraordinary.

A second claim was that Montgomery and Lopez-Ibor had independently analyzed the SmithKline clinical trial databases, and their analyses had demonstrated that Paxil did not induce suicide. Unbeknownst to the plaintiffs, there was an extraordinary set of problems with these figures that became obvious only after the trial.

A third claim was that a report—the Cheng report, which contained the reports to SmithKline of suicides or homicides on Paxil—found similar rates as happened in the population at large.[94] But this defense failed to take into account that the rates at which these events were likely to be reported to SmithKline were at best one in ten of those happening, and perhaps even as bad as one in one hundred of those happening. Reported rates equivalent to the population at large might in fact be consistent with an epidemic of violent deaths.

In the face of SmithKline documents showing that investigators and company personnel had coded clinical trial reactions, including akathisia and hallucinations, as definitely caused by Paxil, the company argued that it is not possible to establish causality in an individual case—this can be done only by randomized controlled trials.

This strategy came through at perhaps the most chilling moment in the entire trial, in exchanges between Ian Hudson and Vickery. Having repeatedly told Vickery that SmithKline could never decide in a case of suicide whether their drug was to blame, Hudson was faced with the following:

Q. Okay. So, your view is: It's simply impossible for SmithKline Beecham to decide whether Paxil did or did not contribute to the homicidal or suicidal behavior of any one given individual; is that your testimony?

A. We would certainly gather all the information, but on an individual case basis it would be impossible to decide whether paroxetine caused an event or not.

Q. Okay. Now—hold on just a minute. . . . If you were to get Exhibit Two there, the Aggression Study [Cheng report]—I've lost my page. Bear with me just a second. Okay. Would you turn to page twenty-one of sixty-three? Are you there with me?

A. Yes.

Q. Now, is it impossible for SmithKline Beecham to determine whether the patient identified in the fifth report on the bottom of that page, whether his behavior was caused or was not caused by Paxil?

A. On an individual case basis, it would be impossible to say whether a drug caused an event.

Q. Okay. Do you know if that patient, that's reflected down there, is the decedent of my client? Is that Donald Schell?

A. I believe it is, yes.

Q. You're telling me, under oath, it's simply impossible for SmithKline Beecham to decide whether Paxil did or did not cause Mr. Schell to murder his wife, his daughter, his granddaughter and then to commit suicide; is that right, sir?

A. It is impossible, on an individual case basis, from individual reports, to assign causality especially in a very complicated area such as this. That's why, when we have issues, we review all the available data and make a determination, on the basis of all the available data, whether there is an issue or not.

Q. Okay. Do you believe that it is possible that Paxil has caused any person, worldwide, to commit an act of homicide or suicide?

A. I have seen no evidence to suggest that at all.[95]

Hudson was opening up an extraordinary black hole here. No matter how many physicians or others reported to SmithKline suicides or homicides they thought related to the drug, SmithKline would deny any evidence for causation while there was no randomized controlled trial evidence. The fact that they had never undertaken any trials and had no plans to do so smacked of washing their hands in the face of a crucifixion. In many internal assessments at the time, companies had, in fact, overridden the opinions of their investigators that the drug had not caused the problem and coded the reactions as caused by the drug—but according to this new defense, even these assessments were not valid.

The jury disagreed with Hudson. On June 6, having recessed for less than three hours after a two-and-a-half-week trial, they returned a guilty verdict against SmithKline and an award for damages four times greater than the biggest previous award in Wyoming—a first-ever verdict against a pharmaceutical company for a psychiatric side effect of a psychotropic drug.

IS FREEDOM IN TORONTO ACADEMIC?

The *Tobin* verdict seemed to have no impact in Toronto. There were no overtures from the university or CAMH to look at the issues afresh.

The position taken by the university and CAMH at this point was that the clinical domain produced its own set of particular issues when it came to academic freedom. The usual rules, it was suggested, couldn't apply when vulnerable patients were likely to be affected by what was said. To allow someone like me to denigrate a treatment like the SSRIs would be like letting a fool cry "Fire!" in a crowded theater.

The need for extra caution in the clinical domain has long been recognized. This is precisely why regulations have been put in place—to limit the abilities of quacks to sell worthless treatments to vulnerable people. But speaking out about the hazards of treatment was exactly why drug treatments were made prescription-only. Keeping quiet about a known hazard *de facto* breaks the spirit of the law.

By this time, the Canadian Association for University Teachers (CAUT) had lobbied the university and others on my behalf. They got no more response than I did. In September, a letter signed by twenty-nine senior figures in the field—including two Nobel Prize winners, former presidents of various organizations such as the American Psychiatric Association, the American College of Neuropsychopharmacology, and a range of other psychiatric and psychopharmacological organizations worldwide—was sent to university president Robert Birgenau, protesting the violation of academic freedom involved in "the Healy case." There was input from Europe, North and South America, Japan, China, and Australia.

Birgenau's response suggested these signatories were not fully aware of the issues in the case. Two weeks later, supported by CAUT, I filed a legal action against the university, involving a first-ever claim for violation of academic freedom, with further claims for breach of contract and libel.[96] This seemed the only way to find out more about the issues in the case.

9

The Tort Wars

THE THALIDOMIDE DISASTER burned deep into our collective psyche. That a drug might produce something much worse than the condition it was supposed to treat was a shock. Early recognition that the power of the new drugs developed after World War II to produce great benefits brought with it new risks came in 1952, when the first book on the side effects of medications appeared.[1] But the new field of drug-induced injury came to public prominence when thalidomide scorched a path through regulators, politicians, and academics into the courts.

Perhaps the new power to cure age-old scourges led the public and physicians to suspend natural caution about drugs. If a therapist is very conscious of the hazards of treatment, the task of persuading someone to take the risks involved becomes more difficult. These problems multiply if employing hospitals or universities discourage clinicians from speaking out about the hazards of new drugs.

The history of psychiatric therapies shows very clearly that these therapeutic and institutional dynamics make it hard for therapists of any persuasion to see the risk in what they are doing. Psychoanalysts blamed their patients' underlying neurosis for their failure to get better. Psychiatrists blamed patients' schizophrenia for antipsychotic-induced problems such as the chronic and disfiguring facial grimacing of tardive dyskinesia.[2] Everyone at present blames the patient's personality or his illness, rather than the agent he is being treated with, for benzodiazepine or SSRI-induced dependence. Lilly and many clinicians have spectacularly blamed depression rather than Prozac for drug-induced suicidality. This history suggests that those delivering a therapy are not the best people to bring the hazards of that therapy to light. But in the wake of thalidomide, it was those entrusted with delivering therapies to whom governments turned to prevent another thalidomide.

Thalidomide, synthesized by Chemie-Grünenthal in 1956,[3] also kicked off a story in which Prozac, Zoloft, and Paxil are the latest installments. It was sold in Europe and Australia under the trade names

Contergan or Distaval, as a sleeping pill, and in Canada as Kevadon or Talimol. In retrospect, the sales campaigns chill. This was supposed to be the new safe sleeping pill. Advertisements showed young toddlers accessing the bathroom medicine cupboard. The message was that if the cupboard contained thalidomide instead of barbiturates, in the event of an accidental overdose, no harm would come. The drug quickly began to sell well.

The first hints of trouble emerged in 1961. An Australian obstetrician named William McBride reported his suspicions that thalidomide was associated with a series of severe birth defects.[4] On November 26, 1961, the German newspaper *Welt am Sontag* published the suspicions of Siegfried Lenz, from Hamburg, under the headline "Malformations from Tablets." Grünenthal labeled the article sensationalist. When the company later withdrew the drug from the German market, it argued that "press reports had undermined the basis for scientific discussion."[5]

In the United States, FDA bureaucracy held up thalidomide, which had not been licensed for use on the American market by the time the crisis broke in Europe. Shortly before these dramatic developments, Senator Estes Kefauver had closed congressional hearings looking at the practices of the newly emerging pharmaceutical industry. These hearings had dragged on for a number of years through the 1950s, looking at the advertising, pricing, and the prescription-only status of drugs; the hearings were talked into the ground.[6] The thalidomide crisis resurrected Kefauver's hearings and led to the adoption of the 1962 amendments to the Food and Drugs Act, which passed both Houses of Congress unanimously on October 10, 1962—the only bill other than a declaration of war to do so in a single day. Something had to be seen to be done.

The crux of the matter lay in pre- and postlaunch testing of new drugs. But the new FDA regulations did nothing to improve safety standards. Instead they mandated a continuing restriction of new drugs to prescription-only status, even though disasters had happened in countries both where thalidomide was available on prescription only and where it had been available over the counter. By maintaining prescription-only status, the FDA made those doing therapy responsible for alerting the public to the hazards of treatment—just the people who, history now suggests, are least able to see or speak out about those hazards.

The new regulations encouraged manufacturers to produce drugs for diseases, rather than for lifestyles or trivial complaints such as bad breath. This was an official recognition that new drugs were inherently hazardous and that the risks of remaining untreated must therefore significantly outweigh the risks of treatment. There was little appreciation then of the possibility that, restricted to marketing drugs for diseases, companies might market diseases and thereby in one sense make us all much more diseased than we had ever been before.

Emphasis on the restriction of drug treatment to disease states carried a hidden subtext. In 1962 the exemplary disease states were bacterial infections. Underpinning the new regulations was the idea that the best of the new drug treatments would act like antibiotics to correct a disease process quickly and effectively, and would do so regardless of the psychosocial setting of patients or their constitutional types. When a clinician prescribes an antibiotic, it makes no difference whether or not she has a good bedside manner. Nor will she need to take into account her patient's gender or social or ethnic status. Treatment goes ahead regardless. The FDA regulations were aimed at just this kind of disease and just this kind of treatment. The triumph of the new amine theories of depression converted "nerves" into an illness that could be observed and treated in this way, and the modern rhetoric of depression insists that its treatment is as value-free as the treatment of bacterial infections, when this simply is not the case.

The post-1962 regulatory system was geared to catering for drugs, which would work ninety-eight times out of one hundred, with perhaps one or two patients experiencing idiosyncratic reactions. It was not a system geared for treatments in which three or four people out of ten might be made worse by treatment, and as many as one out of ten might be made life-threateningly worse. It was not a system geared to a set of drugs whose effectiveness might be significantly affected by the quality of a patient's relationship with his doctor.

Finally, the 1962 amendments endorsed the use of randomized controlled trials as a means of showing that treatments worked. The medical community was pleased to have this piece of "science" incorporated into the regulatory process.[7] However, the RCT may yet come to be seen as a Trojan horse, the petard on which modern medicine has been hoist. RCTs are very expensive to run. Their use forced corporate development on the pharmaceutical industry, so that only those with large development budgets could maintain a place in the new marketplace. As the cost of the work escalated, running such trials ended up beyond the reach of even cooperatives of university departments, particularly when independent federal funding dried up in the 1970s. As a result, the "science" was handed over to the pharmaceutical industry.[8]

From the late 1980s, clinicians and policymakers embraced the slogans of evidence-based medicine, believing that the clinical trial exercise was still a scientific one and hoping that effective treatments would be less costly in the longer run. But as this story demonstrates, there is every ground to believe that, in the process, clinicians launched themselves on a path toward evidence-biased medicine, and that efforts to force a financial camel through the eye of a scientific needle have backfired spectacularly.[9] We are now living with the medico-legal and academic consequences of these developments, but few will link these consequences to their original cause.

THALIDOMIDE AND PROZAC IN THE DOCK

The current academic and legal difficulties center on the problem of deciding when, if ever, a drug can be said to cause an injury. The general rules for proving cause and effect were first worked out by Robert Koch in Germany in the 1880s, to answer the question of whether bacteria could be said to cause infections.[10]

Koch and his group were the first to isolate bacteria, which, by staining, they were able to make visible under the microscope. Pasteur had already claimed these germs caused infectious diseases, but no one believed him. The establishment of the day, the hygienists, believed diseases were transmitted through vapors or heredity. As a result, in the case of tuberculosis, for instance, an illness known to run in families, the hygienists saw no reason not to share a bed with a tubercular relative or friend—the body heat might even help them.[11] When Koch's group claimed the tubercle and cholera bacilli caused tuberculosis and cholera, the establishment challenged him to prove his case. When he demonstrated that there were lots of what appeared to be different kinds of bacteria under the microscope, critics argued these apparently different bacteria might simply be the same bacteria at different stages of maturity.[12]

Koch argued that several principles could point to a link between a cause, such as a drug or a bacterium, and an effect. First, if you challenge with the cause, the effect should appear. Second, remove the cause and the effect should go. Third, the greater the exposure to the cause (the higher the dose), the more likely the effect should be. Fourth, an antidote to a bacterium or a drug should reverse the effect. Fifth, if a cause infrequently leads to an effect, then the effect should not happen in the absence of this cause. Compared with diphtheria, cholera, or tubercle bacilli, for instance, HIV is much less likely to lead to a signature infection after exposure, but none of these diseases happens without the virus or bacterium.

But even in the case of cholera, exposure may not lead to the disease. Koch's bitterest opponent, Max von Pettenkoffer, set out to prove Koch wrong by drinking a brew containing millions of cholera bacilli. As luck would have it, von Pettenkoffer developed only mild diarrhea. Triumphantly, he claimed this demonstrated that disease also depended on the constitution of the individual, as well as soil and climate factors in the area in which they lived. Von Pettenkoffer survived the experiment, but Koch won the argument, and this defeat contributed to von Pettenkoffer's later suicide—an indication of how passionate things can get in the ivory tower.[13]

Most effects of drugs are clearer than those of bacteria, but some may be less clear. For example, it may be harder to show that an antidepressant makes someone who is depressed well. It was certainly much harder to prove that smoking led to lung cancer or heart disease. The smaller the effect of a drug or the longer between the intake of a drug and an effect, the greater the numbers of people who must be investigated to make sure the effect is real, because even the strangest things that drugs can do may also happen normally. The distorted limbs caused by thalidomide also happen naturally, but much less frequently.

This is where epidemiology and RCTs come into the picture. Before Koch, the hygienists had begun to survey populations to establish who was at risk from infections. The early epidemiologists could either survey the entire population of a city like London or else sample the population. In the latter case, they had to show how the samples they picked were representative of the whole population. The epidemiological maps they produced, showing which locations in the city and which classes of inhabitant were more likely to be infected, were later shown to correspond exactly with the sites of known germs, supporting Koch's claims.

Once Koch's argument about bacteria was accepted, laboratory experiments replaced epidemiological studies in courtrooms. Epidemiology was seen as too imprecise. Epidemiology established links but could not show what brought about that link. In contrast, laboratory demonstrations of bacterial growth were universally held to provide firmer evidence of cause and effect. Ronald Fisher, the father of randomized trials, for instance, claimed the epidemiology linking smoking to lung cancer proved nothing—maybe one kind of personality was more prone to both smoking and cancer.

When the effects of a drug are not clear-cut, classic epidemiological methods are too cumbersome to demonstrate a therapeutic effect. In the case of the antidepressants, thousands of subjects would be required to produce a sample representative of the general population, and these thousands would then have to be observed over time. As a way out of this type of difficulty, Austin Bradford Hill, a successor of Fisher, put forward the idea of RCTs in the late 1940s. Where before tens of thousands of patients might have been needed to control for variations for age, sex, and circumstances that might interfere with the outcome of the experiment, randomization allowed experimenters to get away in some cases with fewer than one hundred subjects.[14]

RCTs are, however, essentially a subset of epidemiological studies, which can bring weak effects into focus. If agents have strong effects, such as when an antibiotic saves a child with a life-threatening infection, nobody questions whether it works. But antidepressants never do anything remotely like this. Their beneficial effects—unlike their side effects—are weak to the point where it would be difficult to "prove" to a jury that they did indeed work without relying on the evidence of RCTs.

The best comparison is perhaps with the power of binoculars to bring into focus things that are far away. But using a pair of binoculars to see things close at hand will not work, and far from demonstrating cause and effect, RCTs can obscure just what is going on. They can show associations between antidepressant drugs and responses, but as Fisher might say, they prove nothing—we are left not knowing whether one drug is producing its effect by increasing drive (an NRI) while in another benefits patients by being anxiolytic (an SSRI).

Exclusively practicing in line with RCT evidence would, in fact, "dumb down" clinical practice. It would lead to indiscriminate prescription of antidepressants just because trials have shown antidepressants "work." This is a recipe for disaster, since the same trials have shown a considerable proportion of people get worse on treatment. Ignoring the signs that someone is getting worse during the first weeks of treatment, just because "trials have shown antidepressants work," is a case of being unable to see what is in front of your nose when looking through binoculars.[15]

Applying Koch's rules to the clinic requires challenge, dechallenge, and rechallenge (CDR) relationships; dose-response relationships; and the use of antidotes to minimize or antagonize an adverse response. All these criteria had been met for Prozac and suicide by 1991. Senior pharmacologists, epidemiologists, regulators, and company investigators from Glaxo-SmithKline, Lilly, Pfizer, and others apply these same rules when attempting to establish whether a drug is causing a problem. Over the years, many of these companies applying these methods have coded suicides as caused by their drugs even when investigators hadn't thought so. The rules also have a central place in legal manuals for the Federal Courts.[16]

Nevertheless, things don't work out straightforwardly in court. Even though pictures of the six thousand babies born limbless as a consequence of thalidomide are among the archetypal images of our times, and it would be difficult to find anyone who didn't think the drug had caused this, it was difficult to bring Chemie-Grünenthal to book. In fact, no case has ever been won against the company.[17]

Chemie-Grünenthal were able to find experts to testify there was no conclusive evidence that thalidomide caused fetal malformations. They argued that unborn babies had no legal rights anyway, and that malformations might have been caused by nuclear fallout, television rays, botched abortions by the mothers, or a failure of the body to induce the spontaneous abortions that accompany many deformities. Despite epidemiological evidence that the limb deformities stopped at the Berlin Wall, plaintiffs could not deal Chemie-Grünenthal a knockout blow without evidence of a mechanism of action by which the drug produced deformities.[18]

The American distributor, Richardson-Merrell, was found liable for failures to properly monitor distribution and take due care with a novel compound, not because thalidomide was proven in court to cause abnormalities. Richardson-Merrell also distributed the drug in Canada, where a settlement with some plaintiffs kept others in the dark as to what had happened; this ultimately led to Canadian citizens suing Richardson-Merrell in its home state of New Jersey, an action that in turn led to a settlement.[19]

No one could actually show thalidomide causing limb deformities. The same applied in tobacco-induced lung cancer cases. By the 1960s, large epidemiological studies had shown that smokers had an almost fifteen times greater risk of lung cancer than nonsmokers. The tobacco interests claimed epidemiological studies demonstrated only a link, not the firm cause and effect demonstrable in a laboratory.[20] They demanded a demonstration of tumors growing in human lungs under the influence of tobacco and regressing once that influence was removed. Demonstrating that tobacco smoking directly led to cancer in animals wasn't sufficient to establish the case—using Koch's rules, smoking hadn't been proven to cause cancer in humans.

In the case of thalidomide, the mechanism by which the drug produces deformities can now be demonstrated, so that if a new case were ever to occur, things would be quite different. Something else happened in the case of tobacco. When it became known that companies had concealed evidence that tobacco may indeed cause cancers, that nicotine was addictive, and that smoking did lead to heart attacks, the pendulum swung. Juries finally found against companies, on the basis not of proven cause and effect but on proven failures to warn. It took three decades to arrive at that point. Tobacco companies avoided directly researching the issues; to do so would increase their legal liability. Confidential documents on this issue appear to have been routed through their attorneys where, protected by attorney-client privilege, they remained inaccessible to scrutiny.[21]

THE RESURRECTION OF EPIDEMIOLOGY

The thalidomide and tobacco companies firmly rejected epidemiology as a proof of cause and effect. Only laboratory demonstrations involving CDR relationships and dose-response curves counted as causal evidence. But the next set of cases, involving Bendectin (a morning-sickness pill) and breast implants, set the dial on the medico-legal compass spinning erratically.

In the wake of thalidomide, the use of drugs in pregnancy was a sensitive issue. Bendectin, a combination of vitamin B6, dicyclomine, and doxylamine, was marketed by Merrell-Dow Pharmaceuticals for morning sickness during pregnancy.[22] Claims were made in the early 1970s that it caused birth defects. There were a large number of women who had been on Bendectin giving birth to deformed infants, and many saw a connection between the two events. William McBride, who had first raised the hazards of thalidomide, claimed to have evidence linking Bendectin to birth defects. Legal actions were taken and the plaintiffs were granted substantial awards.

These awards probably stemmed in part from perceptions in court that early laboratory work undertaken by Merrell-Dow should have resulted in more prominent warnings about potential hazards. No company should be convicted on the basis of perceptions alone, but as the tobacco cases were to show, juries convict not just on connections established in court between a drug and an injury but also on the connections established between a company and its attitudes toward profits and people.

Since it is impossible to look at CDR and dose-response relationships between a drug and injury in the course of pregnancy, epidemiological studies offered almost the only way to determine what might be going on. When done, the epidemiological studies suggested that the deformities Bendectin seemed to cause in animals did not happen in humans. This was the first time that epidemiological studies began to play a part in drug-induced injury cases.

The Bendectin cases were followed by breast implant cases.[23] During the 1980s, concern grew that implants, which had become tremendously popular, might be linked to connective tissue disorders such as rheumatoid arthritis and systemic lupus erythematosis (SLE). Implants did lead to problems such as breast scarring and breast-shape distortion in some women; no one needed either laboratory or epidemiological studies to establish this. The problem came with vague complaints of being unwell, which overlapped with the multiple aches and pains and general malaise of conditions such as SLE, in which precise diagnosis can be difficult. The companies claimed the silicone used in breast implants was an inert substance. Possibly so; but it was an unnatural substance, and one that seemed often to leak from implants into surrounding tissues. Connective tissue disorders are relatively common. In a situation where breast implants had become common and leakage from implants was common, there necessarily had to be a number of people with both connective tissue disorders and implant leaks. But were the leaks *causing* the connective tissue disorders?

Evidence was inconclusive. The courts, however, found in favor of the plaintiffs in a number of cases, leading to large settlements and punitive damages that brought Dow-Corning to the point of bankruptcy. Concern over these developments led to the establishment of independent epidemiological studies, which began to feed into the medico-legal arena just as the breast implant story peaked.

The epidemiological studies had to collect data from a large population of women with implants and a further population, identical in terms of age, socioeconomic background, ethnicity, and other factors, who did *not* have implants. The risk for connective tissue disorders should be the same in both populations. If it turned out the risk for the implanted women was greater than twice that of those without implants, an epidemiologist would conclude some basis for a claim of linkage.[24] The epidemiological studies suggested women with implants were not at twice the risk of women without. These results, although contested by many women and their attorneys, provided sufficient grounds to kill the remaining legal cases.

In the wake of this, Marcia Angell, an editor for the *New England Journal of Medicine,* wrote *Science on Trial,* which described a situation in which lawyers and plaintiffs were bringing corporations to their knees using charlatans as medico-legal experts, who engaged with the issue solely in pursuit of money. These "experts" were concocting medico-legal evidence with the appearances of science but not the substance. Tort reform became a political issue. This charade had to be stopped.

But there was a further dynamic in these cases. Although epidemiological studies did not support a cause-and-effect relation between breast implants and connective tissue disorders, the legal controversy over implants heated up once it was realized that implants had never, in fact, been tested by the FDA, any independent body, or even by the companies themselves. It had simply been assumed they were harmless. No one could offer answers on the appropriate level of warnings to accompany breast implants.

FAILURE TO WARN

At the heart of all these cases is the issue of warnings. In the case of thalidomide, the refusal of the company to accept the need for warnings fueled anger. In the case of the tobacco companies, what stuck in the gullet of many people was not that tobacco smoking was addictive or that smoking caused lung cancer or other disorders. It was a free world. But even in a free world, it is appropriate to issue warnings commensurate with the evidence. Warnings are what guarantee relative freedom. But these were exactly what the industry failed to offer. In the case of Bendectin, early laboratory studies had warranted a greater level of warnings than the science finally suggested. The same applied to the lawsuits taken by Vietnam vets after exposure to Agent Orange. It may well be that few, if any, vets developed disorders as a direct result of exposure to Agent Orange, but they were not warned of *any* possible health hazards.

Another set of cases centering on claims about psychotherapy bring out this issue very clearly. Proving cause and effect in the psychotherapy arena provides a real challenge. It is not possible to conduct CDR or dose-response relationships with psychotherapy. Epidemiological studies on the impact of psychotherapies have never been undertaken and may be impossible. How, then, can defendants ever be convicted?

Perhaps the single most famous psychotherapy case involved a surgeon, Rafael Osheroff, who became depressed in 1979.[25] He sought help from a variety of sources and responded inconclusively to a number of antidepressants. In 1981 he entered Baltimore's Chestnut Lodge, a psychoanalytically oriented institution. There he was diagnosed with a narcissistic personality disorder and engaged in therapy. During a nine-month stay he lost fifty-six pounds. He lost his job. His marriage broke up. His feet began to bleed from agitated pacing. Osheroff's therapists reviewed his case a number of times but did not change their approach. He was finally liberated by a family friend and taken to Silver Hill Hospital, where he was diagnosed as having depression. He was put on antidepressants, responded, and was discharged home within three months. He resumed work, remarried, and took legal action against Chestnut Lodge.

The issues in this case hinged not on whether psychotherapy could be shown to injure, nor even on whether it could be shown to work, but on the failure of the Chestnut Lodge therapists to provide Osheroff with information about other therapeutic possibilities. They demonstrated inflexibility in the face of his deterioration and failed to warn either him or others that deterioration of this sort could occur, while other approaches might minimize these risks. In the end, Chestnut Lodge accepted liability.

This matter of responsibly informing patients also lies at the heart of recovered-memory litigation. Plaintiffs charged therapists with wrecking families by "recovering" memories of nonexistent abuse. Juries can never know for certain whether abuse actually occurred. Many may have doubts about the men in these cases. The therapists will usually seem decent citizens concerned to bring to light serious injuries done to their patients. In practice, it is all but impossible to win a case against a decent therapist pursuing a hunch of abuse, provided the therapist behaved reasonably. But what is "reasonable" behavior in this context? It means warning patients or their families prior to engaging on a therapeutic course. It means maintaining an open mind on the issues, especially when a patient deteriorates. The practice of inflexibly explaining away deterioration as a consequence of abuse rather than the therapy was what led juries to convict.

INTO THE PROZAC, PAXIL, AND ZOLOFT MAELSTROM

The SSRI cases happened at a key point in this medico-legal trajectory. Prozac was implicated by a set of CDR and dose-response studies, as well as company documents indicating prior knowledge of injury. But in *Forsyth,* the traditional documents that might have convicted the company were forced out of the trial by Lilly's insistence on their irrelevance to the science at stake. This argument reached its logical conclusion in *Tobin vs. SmithKline,* when Ian Hudson argued for the company that no matter what company personnel might have conceded about cause and effect, their statements were meaningless unless RCTs had proven a link. Against a background of not doing any RCTs or epidemiology to look at this issue, this is a misuse of science of Orwellian or catch-22 proportions.

After *Forsyth,* Lilly, SmithKline, and Pfizer changed tack and contested the validity of my involvement on grounds that CDR and dose-response links between SSRIs and suicide were not the relevant scientific evidence—RCTs and epidemiology were the relevant evidence.

The new company challenge led to a series of Daubert hearings.[26] Daubert hearings stem from the response of the American legal system to the Bendectin cases, a now famous *Daubert vs. Merrell-Dow* ruling.[27] The key issue was how to ensure good science was brought to bear on a medico-legal issue. The case that set the legal ground rules in other areas of science was *Frye vs. United States,* which stated that if a scientific expert's views were to be taken into account in a case, those views had to be "generally accepted" within the expert's field. In 1975, a new set of Federal Rules of Evidence stated instead that expert input had to be "relevant."[28]

Merrell-Dow challenged the new Federal Rules of Evidence, demanding a return to *Frye.* Its argument was that if there had been decent science from the start, many judgments made against the company would not have happened. Merrell-Dow lost the case. The *Daubert* ruling upheld the new Federal Rules of Evidence. This gave district courts discretion to decide whether the scientific evidence brought to bear on the case was appropriate.

But how was a judge to decide this? Lawyers for pharmaceutical companies might repeatedly force a judge to make decisions about relevance, pushing her into territory she would not be familiar with—and where, for a variety of historical reasons, she would find signposts and experts saying that RCTs and epidemiological studies are the way to prove cause and effect. This was the problem facing Kathryn Vratil in *Miller vs. Pfizer.*[29]

The *Forsyth* case against Lilly had looked strong, given the range of company documents, and an extensive series of articles by senior investigators outlined CDR and dose-response links between Prozac and suicidality and the fact that antidotes could block this hazard. Epidemiological evidence from the Jick and other studies pointed in a similar direction. By the time Paxil and Zoloft came to the market, further descriptions of SSRI-induced akathisia or suicidality were no longer scientific news. In any normal scientific universe, the next step was RCTs and epidemiological studies—not to prove something was happening but rather to quantify the *extent* to which it was happening.

But this was not a normal scientific universe. The upshot was that there were no good CDR or dose-response studies between Zoloft or Paxil and suicidality, nor any RCTs or epidemiological studies. Any argument would have to lean heavily on the precedent of Prozac-induced suicidality and, in the *Miller* case involving Zoloft, an article by Roger

Lane of Pfizer that appeared to state very definitely that SSRIs can cause akathisia and that akathisia can lead to suicide.[30]

In *Miller*, Pfizer challenged the plaintiff's lawyers with a set of interrogatories to admit they knew of no RCT or epidemiological evidence showing that Zoloft could cause akathisia, that it could cause emotional indifference, or that it could cause psychotic decompensation; or that akathisia could lead to suicide; or that emotional indifference could lead to suicide; or that psychotic decompensation could lead to suicide; or that Zoloft could lead to suicide.

In addition, Pfizer wanted RCT or epidemiological evidence demonstrating a relative risk greater than 2.0 that any of the above could occur. This requirement had possibly been plucked straight from the pages of Marcia Angell's book. But it was inappropriate. If whooping cough vaccination posed even one-tenth the relative risk of nonvaccination, this evidence would be sufficient to prove that the vaccine *causes* brain damage. In the case of the older antidepressants, the relative risk of suicidality from clinical trials is around half that found with placebo, but even so, a considerable body of clinical opinion holds that while these drugs may reduce the risk of suicide overall, they can trigger suicidality in some. The notion of relative risk is potentially meaningless when a drug can both cause and alleviate a condition. In the case of breast implants, a risk criterion of 2.0 worked because no one ever suggested that implants could *reduce* the risk of connective tissue disease.

The ultimate irony in the SSRI cases lies in the comparison with the tobacco cases. On the one hand, lawyers argue that epidemiological studies "prove" nothing.[31] They want someone to show a jury a cancer growing in front of their eyes in a human lung under the influence of tobacco. Nothing else constitutes proof. On the other hand, in the SSRI cases, suicide is seen to grow under the influence of the drug in front of people's eyes, but (in some cases) the same legal firms who advised the tobacco companies argue this is not proof. What do they want instead? They want epidemiological studies. But these expensive studies put justice out of reach of plaintiffs, as the only bodies that can afford to undertake them are pharmaceutical companies.

In *Miller*, Judge Vratil, faced with Pfizer's arguments, characterized this view as "extreme and incredible. Pfizer's view of the applicable 'science' is heavily slanted towards its self-interest."[32] But Judge Vratil was in a bind. While there are no statements anywhere to say that RCTs are the right way to handle this kind of problem, there are equally no statements anywhere (other than right here) that RCTs are not the gold standard for this kind of problem.

Vickery suggested the court appoint an independent expert. Judge Vratil agreed. Pfizer knocked back a series of suggestions before agreeing to the appointment of John Davis from Chicago, who had been on the original FDA panel approving Zoloft. Pfizer subsequently lobbied for the addition of John Concato from Yale. As Pfizer's challenge was to my inclusion, Judge Vratil asked Davis and Concato to answer a set of very specific questions regarding my suitability to testify as an expert witness. There were no questions about Pfizer's use of the scientific evidence, which she herself characterized as self-serving, extreme, and incredible.

Davis's and Concato's consideration of the issues took a full year, at which point they returned a view that mine was a minority view, and that they had been unable to replicate a calculation I had derived from Pfizer's trials that Zoloft was 2.19 times more likely to lead to suicidality than placebo. This led to a hearing in Kansas in November 2001, at which Dr. Concato agreed that a risk criterion for suicide of 2.0 made no sense in the case of an antidepressant.[33] Despite this, and despite the court becoming aware in the midst of the hearing that Pfizer had manipulated their RCT data, Judge Vratil dismissed me as an expert witness for the plaintiffs. Had it not been for a set of parallel developments, this Daubert hearing might have knocked out all legal actions against the SSRI companies.

The parallel developments came linked to *Tobin vs. SmithKline.* Whereas when my report in *Miller vs. Pfizer* was first written no one had much to go on except a strong case, a Prozac template and an incriminating article from the company, by the time the *Tobin* case took shape, our Zoloft study had led me to Pfizer's and SmithKline's healthy volunteer archives, and a treasure trove of data had turned up from an unexpected source.

In the late 1990s, the FDA was under considerable pressure to scrap placebos in antidepressant trials. Concerns had been expressed about the ethics of exposing patients at risk of suicide to a nontreatment.[34] There was probably at least as great a set of unexpressed embarrassments at how poorly antidepressants did compared to placebo. This led to an article by Arif Khan and colleagues in the *Archives of General Psychiatry* in April 2000,[35] which presented figures for suicides and suicidal

acts from clinical trials submitted to the FDA in the early 1990s as part
of the license applications for Zoloft, Paxil, Serzone, Wellbutrin, and Remeron. Based on the figures they accessed (Table 1), Khan and colleagues were happy to tell the world that placebos did not pose a
threat—the rate of suicidal acts was no higher on placebo than on active
antidepressants. Paul Leber, among others, was invited by *Archives* to
comment and welcomed the findings.

Table I
Suicides and Suicide Attempts in FDA Antidepressant Trials

Drug (Patient No.)	Patient Exposure Years	Suicide No.	Attempt No. Suicide
Zoloft (2053)	508	2	9
Active comparator (595)	91	0	1
Placebo (786)	209	0	5
Paxil (2963)	1008	5	40
Active comparator (1151)	218	3	12
Placebo (554)	72	2	6
Serzone (3496)	1018	9	12
Active comparator (958)	225	0	6
Placebo (875)	204	0	1
Remeron (2425)	672	8	29
Active comparator (977)	195	2	6
Placebo (494)	71	0	3
Wellbutrin (1942)	—	3	—
Placebo (370)	—	0	—
All New Drugs (12879)	3206	27	90
Active comparator (3681)	729	5	25
Placebo (3079)	556	2	15
TOTAL (19639)	4491	34	130

But, insofar as these figures exonerated placebo, they should have
posed a problem for anyone who advocated using SSRIs to detect and
treat depression in order to avoid the risk of suicide. An analysis of
these figures by Tom Laughren from the FDA shows antidepressants
were twice as likely as placebo to be associated with suicide attempts.[36]
Yet the figures didn't seem to bother Laughren or anyone else.

But, in attempting to get Prozac on the market, Lilly had labeled as
"placebo suicides" suicides that occurred when patients weren't actually on placebos.[37] Could SmithKline or Pfizer have done the same
thing? It turned out they had, and no one needed to access any sealed

company archives to find this out. Sitting in FDA files were reviews by FDA officials Hilary Lee, in the case of Zoloft,[38] and Martin Brecher, in the case of Paxil,[39] that made it clear that up to 50 percent of Pfizer's and SmithKline's placebo suicides and suicide attempts had, in fact, occurred when patients had been stopped from prior treatment, and before beginning either the new experimental treatment or placebo. Correcting for this, and adding in comparable data for Prozac,[40] Celexa,[41] and Efexor, leads to Table 2:

Table 2
Suicides and Suicide Attempts in FDA Antidepressant Trials[42]

Drug	Patient No.	Suicide No.	Suicide Attempt No.	Suicides and Attempts as a %
Zoloft	2053	2	7	0.44%
Active comparator	595	0	1	0.17%
Placebo	786	0	2	0.25%
Withdrawal from Prior Drug		0	3	
Paxil	2963	5	42	1.59%
Active comparator	1151	3	12	1.30%
Placebo	554	0	3	0.54%
Withdrawal from Prior Drug		2	2	
Serzone	3496	9	12	0.60%
Active comparator	958	0	6	0.63%
Placebo	875	0	1	0.11%
Remeron	2425	8	29	1.53%
Active comparator	977	2	6	0.82%
Placebo	494	0	3	0.61%
Celexa	4168	8	91	2.38%
Placebo	691	1	10	1.59%
Prozac	1427	1	12	0.91%
Placebo	370	0	0	0.00%
Withdrawal from Prior Drug		1	0	
Efexor	3082	7	36	1.40%
Placebo	739	1	2	0.41%
All New Antidepressants	19,613	40	229	1.37%
All SSRIs	13,693	23	188	1.54%
Active comparator	3681	5	25	0.82%
Total Placebo	4509	2	21	0.51%
SSRI Placebo	3140	2	17	0.61%

What should be immediately obvious from the new figures is that there are far fewer suicides and suicide attempts on placebo. Indeed, given the track record of miscoding in Zoloft, Paxil, and Prozac trials, there can be little confidence that the placebo suicides and attempts in the Celexa or Efexor trials are true suicides or suicide attempts.

With these new figures, the rates for suicides and for suicidal acts on SSRIs or for all new antidepressants is roughly 2.5 times greater than for placebo, and these differences are statistically significantly.[43]

When the issue was the ethics of placebos, it was appropriate for Khan to calculate the data in terms of the length of exposure to placebo, as there was no reason to believe that suicides would happen at any particular point during exposure to placebo. But using patient exposure years for the SSRIs, as the companies have done, produces what can be termed a "space shuttle fallacy." If we estimate the number of deaths per mile covered by astronauts, traveling in space shuttles is probably safer than, for most of us, walking around our houses. This magical transformation of the space shuttle into something ultrasafe is achieved by discounting the fact that there are particular risk periods to being on space shuttles—the stages of exit and reentry.

Just the same applies to the SSRIs, which means that calculating suicidal acts in terms of the numbers of patients going on the drugs is more appropriate. In fact, calculating side effects in terms of the absolute numbers of patients was the traditional means of looking at all side effects until the late 1980s, when the FDA suggested that companies might want to analyze the data in terms of both absolute numbers and duration of exposure. When they did this, Lilly discovered their suicide data looked better when set against duration of exposure.

These figures and the methods of handling the data raise a host of questions. First, FDA officials reviewing the evidence were aware that some of these suicidal acts occurred during the phase of trials involving withdrawal from prior treatment yet did not object to them being categorized as placebo.[44] This presumably applied to European and Canadian regulators also.

Second, given FDA instructions to calculate their data by absolute numbers as well as by exposure, all these companies at some point generated figures that indicated that the risk of suicidal acts on their drugs was double that of placebo. Furthermore, these Paxil and Zoloft data were lying on FDA desks while the Prozac crisis was playing out in the public domain.

Third, the figures point to hazards on withdrawing from antidepressants. The washout period is that point in time after someone agrees to enter a clinical trial where, if they are on other treatment, they are told they must have a week drug-free before they can enter the new trial. This week withdrawing from previous treatment appears to be a particularly hazardous time. Stopping antidepressants is not as innocuous as most psychiatrists would have thought—not at all like switching from vitamin A to vitamin C.

Fourth, ghosts seem to be surfacing in the machinery. In the *Tobin* case, SmithKline appealed to studies—apparently analyzing the Paxil clinical trial data—by Stuart Montgomery,[45] and Juan Lopez-Ibor,[46] a former president of the World Psychiatric Association, to support their case. Montgomery and Lopez-Ibor's articles produced the same figures Khan offered, which seems to indicate that these authors did not see the raw data, had their articles ghostwritten, or were complicit in an unacceptable manipulation of the data.

Companies rationalize the counting of washout suicides as placebo suicides by arguing that placebo is "nothing" and therefore, in some real sense, patients on nothing are equivalent to patients on placebo. If we join the companies in categorizing washout suicidal acts this way, then the number of people who have gone on to placebo in these trials becomes the entire number of people who have gone into the trial. Once the calculations take this into account, rather than double the risk, Zoloft, Paxil, or Prozac becomes three to ten times more likely to trigger suicide than placebo.

These new figures transform the SSRI debate. Previously, the presumption was that only a small group of patients react poorly to SSRIs, while most are helped. Were this the case, in trials of antidepressants, if the number of patients saved from suicide outnumbered the patients made worse, the relative risk would be less than 1.0. In this scenario, working out whether there was a small subgroup of patients made worse by the drug would require a specifically designed clinical trial of the type Lilly and the FDA spent a year working on. These new figures, however, mean that complex trials of this sort just aren't necessary. Simply including sensitive suicidal ideation scales in standard trials would settle the issue.

It turns out there are yet more disturbing figures. In the *Forsyth* trial, Lilly appealed to data from the Drugs Safety Research Unit (DSRU) in Southampton, which, it claimed, showed no problem with Prozac. The DSRU undertakes postmarketing surveillance of drugs following their launch in the United Kingdom, in which they record data from cohorts of twelve thousand to thirteen thousand patients. In the case of the suicides in Table 3, Lilly claimed these figures exonerated Prozac because figures for Prozac, Paxil, Zoloft, and Luvox were essentially the same.

Table 3
DSRU Studies of SSRIs in Primary Care in the United Kingdom[47]

Drug	No. Patients	No. Suicides	Suicide Rate/100,000 Patients
Prozac	12692	31	244 (C.I. 168 – 340)
Zoloft	12734	22	173 (C.I. 110 – 255)
Paxil	13741	37	269 (C.I. 192 – 365)
Luvox	10983	20	183 (C.I. 114 – 274)
Total SSRIs	50150	110	219/100,000

These figures of 219 suicides per 100,000 people treated map almost exactly onto the figures from SSRI trials, which give 180 suicides per 100,000 people treated. This suicide rate of 180 needs to be compared with the rate for primary-care patients, which the Jick and Boardman studies (outlined in Chapter 3) suggest could be as low as 27 suicides per 100,000 patients and cannot be any higher than 68 per 100,000 patients. Company trials also give a placebo suicide rate lying between 44 and 64 per 100,000 patients. There seems, therefore, in primary-care depression to be a suicide rate of approximately 180 out of 100,000 on SSRIs, which, set against with a rate of 60 out of 100,000, suggests a doubling or tripling of the risk on SSRIs compared to placebo or nontreatment.[48]

On every conceivable ground, therefore, from CDR and dose-response relationships to RCTs and epidemiology, along with internal company assessments of causality, the evidence indicates that warnings on the SSRIs would save lives. But, quite aside from the warnings mandated by this evidence, this use of epidemiology, RCTs, and mistaken notions of relative risk by companies and their lawyers is wrong. If the case against the SSRIs had not been so clear-cut, it is difficult to know what the legal consequences would have been. For example, if the drugs did induce suicide in some but saved more than they killed, it is difficult to see how any plaintiff could have ever gotten justice. It is horrifying when expert witnesses parade junk science before juries in order to bankrupt corporations and create mass hysteria. But it is an equal evil—and potentially even more dangerous—for science to be used in a manner that puts justice out of reach of any plaintiff.

Completely unnoticed to most lawyers and academics, following a change in FDA requirements in the mid-1990s, as of 2000, SSRI companies began to report intentional overdose and suicide attempts as adverse effects linked to treatment. Although the evidence for this linkage comes from RCTs, the FDA does not allow anyone to say the drugs have caused these effects and has not required the companies to warn of such effects. Why not? It would seem the FDA has taken a position with significant medico-legal ramifications: namely, that RCTs do not offer evidence of causality in this domain.[49]

When SmithKline mounted a Daubert challenge to the adequacy of my report, both before the *Tobin* trial and again after the trial, Judge Beaman found against them.[50] The resulting trial found against SmithKline, a first verdict against a pharmaceutical company for a psychiatric side effect of a psychotropic drug. Several further Daubert and Frye hearings have confirmed the legal acceptability of the arguments being put forward here, and a large number of cases involving Paxil and Prozac have since settled.

CORPORATE CHUTZPAH

The medico-legal difficulties facing plaintiffs outlined here are compounded by a legal jeopardy that stems from the nonrecording of drug-induced side effects such as akathisia, disinhibition, and emotional blunting, which makes certain side effects all but vanish. We expect marketing departments to make side effects vanish. For example, although nobody thought the figure for sexual dysfunction on Prozac could be as high as 50 percent, everybody knew it was probably more than Lilly's figure of 5 percent.[51] What is unacceptable is for medical experts offering views on behalf of a company to bamboozle courts into thinking that the figure for sexual dysfunction is only 5 percent because this is what RCTs have shown; or for those experts to argue that the absence of figures on suicidal ideation collected with the appropriate instruments means no patients became suicidal.

If Lilly is going to make the side effects of Prozac vanish, in an ideal marketplace competitor companies will make them reappear. The risk with leaving truth and justice to the marketplace is that drugs often come to the market in groups, so that all antidepressants on patent may be SSRIs. This raises the nightmare scenario that no company would have an incentive to investigate a hazard with a particular drug, which appears to be what happened with the SSRIs.

The patenting system was supposed to encourage innovative compounds,[52] but obviously, things cannot proceed any faster than the speed of the science on which developments depend. In the case of the SSRIs, ACE inhibitors, calcium channel blockers, and other agents, patenting in practice leads all companies to produce similar compounds at the same time. In legal terms, this is a disaster. Market forces can safeguard the consumer only if new compounds are up against genuine competitors.

The current patent laws do something else as well. To encourage innovation, patents offer companies the chance to recover their development costs and make a profit. With Prozac and other drugs in the 1990s, this arrangement encouraged companies to recoup their investment costs by developing blockbuster drugs rather a wider range of useful but less profitable compounds. This gives rise to a situation such as that described by a memo from Lilly's Leigh Thompson on February 7, 1990, before the Teicher controversy broke:

> I am concerned about reports I get re UK attitude toward Prozac's safety. Leber suggested a few minutes ago we use CSM database to compare Prozac aggression, suicidal ideation with other antidepressants in the UK. Although he is a fan of Prozac and believes a lot of this is garbage, he is clearly a political creature and will have to respond to pressures. I hope Patrick realizes that Lilly can go down the tubes if we lose Prozac and just one event in the UK can cost us that.[53]

This is not a comfortable situation for consumers or prescribers of the drug, regulators, or even company executives. The current patent system produces great profits, not great innovation.[54] It also creates great responsibilities. Astra, Rhône-Poulenc, Hoechst, and other companies have withdrawn antidepressants from the marketplace because of this. But if a drug is producing a side effect that could be blamed on the illness, what way will the pharmaceutical company executive jump if her company risks going down the tubes? Few people reading this book could say for sure what they would do in the circumstances.

Whether or not Prozac causes suicide, or Lilly overstepped the bounds in defending Prozac, the current system makes it all but certain that at some point a company will overstep the bounds, and a preventable public health disaster will result.

This state of legal jeopardy in which we find ourselves could be solved relatively simply. The IRBs scrutinizing trial protocols might insist that consent forms include a statement that the data on side effects can be used for marketing purposes only, and not for academic or legal purposes. Industry would listen because a great number of people working in companies recognize the wrong in this situation, whatever the legal advice of company lawyers. It would be a simple matter to collect side effects differently and properly—if the confidence of the marketplace depended on it. This would add no extra bureaucracy or red tape. Another solution might be for patient cooperatives to take over the design and management of clinical trials. None of these are likely to happen in America, where private IRBs have sprung up in recent years, often run by the same companies who run the clinical trials for pharmaceutical companies.[55] It may take a European country or Canada to safeguard the legal rights of American citizens.

An alternative might be for companies to allow independent experts access to their data. This is the norm for science. It is expected that investigators can give raw data to any other scientist who asks for it. But requests for such data made to any of the SSRI companies are knocked back.[56] The data are proprietary, owned by the company. According to conventional understandings of science, ownership without disclosure makes all data technical rather than scientific data.

WHO KNEW WHAT WHEN?

The systems Lilly and other companies use to decide on cause and effect require monitoring for CDR and dose-response relationships. These produced internal judgments of a probable relationship between suicide and Prozac, Paxil, and Zoloft by 1990, and at least implicit judgments of a causal relationship in the mid-1980s in the course of healthy volunteer and other studies.

A strategy to handle this was probably settled in Lilly sometime in the mid-1980s. A memo from March 29, 1985, reads:

> The incidence rate [of suicidal acts] under fluoxetine therefore purely mathematically is 5.6 times higher than under the other active medication imipramine. . . . The benefits vs. risks consideration for fluoxetine currently does not fall clearly in favor of the benefits. Therefore it is of the greatest importance that it be determined whether there is a particular subgroup of patients who respond better to fluoxetine than to imipramine, so that the higher incidence of suicide attempts may be tolerable.[57]

The strategy may mistakenly have been to focus on milder depressions, in the belief that these patients were least at risk.

There is scope within the time frame for Lilly to have misread the shift of the sands. When Prozac was being developed, no one anticipated that the depression market would become what it did, or that all the Valium cases would become Prozac cases, or that mildly depressed persons, far from being at no risk of suicide on Prozac, were actually probably most at risk from the drug. It may have been an unfortunate accident that the first reports came from a tertiary referral center such as McLean Hospital, rather than from a clinic with a set of uncomplicated cases. Subsequently, the other SSRI companies had the example set by Lilly beckoning them in one direction.

Could key employees in a company like Lilly have been expected to appreciate the scale of the public health disaster ahead of them, or to demonstrate the wit to avoid getting locked into it? Right up to the end, it would have been possible to persuade oneself that the drug was going to be sold to people not likely to commit suicide, or that even if some people did commit suicide, ultimately more good than harm would be done. At the very worst, the company was making a contribution to psychiatry—rock this boat, and who knew what future benefits to humankind might be lost? Once they were locked into an evolving story, lawyers would have told them there was no way out. The vast majority of company employees will have known nothing about what went on and felt genuinely under threat from fringe groups. They will have found it as easy as psychiatrists did to believe that the greatest tragedy in the Prozac story was all those people denied effective treatment because of protests.

A rapid turnover of people within companies contributed to what happened. Time and again in the *Wesbecker* case, Smith and Zettler handed Lilly employees documents from their own files, only to have them deny all knowledge of the contents or any ability to speak to what they might really mean. Faced with papers he had inherited from Joachim Wernicke's files, Wheadon refused to speculate, as did Wernicke when faced with papers from Paul Stark's files before him.[58] This behavior was not confined to Lilly. During a later consideration of Paxil, Laughren of the FDA denied detailed knowledge of the significance of a healthy volunteer study on Paxil showing problematic side effects, on the basis that he had inherited this file from Martin Brecher.[59]

Does this amount to a conspiracy? This story has everything conspiracy buffs could want: smoking-gun memos that reach into the heart of the FDA; a perfect set of motives; and sets of mirrors that make it difficult to work out who are the good guys and who the bad.

Prozac had licensing difficulties. It was held up for many years in Germany and only finally licensed after some apparently unorthodox lobbying of supposedly independent regulatory panel members.[60] In the United States, difficulties with the Prozac trials gave rise to the new concept of a failed trial. In the course of the various problems before and after launch, executives from Lilly had access to the head of the CNS Division outside work hours and to FDA Director David Kessler at his home.[61] Whether this favored access solved or created further problems is a key issue.[62]

A lot depends on how one interprets what Lilly told the FDA about the assessments of Prozac in Germany. In a letter to Lilly on September 9, 1987, indicating Prozac was approvable, Robert Temple of the FDA wrote:

> We require a review of the status of all fluoxetine actions taken or pending before foreign regulatory authorities. Approval actions can be noted, but we ask that you describe in detail any and all actions taken that have been negative, supplying a full explanation of the views of all parties and the resolution of the matter.[63]

In response, on October 2, 1987, Lilly submitted a series of reports, including one from the German regulatory body, the BGA.[64] The first point (1.0) the Germans made was "the drug is not sufficiently tested . . . and the therapeutic efficacy claimed for [Prozac] is insufficiently substantiated." The second point (2.0) referred to Prozac's: "unacceptable damaging effects." Following this, under 2.1, the BGA noted that "[an] increase in agitating effect occurs earlier than the mood elevating effect and therefore an increased risk of suicide exists." Under 2.2, the BGA noted that during treatment with the drugs "some symptoms of the underlying disease (anxiety, insomnia, agitation) increase, which as adverse effects exceed those which are considered acceptable by medical standards." The letter containing all this was sent to the FDA by Max Talbott, Lilly's regulatory adviser, a former FDA employee himself.

It is not clear what the FDA understood "unacceptable damaging effects" to mean, or whose job it was—Lilly's or the FDA's—to make sure the FDA understood.[65] The FDA routinely sends letters to companies prior to approving drugs, asking to be fully informed about any decisions made by foreign regulators. There were apparently phone calls between Laughren and Richard Kapit of the FDA and members of Lilly, which led to a letter from Talbott on December 4, stating, "In February 1985 . . . the BGA had alluded to 'unacceptable damaging effects.' . . . This phrase was not defined."[66] He went on to say that "the data submitted to the BGA have also been submitted to the FDA, which has reviewed data on more patients using more sophisticated analyses than those submitted to the BGA up to this time."

A memo from Richard Kapit on December 8 records receipt of this letter, the teleconference that had given rise to it, and the assertion that the

> German authorities never defined or documented the phrases "severe organ damage" or "unacceptable damaging effect." The company asserts that all information made available to the BGA has been made available to the FDA. . . . Conclusion: the BGA comments do not appear to reflect clinical events, since no such events have been reported to the FDA and according to the company we have received all information submitted to the BGA. Recommendation: The comments by the BGA should not affect FDA's conclusion that NDA 18-936 is approvable.[67]

By the end of December, Prozac had been approved.

Nearly seven years later, having claimed that if he even overheard someone report a side effect of Prozac in a corridor at a party he would report it to the FDA, Leigh Thompson was confronted by Nancy Zettler with this issue in the course of his deposition in the *Wesbecker* case:

Q. Do you feel that you have an obligation to report the fact that the German government raised the issue and that it was fully analyzed back in 1984 or '85?

A. I would probably call on my legal colleagues to help me interpret it, but under the current NDA [new drug application] regulation, I think the current NDA regulation does request information on negative findings by other regulators. But what that means has never been tested in court in terms of whether that is just a letter that you receive from the BGA saying we're not going to approve your drug, or whether it means everything that you talk about in working up whatever their questions are. I'm not aware that that's ever been resolved.

Q. So let me make sure I understand. You feel it is your absolute duty to report a conversation that you have overheard in the hallway, but you don't necessarily feel it's your duty to report an issue raised by another regulatory agency and the analyses that were done by the drug company in response to that issue being raised?

A. Under the FDA laws and regulations, I think you've stated it correctly.[68]

It seems fairly evident what the "unacceptable damaging effects" were. It is not clear that the FDA sought or received advice from anyone on this point. There is no record of what any of these FDA officials made of the testimony of Joachim Wernicke, a key player at Lilly in steering Prozac through the FDA, who, faced with this very point in the *Wesbecker* trial, acknowledged that a mistake had been made.[69]

In these circumstances, someone who depends on regulators such as the FDA for protection will feel let down and think the agency must have somehow reneged on its duties. But it was never envisaged that the FDA should offer this kind of protection. It is not clear that, if the FDA were to vanish, we would be at any greater risk. The ultimate determinant of what happens lies not in FDA scrutiny but in a company's calculations about how a new drug will be evaluated, and that includes an estimate of how the medical profession is likely to respond. Companies, not regulators, bring drugs onto the market.

This being said, it is worrying to find apparent FDA agreement to let SSRI companies manipulate the figures for suicidal acts. It is worrying that they have apparently not required the companies to present the data in terms of both absolute numbers of patients and patient exposure years, as mandated by their own recommendations. It is worrying to find FDA officials contacting company officers outside official channels on issues such as suicide on SSRIs.

In terms of professional organizational responsibility, DART of the APA and Defeat Depression of the Royal College of Psychiatrists (RCP) began as small, minimally funded campaigns, organized by a few people who really did think that increased recognition of depression might make a difference for the better. None of those involved could have possessed any inkling that far from decreasing suicide rates, their actions might have had the opposite effect. They had almost no reason to think that the relatively small amounts of money they got from pharmaceutical companies such as Lilly compromised them. But if this is true of the small ginger groups of clinicians within APA and RCP responsible for these campaigns, it is not as clear that these professional bodies can be completely exonerated, given that it is our collective duty to speak out about hazards.

One of the many chilling things about the Prozac story is that a mistake or a conspiracy would probably have cost fewer lives. Instead, a sequence of historical events made a poor drug fashionable, made the treatment of an illness all but a matter of public policy, and removed the natural cautions and safeguards that should have saved us. In the midst of this, the one group with a professional brief, because of prescription-only arrangements, to save us from ourselves—physicians—appears to have followed its self-interest as much, if not more, than any other party to the story.

BUSTED FLAT

Methods by which plaintiffs can pursue legal redress differ across nations. The American system involves a "no win, no fee" system that its critics maintain gives rise to frivolous legal actions. Until recently in the United Kingdom, it was possible for the average plaintiff to access free legal aid if in need of such support. Although the UK system led to far fewer legal actions than in the United States, nevertheless the government perceived the cost as excessive, and following the election of a socialist government in 1997, there was a move toward a "no win, no fee" system.

In the United States, "no win, no fee" has meant that when plaintiffs lose, their legal firms have to swallow their costs. These can be substantial. It takes on the order of $250,000 to bring an SSRI case to court, given the Daubert and other motions that must be responded to and the need for a slate of experts to cover the science, from psychopharmacology to drug company data handling and clinical issues. The standard view is that a firm has to lose several such cases before it finds out how to handle one. The price for getting into the game is therefore up to a million dollars. At this kind of price, there will be few, if any, frivolous actions.

If a plaintiff and a legal firm commit to an action, the difficulties they face are anything but frivolous. As Vickery's Web site put it:

> Our responsibility—which we take very seriously—is to discourage litigation in all but the most egregious cases. Involving yourself in a lawsuit with defendants with unlimited resources is a mammoth undertaking, sapping most of your emotional, spiritual and economic resources. In the face of tragedy these resources are already seriously depleted. Our experience is that pharmaceutical companies will do virtually anything to protect their multibillion dollar drugs. When you sue them, their lawyers will open virtually every closet door in your life and microscopically examine every skeleton. Every aspect of your life—a spouse's drinking problem, a daughter's abortion, problems at work—will be blamed for what their drug might have caused. Its not a bit overstating the rigors of litigation to tell you that the process itself might just be worse than the tragedy that caused the filing of the claim.[70]

In the case of Matt Miller, the family had to put up with investigators from Pfizer sampling the carpet and other furnishings for traces of semen in pursuit of a medico-legal kite the company was flying, namely, that this 13-year-old boy had in fact died when the autoerotic asphyxiation he was engaged in went wrong.

Under the UK, Canadian, and European systems, when plaintiffs lose they are liable for not only their own costs but those of the defendant as well. In the case of pharmaceutical companies, who typically retain the services of ten or more experts and may have several legal offices involved in filing sheaves of briefs, the costs are so great that simply insuring a legal office against losing a case might require a premium of millions of dollars.[71] This system appears designed to maintain a tradition, in Europe and the English-speaking world, of never recording verdicts against pharmaceutical companies.

Vickery had been profoundly depressed after the *Forsyth* case. In the *Miller* case, his idea of commissioning an independent report backfired and nearly sank any further legal actions. While he won the *Tobin* verdict, SmithKline appealed to the U.S. Tenth Circuit Court and was entitled to appeal to the Supreme Court if they lost in the Circuit Court. An appeal process can take several years. There was no onus on the company to pay any monies until all appeals were exhausted. It was obvious that Vickery's resources to fight actions were limited, given that experts working for him were unpaid. To keep his partnership with Paul Waldner going, he and Waldner cashed in pension plans and raised money in other ways. One option for Vickery in these circumstances was to sell part of his verdict on a greatly reduced basis to companies that make a living out of buying portions of verdicts. He did this. Nevertheless, in mid-December 2001 the Vickery-Waldner partnership dissolved. He let his paralegal, Rhonda Hawkins, go. His tax liabilities looked likely to force him to file for bankruptcy.

After the *Tobin* verdict, Vickery filed a collateral estoppel motion, which, had it succeeded, would have meant he would not have had to argue for general causation in any further Paxil cases. It would have greatly reduced his legal overheads. But he lost this motion in the face of SmithKline's argument that suicide on SSRIs was a class effect and, since the *Forsyth* trial had ended in a verdict for the defendant, collateral estoppel was inappropriate. This was ironic in that the key to SmithKline's defense in *Tobin,* and Pfizer's defense in *Miller,* was that a phenomenon claimed to occur on Prozac should not be assumed to occur on any other drugs in the SSRI group.

But in December 2001, SmithKline withdrew their appeal in *Tobin* and settled this and a number of other cases with Vickery and other lawyers. While the terms of the settlement involved a return of all confidential material, the fact of a settlement meant that legal actions would continue, including my action to find out what had happened in Toronto, filed in September 2001.

10

Let Them Eat Prozac

IN 1966, the *New England Journal of Medicine* published an unusual article. The author, Henry Beecher, was a professor of anesthesia at Harvard. The article had previously been rejected by the *Journal of the American Medical Association*—not on scientific grounds, because this was not a scientific article. This was an article about ethics.[1]

THE END OF INNOCENCE

In the 1960s, there were no institutional review boards, nor ethics committees in hospitals, nor procedures to inform patients what would happen to them or to obtain their consent to participate in research or treatment. The relationship between doctors and their patients was paternalistic. Doctors were assumed to have their patients' best interests in mind and could volunteer their patients for research or for treatment without consultation.[2]

Beecher's article outlined twenty-two projects whose subjects did not know they were participating in research rather than receiving routine medical care. He was not describing bad or unfortunate incidents in the back wards of obscure rural hospitals. He was describing normal practice in some of the best hospitals in the country, carried out by distinguished professors of medicine or surgery. One such professor later became the president of the American Association for Cancer Research, and another won a Lasker prize.

Beecher did not claim any specific wrong had been done in any project. He simply put it as a matter of near statistical certainty that in at least one—and perhaps all—of these projects, harm was done to the patients by their not being informed.

The impact was immense. Things changed, for better and for worse. Hospitals, universities, and the NIH designed consent forms and set up

IRBs. Regulators worldwide were forced to insist that all research document the informed consent of participants.

Beecher had crystallized a growing worry about research that soon spilled into the rest of medical care. Patients began to question the everyday decisions of their doctors. Patient support groups sprang up as routine medical care began to make headlines. Doctors were turning off incubators on handicapped children: Who gave them the right to do this? Doctors were refusing to turn off the life-support machines of patients whose families wanted them to die in peace: Who gave them the right to deny the wishes of the family? Increasingly health-conscious patients began to demand a say in things done to them and for them.[3]

As medicine became more high-tech and impersonal, the public felt increasingly alienated from it. Where the relationship between physician and patient had often been sustained and complex, with much left implicit, things now had to be spelled out. Physicians who saw only the tremendous benefits of modern medicine resisted this new literalism. Society's ingratitude and the steps it took to control medical power and limit medical discretion astounded them.

These physicians failed to see that the corporations producing new technologies answered to shareholders instead of the community. A process had begun whereby medical research would follow the money. It would become selective, potentially benefiting the favored few rather than the community at large. Genetic research might now be preferred to social and preventive research. This research, which might pinpoint the genes responsible for lung cancer, would ignore the question of whether smoking was a preventable cause of lung cancer. Few were aware that the new pharmaceuticals, especially psychopharmaceuticals, would fit squarely into the eugenic tradition of offering "biological" solutions to social problems.

Beecher's revolution had its immediate drawbacks. It gave rise to bureaucracy and red tape. Quickly, doing good for people became harder in some circumstances; sometimes, it would be hard to do anything at all. Despite paternalism, health care at its best had been conducted in an atmosphere where patients and doctors shared unspoken information. But the new revolution required that things be done by the book. As the joke went, if doctors and their patients weren't feeling what the book said they should be feeling, they must be mistaken.

AN ARRANGED MARRIAGE

The relationship between companies and physicians mirrors the doc-tor-patient relationship. No one paid much heed to this relationship until recently, since in the early days pharmaceutical companies were small enterprises. What are now giant corporations began life shortly after World War II as small divisions of chemical companies. It was a small world where people knew each other and a great deal could hap-pen without too much having to be said. It was a far cry from the mod-ern world of glass and steel corporations, where I regularly have to in-troduce people from one division of a corporation to others from dif-ferent divisions of the same corporation. Whatever mistakes pharmaceutical companies could make in the past, given the all too human mixture of motives—greed, short-termism, and power, allied to simple venality, which all organizations will always suffer from—there wasn't the vacuum that is now present in many pharmaceutical corpo-rations.

People now move between departments and companies with be-wildering speed. This being the case, it may seem a good thing from a company point of view that they can't take too many secrets with them. But the resulting situation echoes a famous Tom Lehrer song: "Once the rockets are up, who cares where they come down, that's not my de-partment, says Werner von Braun."[4] We return to the deposition of Catherine Mesner in *Fentress vs. Eli Lilly*, taken by Nancy Zettler:

Q. Why did they not pursue the rechallenge protocol?
A. I don't know.
Q. You weren't curious as to why they wouldn't pursue it after they worked on it for two months? [Mesner had ordered clinical trials materials because she had been certain the pro-tocol would proceed.]
A. No.
Q. Did you ever ask anybody why they didn't pursue the rechallenge protocol?
A. No, I moved on to the next step.
Q. What was your next assignment after the rechallenge protocol?
A. I continued to work on scale validation protocol [on the MSSIR, a scale to detect suicidality, which Lilly had told FDA it would develop.]

Q. What was the result of the scale validation protocol on MSSIR?

A. I left my responsibility behind on that before it was ended.[5]

Or consider Richard Wood, the chief executive of Lilly up to 1991, in a deposition littered with acknowledgments of ignorance and fogginess:

Q. Do you know how many patients were covered by Protocol Number 27? [This was the key study submitted to the FDA in the license application for Prozac.]

A. I haven't the foggiest idea.

Q. Do you have any reason to suspect that Protocol Number 27 was not done in a good and scientific manner?

A. I haven't the foggiest idea.

Q. Do you know if it was done by Lilly?

A. I never heard of Protocol 27.[6]

Mistakes could happen in the "good old days," as thalidomide demonstrated horrifically. But medicine was still in control of its pharmaceutical partner. This was why the 1962 amendments to the U.S. Food and Drugs Act made new drugs available on prescription only. Patients couldn't know about the hazards of these new modern miracles, or even the right questions to ask; but their physicians would. The expectation was that physicians would act as consumer advocates. They would harass the drug companies and quarry information out of them. They would be in a position to force companies to do what needed to be done.[7] When it comes to pharmaceuticals, the public generally thinks that the regulators are looking after them; but the mechanism the regulators have put in place to do this is prescription by a physician.

This arrangement depends on two things: inquisitive doctors and honest and genuine pharmaceutical companies. The relationship is one of trust, very like the relationship between physician and patient. A trust-based relationship can produce the conditions that make serial killings easy, so that the physician Harold Shipman, with over two hundred deaths attributed to him, now stands as perhaps the greatest serial killer of all time.[8] In just the same way, the relationship between physicians and companies could conceivably make even greater and more systematic drug disasters than thalidomide possible, if companies fail to respect the vulnerable position physicians occupy in this relationship.

By the 1960s, the pharmaceutical companies had become sufficiently profitable to be hived off by their parent companies. Where chemists or physicians had been in charge, the new companies brought in business managers with MBAs. These new professionals took a standard approach to business management. Doing things by protocol became the order of the day. But the hugely creative process of pharmaceutical development cannot be made routine or fitted within protocols. It requires an ability to think laterally, the opposite of assembly-line production. Nevertheless, the efforts of chemical, marketing, and pharmacological departments were increasingly strapped down to protocols.[9]

Clinical trials of drugs became bound by protocols. North American researchers in the 1950s and 1960s had devised randomized controlled trials and rating scales that had made it possible to assess whether psychiatric drugs worked or not. Part of their concern was to contain the pharmaceutical industry; but their very success created clinical trial templates that companies could now use without going back to those who really knew what clinical trials did and did not show. The expansion of psychiatry in the 1960s and 1970s meant companies could hire investigators who would do it simply for the money.

When independent investigators ran the clinical trial programs for the first psychotropic drugs, they analyzed their own results. By the time the SSRIs came onstream, companies ran multicenter trials, collecting results and analyzing them in-house. The clinicians involved in these trials lost any overview as to what the new drugs did.[10] The drugs might be shown to work, but in an important sense there was no longer a hands-on feel for *how* they were working. As the German regulatory assessment of Prozac put it:

> [A] condition for a promising therapy is the choice of antidepressant with a profile of action, which is right for the clinical picture. On grounds, of the submitted studies the profile of action of the preparation [Prozac] is hardly identifiable: perhaps it possesses a slight anxiolytic activity.[11]

This assessment, which points out that no one seemed able to tell these regulators what Prozac really did, points to a vacuum at the heart of modern clinical practice to parallel that at the heart of pharmaceutical companies.

Even at this stage of incoherence, it was necessary for a clinical figurehead to write up the results. No one would believe results from an off-the-peg clinical trial protocol and in-house analysis if the final papers were written up by company people. A convenient fiction was adopted until the 1991 Beasley article in the *BMJ* legitimized the company article. Many articles, however, continue to carry the bylines of well-known clinicians, despite the fact that perhaps as much as 50 percent of the therapeutics literature is now ghostwritten.

FROM TOBACCO TO PHARMACEUTICALS

Through the 1980s, business management's participation in the running of growing pharmaceutical companies led to the appointment of businesspeople as chief executive officers.[12] SmithKline Beecham ended up with Jan Leschly, a former international tennis player, and Eli Lilly with Randall Tobias, a former CEO at AT&T. They could equally well have rotated in from Philip Morris or British American Tobacco. These new executives were paid partly in share options; when company shares went up, so did their personal fortunes. If the price of the stock fell, they lost money. In 1999, Leschly's net worth under these arrangements was cited by Britain's *Guardian* newspaper as $150 million.[13]

Lawyers presumably advise all corporate clients in a similar fashion. It is not clear whether lawyers make any allowance for the special relationship between companies and clinicians. In the case of Upjohn and Lilly in the 1980s and 1990s, one of the legal firms used was Shook, Hardy and Bacon, legal advisers to major tobacco companies.[14] As Ian Oswald's libel lawyer, David Hooper, would later put it:

> Upjohn's legal tactics were honed by a United States law firm renowned for its successful defense of tobacco firms. It is a moot point whether the tobacco companies have learnt from the drug companies how to fight product liability cases or vice versa.[15]

Certainly, some tobacco executives got the message that conducting research on the effects of smoke on human lungs and hearts or on the addiction potential of nicotine could only increase a company's legal liability.[16] This apparently extended to closing down research on a safer cigarette, which would legally have been problematic. Lawyers advised which research could be published and which not.

Interestingly, in the twelve years following the public emergence of concerns over Prozac, there is not a single study designed to answer the question of whether Prozac or any other SSRI can induce suicidality.[17] Lilly spent a year designing one, but it was never undertaken.[18] Simply mentioning this point appears to have brought the Toronto house down.

What about closing down programs to produce a safer Prozac? Consider this: As early as 1986, Stuart Montgomery had reported that once-a-week Prozac was as effective as daily Prozac.[19] This would have probably reduced the risk from key side effects such as the induction of agitation.[20] It would probably also have reduced profits.

In 1988, a further study showed that 5 mg of Prozac once a day was as effective as the 20 mg tablet.[21] This lower dose could have been expected in clinical practice to produce less agitation—but it would have meant introducing multiple different doses of Prozac, which would not have suited the "one size fits all" marketing strategy that Lilly ultimately adopted.[22]

Finally, while the fact that Lilly held the patent on R-minus fluoxetine hit the front page of the *Boston Globe* in 2000, there is another story behind this. The R-fluoxetine patent laid the basis for an action for fraud on the court in the *Forsyth* appeal. The fraud action then uncovered the fact that Sepracor had also patented S-fluoxetine as less likely to produce agitation than Prozac. Lilly considered buying S-fluoxetine in 1992. But buying S-fluoxetine, whether in fact it was safer or not, risked difficulties in the close to two hundred legal cases Lilly faced, rather like the difficulties a safer cigarette would have posed for the tobacco companies.[23]

There are strikingly few publications available on these alternative formulations of Prozac, but not because the data do not exist. Montgomery's study appeared in the program for the CINP meeting in 1986, but the abstract did not, and no article has since appeared. Some publications on S-fluoxetine might have been expected. One possible explanation for this unusual situation, based on precedents in the tobacco litigation, is that company lawyers' blocked publication.

Against this background, the words of former U.S. Attorney General Janet Reno, applied to the tobacco story in 1999, become even more unsettling:

The companies that manufacture and sell tobacco have waged an intentional and co-ordinated campaign of fraud and deceit. . . . It has been designed to preserve their enormous profits whatever the cost in human lives, human suffering and medical resources. . . . The truth represents a mortal threat to their business. At every turn, they denied that smoking causes disease and denied that it is addictive.[24]

On April 8, 2000, *The Lancet* published a study showing how the tobacco industry spent large amounts of money on coordinated efforts to discredit studies on passive smoke inhalation.[25] A *Lancet* editorial stated:

Tobacco is not the only aspect of medicine open to twisted corporate communication strategies. A 1998 study reported that published opinions on the safety of calcium-channel blockers were related to the financial rewards bestowed by pharmaceutical companies on those giving such opinions. All policymakers must be vigilant to the possibility of research data being manipulated by corporate bodies and of scientific colleagues being seduced by the material charms of industry. Trust is no defense against an aggressively deceptive corporate sector.[26]

Of course, the pharmaceutical and tobacco industries differ—but by how much today? In 2000, Richard Smith, the editor of the *BMJ*, famously resigned from Nottingham University because it took tobacco money as research support. At what point would the *BMJ* feel obliged to stop taking pharmaceutical company advertisements?

Prescription-only arrangements cannot tolerate even a fraction of the lack of company-sponsored genuine research on the product that exists within the tobacco industry. Given the way tobacco companies behaved, there was an ethical onus on medical people to research the hazards of tobacco, and independent funding was forthcoming to support them. Tobacco companies did not control researchers as pharmaceutical companies now control clinical researchers. In the case of tobacco, the community was never in a position where all *its* experts were beholden to a corporation for research monies, speaking opportunities, or consultancy fees; where all its researchers could be body-snatched.

Pharmaceutical companies need senior clinicians in the field to advise on clinical trial research. They need senior clinicians to explain the advances to others. And these clinicians must be able to sup comfortably with these companies. The world wouldn't work if physicians and other health care researchers viewed pharmaceutical corporations the way they view tobacco companies.

There is a growing urgency here. In recent years, we have come to the verge of breakthroughs in genetic technologies. The mapping of the human genome is one of the greatest projects undertaken by mankind, a project that could hugely benefit the health of all of mankind and answer some age-old questions about human nature. The very prospect of success in these projects has made pharmaceutical stocks the magnet they have been. These genetic revolutions, however, won't give rise to new genes corporations. Genes can be patented, but these genes give rise to protein products, and the next generation of drugs will come from these proteins, made directly into drugs or from agents targeted to act on these protein products. The winners in this genetic revolution will be the pharmaceutical corporations.

It is natural to be concerned about what these new developments will bring. But does the problem lie with further scientific advances, or in the risk that chief executives, advised by lawyers answerable only to shareholders, will control the new knowledge? Does the problem lie in new knowledge or in already proven nonreporting of deaths and other adverse outcomes in gene therapy studies? Should we be more worried about the new research or about a lack of accountability in this critical area of human endeavor?

Some of the issues were caught by Jonathan Quick of the World Health Organization (WHO):

> If clinical trials become a commercial venture in which self-interest overrules public interest and desire overrules science, then the social contract which allows research on human subjects in return for medical advances is broken.[27]

Getting the arrangements right for the new world we face doesn't mean ensuring equal health care for the poor and the rich. Perhaps only the rich will be able to afford these new developments at first. But if the wealthy are going to be the guinea pigs for the rest of society, they must give informed consent to what is happening. Given that pharmaceutical corporations at present target the United States with their new products, there is the further question of whether American society has given consent to the experiment being conducted upon it.[28]

THE SEROTONIN CULTURE

Many readers of this book will not have taken an SSRI. Many never would. Despite this, everyone is at risk for a series of side effects from the SSRIs. Prozac, Zoloft, and Paxil were not put in the drinking water, but they were put into the cultural air we breathe.

In a way unimaginable ten years ago, popular culture takes it for granted that serotonin is low in depressed people. Talking about her depression in 1999, Tipper Gore told *USA Today*:

> It was definitely a clinical depression, one that I was going to have to have help to overcome. What I learned about it is your brain needs a certain amount of serotonin and when you run out of that, it's like running out of gas.[29]

Similarly, in the mid-1990s a cover for the review section of Britain's *Guardian* newspaper carried an image of a Britain where everyone had become depressed. Inside, a psychologist claimed the British had become a "low serotonin people."[30] Less high-powered magazines say similar things with no attempt to justify them. The belief system has become pervasive.

In the *Observer*, another British broadsheet, the health section stated:

> [S]erotonin and norepinephrine are derived mainly from sugary and carbohydrate-rich foods, which is why some people feel happy after they have eaten chocolate, bowls of mashed potato, tubs of ice-cream or thick slices of crusty white bread. It also explains why we crave steamed puddings or malted chocolate drinks and gravitate towards bowls of pasta during dark and dreary months.[31]

But, we are told, these rapidly absorbed sugars cause an initial boost in serotonin levels that is then shut down by insulin, causing us to feel worse than ever. Our bodies will try to keep up these sugar swings by tempting us to eat another biscuit, but the "more sweets you eat, the more you'll need to make yourself feel happy and your moods will swing all over the place." Taking a similar line, books sell themselves as offering information about "nature's Prozac." But as a man on a charge of murder, after killing someone nine days into a course of Prozac, put it to me, "You read about feeling good after chocolate or exercise and I feel good after these, but this is nothing like the way you feel after Prozac."

Talk-show hosts kick off programs by mentioning the recognized serotonin deficiency in depression. I have repeatedly brought such shows to a crashing halt by saying there is, in fact, no truth in this. Neither the questioner nor I know what to say next. How do I even begin to explain how there never was any basis for this idea? How can the host cope with someone breaking one of the fundamental rules of the game?

Part of the problem is the widespread use of "biobabble." During the middle years of the twentieth century, Freudian ideas leaked out into popular culture—partly because Hollywood found the new scripts irresistible, partly because people have an insatiable appetite for books that explain/excuse their personal predicaments. A pidgin psychoanalysis was created, a psychobabble in which terms such as *complexes* and *transference* bore little relationship to their original theoretical framework. This was not a harmless development. It had incalculable consequences for how we view ourselves, how we bring up our children, and how we view issues such as moral and criminal culpability.

Now this psychobabble has been all but replaced by an equally vacuous biobabble, which in turn has consequences for how we view ourselves, how we view the turmoil of adolescence or school underachievement or, finally, moral and criminal culpability. This cannot be blamed on Eli Lilly, but it does stem in great part from the marketing of Prozac and other SSRIs—and it affects the lives even of those who have never heard of Prozac.

The book that made serotonin a subject of after-dinner conversation was Peter Kramer's *Listening to Prozac*.[32] The message that you can be better than well, that these drugs can be used cosmetically, made Kramer's book a publishing phenomenon. He was offering a lifestyle option, and his success suggests this must have been something people were looking for. Why?

A few years later, Viagra appeared, now openly referred to by Pfizer as a lifestyle drug. But where the public saw one meaning for the word *lifestyle,* companies saw another. Drugs can become lifestyle agents only if they reliably produce the responses promised by their makers. Good-quality health care for most of us means a sympathetic and respectful interaction with another human being. For industry, good quality means reproducibility. Big Macs are quality hamburgers because they are the same every time. This logic is increasingly leading to health care and academia with all the quality of a Big Mac.

The difficulty was that antidepressants simply don't work regularly. Prozac could indeed produce a better-than-well response—but not *reliably*. When responses are not reliable, a disease concept is vital for companies. The background of a disease excuses poor reliability in the product. If they could produce Viagra-like reliability with antidepressants, with a response that was predictable ninety-five times out of one hundred, companies could afford to ditch the disease concept of depression. The possibilities that this could be done are tantalizingly close. The healthy volunteer study outlined in Chapter 7 inadvertently did more than almost any other study to prove Prozac and Zoloft could, in fact, produce "better than well" responses even in normal subjects.

To move from antidepressants to lifestyle drugs will require pharmacogenetic tests and neuroimaging technologies to provide a readout of people's temperaments and personalities. This would get us close to producing Viagra-like responses, even from current drugs such as the SSRIs, by ensuring those likely to respond poorly are detected beforehand. But if those not suited to Prozac are less likely to get it, companies will need to ensure that all those who could conceivably benefit are identified and persuaded of the benefits, if the companies are not to lose sales. Direct-to-consumer advertising will play a part. Employers could be persuaded that productivity is at stake. But the biggest untapped market is children. Who will protest? Have physicians protested the thousandfold increase in the diagnosis of depression in the psychotropic era?

In the meantime, the idea that depression is a state in which serotonin is lowered does a great deal to legitimate the taking of Prozac. When comparisons are drawn between Prozac and Valium, Valium is seen as a darker and more dangerous drug. While pill taking poses problems for many, the fact that Prozac supposedly corrects an abnormality, and by implication restores people to normal, overcomes many scruples. Categorical statements that it is nonaddictive overcome others. And statements that it doesn't work for several weeks deflect many from making any connections between the drug and the emergence of suicidality in the first few weeks of treatment.[33] But in fact, the SSRIs and the benzodiazepines are similar in many respects. They are given to the same groups of patients. Both sets of drugs cause physical dependence—the SSRIs probably more so than the benzodiazepines. And, unlike the benzodiazepines, the SSRIs trigger suicidality in a significant proportion of those who take them.

THE GLOBALIZED INDIVIDUAL

The idea that Prozac is correcting an abnormality does something to explain why we now give SSRIs so commonly to our children. Only a generation ago, the idea of exposing their developing brains to powerful psychotropic drugs would have seemed anathema. But giving drugs to children is powerfully mandated from another source—clinical trials.

The trials showing that Prozac, Paxil, and Zoloft "work" have been interpreted as providing results that generalize to all individuals in all places. RCTs are key to pharmaceutical companies' globalization efforts. The message is that these results hold for all ethnic groups, both sexes, all ages, all cultures, and across time. If the diseases being treated vanished after treatment, there might be something to this implicit claim. In the face of a steadily mounting burden of nervous disorders, it is alarming that the discrepancy between the claims of trials and the reality has not been subject to critical scrutiny. When asked to rate the strength of influences on them, clinicians smugly put marketing at the bottom of the list and rate evidence as their main guide, not realizing clinical trials are now drawn up, written up, and talked up in marketing departments.

In the case of children, the message is that these drugs will bring deviant children back toward a behavioral norm that carries fewer risks for their future. We are seeing a replay of the development of IQ testing in the early twentieth century. As a result of these new tests, parents who discovered their children fell outside norms created a huge market in educational and child psychology.

Before the mid-twentieth century, children were given far more psychotropic drugs than in the decades following World War II. In the nineteenth century, for instance, they were often kept quiet with opiates. These drugs could be seen to work in the short term. In the second half of the twentieth century, however, behavioral methods were the preferred treatment. Giving children psychotropic drugs became taboo in many circles. Now we have entered a new phase, based on the promise of clinical trials to help us manage risks in our children's development.

Management of hypertension gives a good example of a new creeping medicalization of risk. Antihypertensives were initially used to treat malignant or life-threatening hypertension. Success was a triumph of modern medicine. The contemporary antihypertensive market, the biggest in pharmaceuticals, however, is based on reducing future risks through treatment of ever-more-debatable elevations of blood pressure. Blood pressure that lies even slightly above the norm can be shown to carry some risks. But the risk minimization gained by treating mild hypertension is so small that, with the agents available in the 1980s and 1990s, up to 850 patients would have to be treated to save one life.[34] Companies and physicians nevertheless united in efforts to treat such patients, even though the results in terms of quality of life, and of the illness behavior that results from telling people they are ill, makes such efforts morally ambiguous.[35]

The mythologies underpinning Prozac cast it as an antibiotic of the mind, raising lowered serotonin levels to normal, when its use is in fact more like treating mild hypertension. Today's best-selling drugs do not correct a condition but rather are longer-term, even lifelong agents administered for almost virtual rather than real reasons—to reduce possible risks. Few taking these agents appear to appreciate the nature of the treatment they are receiving or the slender basis on which that treatment is predicated. In the case of the SSRIs, sales are geared to lowering suicide risk—without any factual demonstration of lowered suicide risk.

Far from yielding evidence that SSRIs work, RCTs of psychotropic drugs give evidence of treatment effects in samples of convenience. SSRIs can be shown to do something. But whether doing what SSRIs do is a good thing, or is something that will work in the longer run, is not answered by these trials. The decision to employ the benefit that SSRIs might confer should be a matter of clinical wisdom. It may, in fact, be a practical impossibility to do independent trials that will show whether it actually is a good thing to treat children or adolescents or even adults with SSRIs in the longer term. The answers to questions like this are likely to come only from the gigantic uncontrolled experiment we have been conducting with these drugs from the early 1990s onward. We may learn the answer only when these drugs go off patent and there is a new market for a set of very unpalatable findings.

These drugs reached the market after a demonstration of treatment effects in a minority of the trials undertaken with SSRIs. This provided a basis for using these drugs judiciously. It does not provide a rationale for widespread indiscriminate usage. Neither patients nor parents appear to understand this. The startling thing is that few patients seem to be faced with *clinicians* aware of this either.

Since the development of anesthesia, physicians have been prepared to do harm to a few patients in order to benefit a majority of patients. The *de facto* Hippocratic Oath has always been "Do no harm to *a majority* of your patients." In the case of the SSRIs, the clinical trial evidence indicates that we may benefit some patients. None of this evidence shows us what proportion of patients benefit from SSRI treatment and what proportion are harmed by it. In the case of anesthesia, much less than 1 percent of takers are at risk. In the case of the SSRIs, there is a serious risk to more than 1 percent of takers, but neither society nor the psychiatric profession has expressed a view as to what constitutes an acceptable minority of harmed patients.

Weighing scales offer an example of the tyranny of numbers. Shortly after scales to weigh people were invented in the 1870s, norms for weights developed. The insurance industry realized that excess weight, far from being healthy as was previously thought, was in fact risky. Over the following half a century, the scale moved into drugstores—where the most common model had a metal plate fixed to it, engraved with norms for height and weight. Then it transmuted into the portable device most people keep somewhere in their home. In this process, our ideas of beauty—how we view ourselves—quite literally changed.

Anorexia and then bulimia emerged and reached epidemic proportions in those parts of the world using domestic scales. There are biological, psychological, and sociological theories about the origin of the eating disorders, but none of these theories pays any heed to the role of the scale as a source of feedback in creating and maintaining these syndromes, even though it is almost impossible to imagine an epidemic of eating disorders without the self-imposed tyranny of the scale.[36]

This illustrates the effect quantification may have on us. If some set of figures demonstrates a risk, it is difficult not to want to do something to minimize that risk. If there are no figures from other areas of our life to show what we might lose in the process, or the risks we run in paying too much heed to figures on the scales, we risk becoming slaves to those figures we can see. The introduction of clinical trials for psychotropic drugs brought a welter of checklists such as the HAM-D, complete with norms. Checklisting spread from there into all areas of life, from the school playground to the pages of magazines, covering anything from personality features to sexual behavior and activity levels. Finding that we, or our children, fall outside some norms impels us to take action to minimize the risks we now "know" we run.

If we want to get some balance among these figures, in the case of drugs we need two other sets of figures. One is the number of people who must be treated in order for even one person to benefit significantly. If one in ten of us needs to be treated to save a life, then most of us would opt for treatment. But if the figure were 1 in 850, as in mild hypertension, few would opt to take the pills. Whether or not we would be happy to have treatment might also depend on a second set of figures reporting the impact of treatment on our sex lives, vitality levels, or other aspects of our selves. Neither set of figures is routinely given to someone prescribed an SSRI.

A clinician who has only a set of HAM-D scores and operates on the basis of those figures is like an adolescent trapped by the figures on the scale dial. No one would argue that the figures on the scale should be the most important set of figures in a life, but this effectively is what is happening in health care at the moment. And there is a weird twist that stems from prescription-only arrangements: The clinician watching the figures makes someone else's life a misery, rather than his own.

What alternative is there? Trials are now so expensive, we want pharmaceutical companies to run them. They must take place in so many different centers that no one clinician gets a good feel for what lies behind the figures. But we have this difficulty only because the effects of the current generation of drugs are so weak. If the antidepressants were anything like their hype leads people to think they are, a clinical trial could be run in a single university center and give results so clearcut that rating scales would not be needed. The fact that this is not the case screams out that these drugs should only be used judiciously.

THE DOGS BARK, THE CARAVAN MOVES ON

Given company success in shutting down concerns about SSRIs and suicide, no one can be sanguine that the truth will out. As Ed West said at the end of the *Wesbecker* trial, "The verdict demonstrates the futility of blaming medications for harmful and criminal acts."[37]

For companies, protests are dogs barking at a passing caravan in the desert.[38] Once you lose your grip on power, however, the dogs become more threatening. The SSRIs are an old group of drugs coming off patent. Were new antidepressants coming onstream, the companies marketing them would have every incentive to do the SSRIs in. But drug development in psychiatry has slowed to a trickle, and there are no new antidepressants in sight.

Nevertheless, a specter stalks the SSRIs. Most people feel that suicide on treatment is not something that could happen to them. But almost all of us believe we could become dependent on drug treatment. This makes us skeptical of claims by the DART and Defeat Depression campaigns that antidepressants are not addictive.

Prozac packets still contain the message "Don't worry about taking Prozac over a long period of time—Prozac is not addictive."[39] Until very recently, Glaxo-SmithKline said "withdrawal" reactions are rare on Paxil, and when they do happen, they are mild and self-limiting. But now it seems that these drugs, which were not supposed to cause dependence because they were "antidepressants," cause a more serious dependence than the benzodiazepines ever did.[40]

In the face of concerns, one company line is to claim that it is not possible to distinguish between withdrawal and the symptoms of the original illness. This, too, is a straight replay of the benzodiazepine script.[41] Long before Paxil came to the market, as I became aware while accessing SmithKline's archives in the *Tobin* case in March 2001, SmithKline was aware that healthy volunteers who had only been taking Paxil for a few weeks had difficulties on withdrawal.[42] In the mid-1980s, SmithKline had run healthy volunteer studies in which a large proportion of the volunteers had distinct withdrawal syndromes after a brief exposure to paroxetine. These details, including the death of one volunteer, have not been published. Despite this, SmithKline designed long-term treatment trials in which patients who had responded to Paxil were re-randomized to either continuing Paxil or a switch to placebo.[43] Similar studies were carried out on Zoloft. The difficulties of those switching to placebo were interpreted as new illness episodes, and on this basis the companies were granted licenses to claim that Paxil and Zoloft were prophylactic in depression. And these licenses stand, even though SmithKline repeatedly, in public, has said that it's not possible to distinguish between withdrawal and the underlying illness.

Here the companies are playing on the fact that SSRIs will not transform patients into junkies, and that psychiatrists will line up to support them on this. But not becoming addicted in this sense does not mean takers will be able to stop treatment whenever they want. For the better part of ten years, regulators and others have told the public that any difficulties on withdrawal are mild and last no more than a week or two. But the scientific data are from patients who discontinue early from trials or are discontinued after a few weeks in a trial. There are no data on what happens to patients who, having been on treatment for some months, try to stop. Many simply cannot stop, and some may never be able to stop.

The most common symptoms on withdrawal are depression and anxiety. A host of other bizarre symptoms appear to map better onto conditions such as tardive dyskinesia, a feature of antipsychotic withdrawal, than onto the withdrawal from opiates or alcohol. In contrast to opiate or alcohol withdrawal, which is usually over in two or three weeks, tardive dyskinesia can last for months or years, as can SSRI withdrawal.[44]

A growing number of patients refuse to credit the myth that their difficulties upon halting are the reemergence of their original disorder. Indeed, these withdrawal effects were so obvious on the ground that as early as 1997, Lilly ran a set of advertisements, convened meetings, and sampled psychiatric opinion on the issue of discontinuation syndromes—hoping, it would seem, that it would be difficult to link these effects to Prozac, given its long half-life.

The issue of dependence on and withdrawal from Paxil led Baum, Hedlund to file a legal action against SmithKline in August 2001, alleging fraudulent deception.[45] In January 2002, SmithKline amended its product label for Paxil to reflect the fact that difficulties could occur on halting treatment.[46] This did not stop lawyers in Canada and the United States from filing class action suits against Glaxo-SmithKline.

Psychiatrists continued to deny that Paxil or other SSRIs could cause difficulties and to denigrate anyone who referred to the problems in public. This is hard to understand. There are differences among the various drugs in the antidepressant group and among the various SSRIs in their likelihood of producing dependence. Accepting that dependence can be produced has to be the first step to exploring the differences between compounds, and exploring the differences is the only way to find out what causes dependence. Until the basis of dependence is understood, it will not be possible to design treatments that avoid it. Refusal to accept that dependence happens has a proven track record in leading to the use of treatments being restricted. Faced with this calculus, organized psychiatry has consistently jumped the wrong way.

STEPS IN SEARCH OF A SOLUTION

The regulations that set up physicians as advocates for consumers have meant there are no consumer groups in medicine or psychiatry with the power to force change. The public falls back on the illusion that we do not need consumer groups—the regulators are looking after us. The regulators, ill equipped for this purpose, depend for advice on experts who increasingly claim independence on the basis that they have consultancies with *all* the companies. Besides, as Paul Leber intimated, if a regulatory agency acts other than in response to public clamor, it risks being sued by those who will claim they have been injured by the removal of the drug in question. Companies are not above threatening regulators in just this way.

Is Prozac too dangerous at any price? This returns us to the dilemma facing the FDA in 1991. Warnings may make some difference to some prescribers and some consumers, but there will still be cowboy prescribers and rogue consumers. Unless a drug is absolutely safe, no warnings can protect everyone. What is an acceptable number of problems?

It is difficult to find any evidence in the psychotropic story that further regulation might be the answer. To date, regulation has all too often handed companies an easy means to show that they are playing by the rules while, in fact, they buy the rulebook. Far from containing companies, regulations are likely to become a hazard to the consumers they are designed to protect. Civil actions by lawyers on a contingency-fee basis may be as good a method as any to get to grips with companies. In the United States, however, Republicans and Democrats alike have pledged themselves to weight the legal balance in tort cases in favor of corporations and against plaintiffs. In Canada and Europe, consumers are even less well placed.

But for the legal system to work properly, it needs a set of experts to whom plaintiffs can turn. Once upon a time that might have been their physicians. Sadly, a further lesson of the Prozac story is that this no longer seems possible.

OVER THE COUNTER?

Were medicines made available over the counter rather than on prescription only, medical practitioners would become more independent of the pharmaceutical industry. Industry would court consumers directly. This might mean at least some expert physicians would be prepared to testify in court on behalf of plaintiffs injured by pharmaceutical products. How much would medical people have done to establish the harmful effects of cigarettes and nicotine if tobacco products had been available on prescription only and under patent? Both physicians and researchers earn a living by opposing tobacco. What if they earned their living out of making it available? How long would it have taken the truth to come out in these circumstances?

Prescription-only arrangements were intended to protect the consumer. At first, pharmaceutical companies lobbied against them. Now these same arrangements all but guarantee legal immunity to companies faced with medical misadventures. Elsewhere, whether it be through warnings on tobacco products or on computer games, companies must inform the public of the possible dangers posed by consumption of the product. Prescription-only arrangements, product inserts notwithstanding, enable companies to avoid posting warnings on the basis that it is the doctor's duty to educate and warn the patient. They wouldn't want to tamper with the sanctity of the physician-patient relationship. Put it under great stress by direct-to-consumer advertising, yes—but tamper with it? No, never!

Is it possible to contemplate the alternative, making drugs like Prozac available over the counter? The surprising answer is that they might be less dangerous. Anyone buying Prozac over the counter would quickly decide if it was helping them or not and stop if need be. In contrast, at present the giving and taking of drugs is embedded in a highly dynamic patient relationship with the doctor that makes it more difficult to stop a drug in the face of adverse events.

There is no problem when the person given an SSRI has a better-than-well response. But when things go wrong, the situation can escalate rapidly, and the dynamics that shape this escalation are the same as those in any hostage situation. The doctor who has probably unwittingly trapped the patient becomes the only way out. The patient may be too frightened to stop treatment or do anything other than what the doctor advises. A patient "going mad" really does need skilled help. When the doctor says to keep on taking the tablets, it takes a brave patient to do otherwise.

Take Anya, a 71-year-old woman who suffered from a number of physical illnesses but who had never had a nervous disorder in her life. Overwhelmed by a combination of stressors, she took an aspirin overdose. Given her physical problems, and in the light of the fact that her daughter had responded to Prozac for a nervous condition, I suggested Zoloft in a note to her primary-care physician. She rapidly developed breathlessness and chest pain. She ended up in the hospital on medication for heart failure. Her doctor continued the Zoloft because there was no mention of adverse cardiac or respiratory effects in the *Physician's Desk Reference*. I finally got to see her again and stopped the Zoloft. It seemed likely her breathlessness was a Zoloft-caused respiratory dyskinesia, not mentioned in the data sheet, and I had seen a number of cardiac complications on Zoloft. Her fluid retention and wheezing quickly cleared up. She, too, put all these problems down to Zoloft. Why hadn't she stopped it? Because, even though she knew it was ridiculous, she increasingly felt she might need her doctor for a real emergency some night and was concerned he wouldn't respond if it appeared she had disobeyed him.

The hostage bind is even worse for children, who are trapped by both doctors and parents who have no idea what the child is experiencing. No one believes a doctor would knowingly put children on a medication that might make things worse. What do "guilty" doctors do after disaster strikes? They blame the terrible illness. This is not a rare occurrence: One-quarter of all deaths in health care are now caused by treatments of one sort or the other. Doctors would find it very hard to function if forced to face up to all the damage they cause in their efforts to do good.

One consequence of the recent "biological" turn is that psychiatrists increasingly fail to appreciate the dynamics of their relationships with patients.[47] There is a growing split between pharmacotherapy and psychotherapy that is most evident in North American psychiatry. Actual time spent with patients is shrinking rapidly. Psychiatrists now commonly prescribe medications after only a brief encounter with the patient, and with only occasional follow-ups. There is an almost complete reliance on RCTs, which owes something to a perception that going by evidence other than RCT evidence is just not scientific—that's what we used to do back in the bad old days. Prescribing an antidepressant has become as antiseptic a therapeutic encounter as giving an antibiotic.

Making drugs available over the counter might have another surprising consequence: the disappearance of this terrible illness, depression. If companies could sell direct to consumers, they would market their products the way St. John's Wort is marketed: for stress, or burnout, or as a tonic. We would all pretty quickly find ourselves interpreting our nervous states in terms of being "out of sorts" or "burned out." We would see ourselves as being in need of a tonic rather than an antidepressant, and depression would shrink back to the levels at which it occurred in the 1960s.

Is medical business just another business? If not, then companies cannot simply play by business rules and aim at maximizing profits. At some point, the patient must come first. The alternative is that prescription-only arrangements are arguably out of place. They anesthetize the "consumers" and lead them to set natural caution aside.

For reasons completely unrelated to the dynamics outlined above, there is, in fact, a substantial movement at government and corporate levels to move toward a greater over-the-counter provision of medicines.[48] One indicator of this is the advent of direct-to-consumer advertising.

"SHRINKS"

If prescription-only arrangements are to stay, the medical profession must take its responsibilities more seriously. Even without being a shareholder in a pharmaceutical company, as a prescriber, I would want senior scientists in a pharmaceutical company to mount a vigorous defense of the company's product. I can also appreciate skillful legal footwork, but it is harder to defend the deafening silence of psychiatrists faced with published clinical trial evidence that the relative risk of suicidality from newer antidepressants is greater than placebo. This silence gives a whole new meaning to the term *shrink*.

One means of strengthening the nerve of physicians might be to put in place a new division within the regulatory apparatus, aimed specifically at managing hazards that emerge after products are launched. A recent study of the controversies surrounding the sleeping pill Halcion suggested that when it comes to investigating postmarketing adverse events, the field needs a body independent both of the companies and of the regulators responsible for licensing a compound.[49] This would mirror the distinction between the Federal Aviation Authority, which regulates air travel, and the Aviation Safety Board, which investigates and draws lessons from crashes.

When the SSRIs were first licensed, regulators faced clinical trial data that others might well have considered insufficient to permit these drugs to be licensed as antidepressants. Paul Leber's position on the results was that these drugs could be shown to do something, and that to believe they might have beneficial effects in certain cases of depression was not unreasonable. In my opinion, this was a brave and correct decision. Neither Leber nor the FDA is responsible for subsequent company efforts to market the SSRIs aggressively. Neither Leber nor the FDA can be held responsible for the failure of clinicians to contain the pharmaceutical industry.

But the SSRI and Halcion stories suggest that individuals responsible for recommending a product for licensing should not be those who afterward sit in judgment on that product's hazards as revealed in clinical practice. In the face of later hazards, critics of a drug are prone to misunderstand earlier judgment calls. If this misunderstanding fuels *ad hominem* attacks, it will further confound any appeal process and bias the future efforts of those who supported the product. If only for this reason, there should be a separation of powers within the regulatory apparatus. In comparison to the United States, the situation is even worse in Britain, where the regulatory agency responsible for monitoring difficulties with drugs after licensing is part of a department whose brief includes fostering the development of Britain's pharmaceutical sector.

A separation of powers would increase the sophistication of postmarketing surveillance. RCTs now prevent completely inefficacious compounds from making it to the marketplace. But the success of RCTs obscures the fact that there is much less understanding of how to handle postmarketing adverse events, an issue at least as important as the need to ensure that compounds work. The Prozac story shows that our regulators sometimes know little about what is going on. Obliging some department to know something might help.

WHOSE DATA?

A last solution lies with the volunteers for clinical trials. Pharmaceutical corporations have become among the most profitable companies on the planet. This is because we volunteer for clinical trials.

Many physicians who recruit patients into trials would not volunteer themselves or their family members. But patients who come to medical settings are in a hostage situation—the doctors are the way out, so keeping them happy is important. Agreeing to participate in trials, we donate samples of our bodily fluids, personal details, and other data, assuming the risks necessary to determine that some drugs simply don't work or may be too hazardous to market. Using our lives, companies find out some drugs are too hazardous to market, or they find out about hazards we are not then told about, or they use us to determine the right marketing niche for their compounds. We take these risks for free, and it is our voluntary efforts that produce the enormous market capitalization of these companies.

The companies take these data and call them proprietary. They select the good bits and market them back to clinicians and the public as science. When anyone else in any other area of science refuses access to data, scientists usually pay no further heed to the claims being made. But these rules of science are suspended when it is a pharmaceutical company that refuses access.

We are persuaded that it is an act of good citizenship for us to engage in trials. Without trials, we are told, development of new and breakthrough agents would not happen. This simply isn't the case. The majority of clinical trials now are marketing studies. Achieving blockbuster status for drugs has become the priority for pharmaceutical companies, rather than genuine medical breakthroughs. The actual flow of new breakthrough drugs is falling.

The question of whose data these are underpins a growing string of academic freedom cases, the most famous being the *Olivieri* case, which have sparked fierce debate between universities and pharmaceutical company sponsors on one side and academics on the other.[50] The university and company side suggests that traditional university and scientific values have to be weighed in the balance with the clinical values of concern for patient welfare. Speaking out about the possible hazards of treatment would supposedly worry too many patients unnecessarily. In Toronto, university spokesmen compared speaking out about the hazard of drugs to someone screaming, "Fire!" in a crowded theater. The implication is that people may be hurt in a stampede to the exit. But if there is indeed a fire in the theater, those who do not shout a warning are likely to be responsible for a greater number of deaths.

This supposed contrast between the values of science and the values of clinical care is an artificial one. What is involved in many of these academic freedom cases is a clash between the values of science and the values of business. As long as the clinical trial data from pharmaceutical company trials remain proprietary data and unavailable to public scrutiny, they cannot be called scientific.

Making the raw data available would do more to keep researchers and universities honest than any of the research safeguards or ethical frameworks that universities are busily trying to put in place to manage links between industry and academia. If the raw data were available, conceivably a large proportion of the articles in key journals could be ghostwritten and researchers could have links to many companies without there being the same problem as there is now.

What needs to be done to make these data available? One possibility might be for participants in clinical trials to transform the informed consent forms they sign into a contract between them and the company. Contract law trumps every other form of law. In this case it would give patients, volunteers, or consortia of patients and volunteers equal rights over the data. It would be possible for those who are being experimented upon to insist on access to the resulting data.

Dancing with a python is a traditional entertainment in Malaya. Part of its fascination lies in the skill employed by the woman to ensure the python cannot hook its tail onto some fixed object; otherwise, it can squeeze the life out of a dancer. The point at which industry gets to hold onto the data we generate is the point at which they begin to squeeze the life out of us. When their trials were run by academics in just a few centers, this wasn't possible. When clinical trials became multicentered, the dynamics changed, and suddenly only companies had access to the full picture.

It is argued that we have little option—if we want new treatments, we must have multicentered trials. But multicentered trials are needed only if a treatment is comparatively ineffective. If a newer treatment were significantly more effective, its benefits could be shown in a single-center study. Precisely because the gains to all the rest of us are so minimal, if such trials are going to go ahead, there is an overwhelming case for insisting on contracts between us and the companies experimenting on us. In the dance between academia and the pharmaceutical industry, the industry needs the public and the public's academics far more than we need the pharmaceutical industry.

A CONSPIRACY OF GOODWILL[51]

Introducing the possibility of making antidepressants available over the counter is a thought experiment aimed at alerting readers to hidden aspects of the current situation. Offering a more realistic alternative to the current situation than an over-the-counter option for all psychotropic drugs is not a job for one person.

The history of the psychotherapies, from psychoanalysis to the recovered memory stories, shows a dynamic similar to the Prozac story. Treatments or techniques that could do good are overenthusiastically adopted as solutions to the complexity of life, rather than advances that may provide limited benefits if used judiciously. A conspiracy of goodwill gives those offering new treatments the benefit of the doubt. Both therapists and patients want new treatments to work. In the case of the pharmacotherapies, companies, regulators, and governments also want the treatments to work.

The rise and fall of psychoanalysis is particularly sobering. If ever a group of therapists should have been able to manage the dynamics of therapy, psychoanalysts were that group. But even analysts were seduced by our need for solutions. Sometimes all that can be done is to document the situation and move on. Conspiracies are not easily dismantled.

The Prozac story joins the Halcion story in psychiatry as an example of such "conspiracies" supplemented by vigorous company defenses of a product. There are comparable stories from elsewhere in medicine. One of the earliest involved beta agonist drugs used in the treatment of asthma, and later the use of fenoterol.[52] The presentation of scientific data about fenoterol was met with threats to sue and successful efforts to block publication in *The Lancet*. The integrity of the researchers was impugned, and the company mobilized a supposed "expert consensus" to support its position.

But the uncritical adoption of psychoanalysis in the 1950s and 1960s contains a further lesson in that it was followed by its uncritical rejection in the 1990s. In psychopharmacology, the benzodiazepines suffered a similar fate. The SSRIs may be headed for the same rocks. This would be a tragedy, because these and other antidepressant drugs have the potential to help many patients.

One quirk to the SSRI story is that but for the fact that companies have become much less adept at making new drugs than they are at marketing comparatively poor drugs, these same companies—Lilly, Pfizer, and SmithKline—might have used me to help bring about the demise of generic fluoxetines and sertralines in favor of new agents. Another is that, while I may be criticized for contemplating over-the-counter compounds, the companies sponsoring these criticisms will be lobbying actively for just that. A final glitch is that no one knows where legal liability for adverse events on generic fluoxetine, sertraline, or paroxetine may lie. No other drug has ever come to the end of its patent life with major issues about its side-effect profile still undetermined.[53]

Meanwhile, the antidepressant market is now worth $10 billion a year and projected to grow further, especially among children and teenagers.[54] In 1999, eighty-four million prescriptions for SSRIs were filled and $5.5 billion spent in the United States alone. Far from being the most researched drugs in history, these drugs have been tested only to the minimum extent needed to get on the market and to develop that market. This leaves us a long way from knowing what the drugs do. The use on this scale of a set of drugs about which so little is really known would seem almost certain to produce a blowout somewhere in the system.

While a conspiracy of goodwill has a nice ring to it, that goodwill has never extended to anyone who has attempted to unpick the conspiracy. The outlines of a backlash are easily drawn. We can predict that media outlets will receive "independent" views about how dangerous this book is. These views may cite the thought experiment about over-the-counter prescribing to illustrate just how far I am from the mainstream. The independent views will come from a relatively small number of people who will be portrayed as constituting an expert consensus—people who have not heard me talk to the data involved, who have not tried to discuss the issues with me, and who would refuse to provide a platform for debate on the issues.

SEPTEMBER 11

The Prozac story hangs between one September 11 and another. Given the name fluoxetine on September 11, 1975, it was poorly placed to compete when the world changed on September 11, 2001.

The SSRIs had come to the market as antidepressants. This was a business rather than a scientific decision, dictated by public concerns about dependence on the benzodiazepine tranquilizers. It was easy to predict in 1990 that the new drugs would initially be marketed as antidepressants, but that companies would strike out from the beachhead of depression to try to capture the hinterlands of anxiety—where the real money is.[55] The surprise was that depression proved such a profitable intermediate step.

The market development of Paxil, Zoloft, and Efexor followed this script rather precisely, with these companies picking up licenses for generalized anxiety disorder (GAD), post-traumatic stress disorder, social phobia, panic disorder, and anxious depression in the course of 2000 and 2001. Prozac, in contrast, went off patent with no indications for anxiety disorders, when the World Trade Center towers collapsed and pharmaceutical companies discovered we were, in fact, anxious rather than depressed.

After September 11, magazines, broadsheets, and tabloid newspapers told us we now had generalized anxiety disorder or post-traumatic stress disorder. GSK, Wyeth, and Pfizer had all received licenses for their compounds for these anxiety indications during the course of the previous year. The S-isomer of Celexa, S-citalopram, also had already been moving toward the market in early 2002—for anxiety disorders in addition to depression.[56]

This ratcheted forward development plans that had been laid for a succeeding generation of compounds stubbornly slow in coming onstream. It was thought that sufficient time had elapsed that the "tranquilizer" bogey could be overcome by simply rebranding the new drugs as anxiolytics. Nobody would point out that the benzodiazepines were anxiolytics.

Could this simple trick have been pulled off? Would psychiatrists and primary-care physicians have swallowed it? Why not, if they were prepared to swallow the Paxil advertisements for GAD in the wake of September 11?

> Paxil . . . works to correct the chemical imbalance believed to cause the disorder. . . . Most people who experience side effects on Paxil are not bothered enough to stop taking Paxil. . . . Talk to your doctor about non-habit-forming Paxil today.[57]

What chemical imbalance is this? It's a lowering of serotonin. The advertising copy for Zoloft, Paxil, and Efexor likewise contains this key commercial message: Anxiety involves a chemical imbalance in serotonin systems.

It is true that in clinical trials the majority of people taking Paxil hadn't dropped out. But even SmithKline volunteers tested on it before it came to market had dropped out at higher rates than volunteers taking amitriptyline, generally seen as the worst of the older drugs for side effects.

A second key commercial message put out by all these companies is that anxiety can also be treated by benzodiazepines, but that the benzodiazepines produce dependence and these SSRIs are not benzodiazepines. The clear implication is that SSRIs will not cause dependence. As for denying dependence, this seems one habit-forming property of psychotropic drugs that psychiatrists do nothing to prevent.

FROM *FORSYTH* TO TORONTO

In the face of the smoking isomers of S- and R-fluoxetine, Lilly resolved the *Forsyth* case in 2002.[58] The *Berman* case and a string of other cases involving Prozac and Paxil have since been resolved.

October 10, 2002, was the fortieth anniversary of the passage of the 1962 amendments to the Food and Drugs Act. The annals of U.S. public safety and U.S. government history may yet register this date for other reasons. On that day, following representations from the most senior level of the FDA, a court in the United States upheld Glaxo-SmithKline's right to label Paxil as non-habit-forming—on the basis, it would seem, that if the FDA had approved this wording, even if it flies in the face of common sense, then the courts are powerless. The fact that the FDA chose to get involved in a court case appears to call into question the separation of powers—the separation of the judiciary from the government—that is at the basis of modern polity.

On the same day in the United Kingdom, in contrast, a pharmaceutical industry complaints procedure found representatives of GlaxoSmithKline in breach of the industry's code of practice for claiming that withdrawal problems from their drug were rare and invariably mild. This was not the first such ruling against the company on this issue. And furthermore, the industry's code of practice in Britain states clearly that no company should ever state their drug is not addictive. A series of *Panorama* programs were also about to air on BBC that would transform the SSRI story.

In 2002, between one September 11 and another, CAMH and the University of Toronto reached a mediated settlement in the Healy affair. The original action involved claims for breach of contract, libel, and breach of academic freedom. This action was drawn up by Peter Rosenthal, a professor of mathematics at the University of Toronto, and also a lawyer noted for his role in legal cases involving cutting-edge social issues.[59] My primary concern was to find out just what had happened. Contract law trumps pretty much everything, and the university settled the breach of contract. It repaired its libel by making me a visiting professor. Nothing I found out led to any change in the account two chapters back of what happened when my job vanished.

In an almost certainly well-intentioned move, the University of Toronto has since put clinical trial and other research safeguards in place. Another set of rules and rulebooks for industry to master?

Epilogue

Anecdotal Deaths

IN A BBC *Panorama* program in October 2002, Alastair Benbow, a senior medical spokesperson for Glaxo-SmithKline, was quizzed by Shelley Jofre about the only published trial of Paxil in children. This trial shows dramatically higher rates of suicidal acts in children taking Paxil (Seroxat in Britain) than in those taking placebo.[1] When challenged on the use of Paxil for children, Benbow responded:[2]

> There are a number of allegations that you made there, none of which are correct and in terms of whether we think Seroxat should be made available to children? Absolutely. Two per cent of children, 4 per cent of adolescents will develop depression. The adolescents are at particular risk of suicide.
>
> We have an obligation to make our medicines available to those patients at need. Adolescents are some of the patients who are most at need of anti-depressants. Suicide in adolescents is the third leading cause of death. . . . We have a strong obligation to study our medicine in these patients to see if we can help them.
>
> The vast majority of these patients did not have side-effects significant enough to withdraw from the treatment. The reality is that in this population depression is an extremely serious condition and in many cases leads to suicide.

Benbow made these statements knowing that GSK had a total of nine studies of Paxil in children and adolescents, eight of which were unpublished. When the British regulators got to see all these studies in June 2003, they concluded that, combined, they pointed to a 1.5 to 3.2 times greater risk of suicidality on Paxil than on placebo. An immediate warning was issued against the use of Paxil in children and teenagers, but a company circular to health care professionals cautioned against abrupt discontinuation of treatment, as withdrawal could precipitate depression and suicide.[3]

When faced with the fact of a ban in Britain, Glaxo-SmithKline spokespersons in the United States refused to concede there was a problem, stating that their interpretation of the data differed from that of the regulators. Experts such as John Mann from Columbia, who have featured as legal experts for the company, publicly supported GSK. In Britain, there were complaints in the House of Lords about the unfortunate consequences of *Panorama* journalism. Nowhere were any voices raised questioning GSK's practices. No academics protested about the fact that highly relevant data on a key issue to do with patient safety remained inaccessible. When the data Jofre had faced Benbow with had been presented to thousands of psychiatrists, no one had raised a peep. Echoes of the Emperor's New Clothes are hard to ignore.

This doubling of the relative risk of suicidal acts on Paxil in children parallels the doubling of the relative risk of suicidal acts in adults on Paxil and other SSRIs. There is no reason to believe that where children are concerned this hazard is unique to Paxil, and indeed, shortly afterward Wyeth, the makers of Efexor, warned that Efexor, too, might cause suicidality, and British regulators followed their warning on Paxil with a warning against the use of Efexor (venlafaxine).

A number of key issues fell out from this. One was the fact that the few publications that emerged from these clinical trials in children had managed to conceal the problem. Some of the children were described as becoming "emotionally labile" on treatment, when this almost always appears to have meant suicidal. Others were described as "hostile," when this term can mean actual homicide, homicidal acts or ideation, or other aggressive behavior, raising the question as to how much of the academic silence can be linked to this very particular use of language. A second point is that a number of the key trialists and authors of the papers writing up these studies, such as Karen Wagner, were among the authors coordinated by Current Medical Directions for Pfizer's publications on Zoloft. At least some of the trialists in these studies appear themselves not to have known what the underlying raw data looked like.[4]

A further point that emerged concerns the regulators. They had to be told to ask the companies what emotional lability actually meant. When the details emerged, the British regulators asked GSK for all their clinical trials data on Paxil. The regulators ended up with rooms full of material and didn't know what to do with it. Apparently, when faced with fewer data for the original licensing of a drug, they had become used to working from the company summaries; but all of a sudden it appeared that the company summaries were the problem.

Except for the ends of the last three chapters, I wrote this book in the midst of also writing *The Creation of Psychopharmacology* in 2000.[5] *Creation* outlines in general terms the emergence of a picture, whereas this book gives a specific case in as much detail as possible. The plan was to present the SSRI issues as unresolved, in order to focus as much as possible on why it can fall to a journalist rather than the experts to comment on the latest imperial nakedness.

The story has moved on and is now less of a puzzle and more clearly a problem, perhaps a scandal. One of the chilling things about these events, whether a puzzle or a scandal, is how a very few people in key positions can determine the course of events and shape the consciousness of a generation. I was publicly on the record before the drugs were called SSRIs, stating that companies would market these new anxiolytic drugs as antidepressants and would branch out from there to seek markets in anxiety.[6] A raft of company material has since confirmed what seemed obvious then. It only took a few advisers to start companies on doing discontinuation trials and using the effects of withdrawal from treatment to justify campaigns to put people on maintenance treatment for years. It only took a few people to start a trend for getting the need for long-term treatment written into guidelines for the management of depressive disorders. These guidelines were completely at odds with what most clinicians thought before Prozac, and at odds with the most recent evidence, which suggests that far from requiring treatment for months or years, depressions on average last for three months.[7] Treatment accordingly need not last any longer in many cases—unless the drugs in fact cause withdrawal.

This story also brings out the fact that there is something about the current setup that enables a handful of shrewd advisers and marketers to infect health care with a clinical immune-deficiency virus (CIV). The defense reactions that might have been expected from prestigious journals and professional bodies just don't seem to have happened. Quite the contrary, the virus seems to have been able to subvert these bodies to its own purposes, so that when hazards are raised, they have reacted almost as though it was their programmed duty to shield a few fragile companies from the malignant attentions of a pharmacovigilante.

But this is not just a story about SSRIs and depression. Within psychiatry, there is a comparable marketing of ADHD, bipolar disorders, stimulants, and antipsychotics, and this looks like the norm for all future developments. In other areas of medicine a similar dynamic applies, from the marketing of hypertension to the lipid-lowering statin group of drugs and female sexual dysfunction, as well as to many other new pharmaceuticals; and it will apply to developments in genetics. Beyond medicine, the development and marketing of genetically modified (GM) foods follows a comparable template.

The Prozac story is therefore ultimately about cultures and the limits of propaganda. We are facing a future of real biomedical developments, but these will take place in a world in which corporate capacities to colonize the consciousness of citizens, physicians, regulators, and others outstrip their capacities to bring real benefits onstream. A world in which corporate capacities to get us to ignore naked emperors will greatly outstrip their ability to produce something genuinely beneficial for the emperor. A world in which a new totalitarianism and newspeak have replaced the old totalitarianisms and newspeak of communism.

In psychopharmacology, the trinkets and junkets of influence are an obvious part of the culture. Psychiatrists look at this and deny being influenced by company propaganda, when we probably mean that we deny being compromised by such. Responsible adults recognize that even university departments are businesses these days, and that practitioners are heavily influenced by the government and third-party payers, in addition to pharmaceutical companies. Being a professional, it is implied, means being able to balance these pressures, and of course we fall back on the bedrock of scientific evidence as the guarantor that while we may be influenced, we are not, indeed almost cannot be, compromised.

But the SSRI story sees this supposed bedrock against influence crumble into quicksand. RCTs have become one of the key weapons in the propaganda bag. Only when hazards are demonstrated in trials do they exist. And even then, if suicidal acts are coded as emotional lability, subsequent readers of a scientific article simply may not understand what that trial really showed.

The other side of this coin echoes a theme of Milan Kundera's *Unbearable Lightness of Being*—how can we know what life is all about as we only live it once? For GSK, Lilly, and Pfizer, the deaths of people from SSRIs have become anecdotal deaths.

Applying this logic across the board would make my sacking an anecdotal sacking from which it is impossible to draw lessons. Who knows what the key players had in mind, or what role pharmaceutical company influence might have had? Even the version that key players offered of what they did would be meaningless. Just the same logic would anesthetize us in the face of a drug disaster—what lessons can we draw from an anecdote?

Kundera's book was a response to communist totalitarianism. Both it and Orwell's *1984* suggested that a triumph of propaganda was in fact the true end of that ultimate anecdote—history. In Eastern Europe during this period, Stalin was referred to as the "Engineer of Human Souls." But with their capacities to control the media and their abilities to reshape our most intimate thoughts and experiences, from sex to the turmoil of adolescence, and the language in which we express our nervousness, GSK, Lilly, and Pfizer have become the new engineers.

This is not a story of ineluctable doom. The arrangements under which we operate are human arrangements, and human wit can adapt them. The environment has not yet been destroyed completely by these chemicals from which money can be made. But if we are not to poison a generation and produce a Silent Spring in our academic institutions, we need to resist the effects of the anesthetic, we need to recognize the hazards, and we need to act.[8]

Notes

NOTES TO THE PREFACE

1. There can be legitimate differences of interpretation on many of the points raised in this book, and hence the background documentation is being made available on a Web site, www.healyprozac.com.

2. Eli Lilly, AstraZeneca, Organon, Lundbeck, Rhône-Poulenc, and Pharmacia and Upjohn have retained me as a consultant. I have, in addition, chaired or spoken at international symposia for Pfizer, SmithKline Beecham, Roche, Pharmacia and Upjohn, Pierre Fabre, and AstraZeneca. I have been involved in clinical trials for SmithKline Beecham, Janssen Pharmaceuticals, Solvay-Duphar, Lilly, and Knoll Pharmaceuticals. Finally, I have been expert for the defense far more often than for plaintiffs in medico-legal cases.

NOTES TO THE INTRODUCTION

1. K. R. Jamison, *An Unquiet Mind* (New York: Alfred A. Knopf, 1995).

2. F. K. Goodwin and K. R. Jamison, *Manic-Depressive Illness* (Oxford: Oxford University Press, 1990).

3. "Spirit of the Age: Malignant Sadness Is the World's Great Hidden Burden," *The Economist,* December 19, 1998, 123–29.

4. D. Healy, M. Savage, P. Michael, M. Harris, D. Hirst, M. Carter, D. Cattell, T. McMonagle, N. Sohler, and E. Susser, "Psychiatric Bed Utilisation: 1896 and 1996 Compared," *Psychological Medicine* 31 (2001): 779–90.

5. Letter to the author from Linda Hurcombe. Caitlin Hurcombe's suicide note was delivered to her mother, Linda, on April 6, 1998.

6. This was Drinamyl in the United Kingdom.

7. For the Miltown story, see E. Shorter, *A History of Psychiatry: From the Era of the Asylum to the Age of Prozac* (New York: John Wiley and Sons, 1996); F. J. Ayd Jr., "The Discovery of Antidepressants," in D. Healy, *The Psychopharmacologists,* vol. 1 (London: Arnold, 1996), 81–110; M. C. Smith, *A Social History of the Minor Tranquilizers* (New York: Haworth Press, 1991).

8. This term was probably originally coined by F. Yonkman, working for

Ciba to describe the effects of reserpine. See H. Bein, "Biological Research in the Pharmaceutical Industry with Reserpine," in F. J. Ayd and B. Blackwell (eds.), *Discoveries in Biological Psychiatry* (Philadelphia: Lippincott, 1970), 142–52.

9. M. C. Smith, *A Social History of the Minor Tranquilizers* (New York: Haworth Press, 1991).

10. Ibid.

11. The benzodiazepine story is covered in greater detail in D. Healy, *The Creation of Psychopharmacology* (Cambridge, Mass.: Harvard University Press, 2002). See M. Lader, "Psychopharmacology: Clinical and Social," in D. Healy, *The Psychopharmacologists*, vol. 1, 463–82; D. Sheahan, "Angles on Panic," in D. Healy, *The Psychopharmacologists*, vol. 3 (London: Arnold, 2000), 479–504.

12. M. Bury and J. Gabe, "A Sociological View of Tranquillizer Dependence: Challenges and Responses," in I. Hindmarch, G. Beaumont, S. Brandon, and B. E. Leonard (eds.), *Benzodiazepines: Current Concepts* (Chichester: J. Wiley and Sons, 1990), 211–25; J. Gabe and M. Bury, "Tranquillisers and Health Care in Crisis," *Social Science and Medicine* 32 (1991): 449–54.

13. See interviews with Teruo Okuma, Michio Toru, and Toshi-Hiro Kobayakawa in Healy, *The Psychopharmacologists*, vol. 3.

14. Sheahan, "Angles on Panic," 479–504.

15. Buspirone was marketed by Mead Johnson in the United States and by Bristol-Myers Squibb elsewhere.

16. This section depends heavily on chap. 2 in D. Healy, *The Antidepressant Era* (Cambridge, Mass.: Harvard University Press, 1997).

17. F. J. Ayd Jr., *Recognizing the Depressed Patient* (New York: Grune and Stratton, 1961).

18. D. Healy, "The Three Faces of the Antidepressants: Critical Comments on the Clinical-Economic Framework of Diagnosis," *Journal of Nervous and Mental Disease* 187 (1999): 174–80.

19. See R. Battegay, "Forty-four Years in Psychiatry in Psychopharmacology," in Healy, *The Psychopharmacologists*, vol. 3, 371–94.

20. M. Shepherd, B. Cooper, A. C. Brown, and G. Kalton, *Psychiatric Illness in General Practice* (London: Oxford University Press, 1966).

21. The most significant were the epidemiological catchment area studies (ECA).

22. M. Shepherd, "Psychopharmacology: Specific and Non-Specific," in D. Healy, *The Psychopharmacologists*, vol. 2 (London: Arnold, 1998). For the evolution of this story, see D. Goldberg and P. Huxley, *Mental Illness in the Community: The Pathways to Psychiatric Care* (London: Tavistock Press, 1980).

23. D. Rosenhan, "On Being Sane in Insane Places," *Science* 179 (1973): 250–58.

24. DART update, October 1989. Depression—Awareness, Recognition,

and Treatment. National Institute of Mental Health. Includes quote by Lew Judd, below.

25. Results of the 1991 Defeat Depression poll survey of public opinion and the thinking behind the campaign can be found in E. S. Paykel, A. Tylee, A. Wright, R. G. Priest, S. Rix, and D. Hart, "The Defeat Depression Campaign: Psychiatry in the Public Arena," *American Journal of Psychiatry* 154, supplement (1997): 59–65.

26. E. Shorter, "Depression," in A. Dawson and A. Tylee (eds.), *Depression: Social and Economic Timebomb* (London: BMJ Books, 2001); Healy, "Three Faces of the Antidepressants," 174–80.

27. C. Murray and A. Lopez, *The Global Burden of Disease* (Cambridge, Mass.: Harvard University Press, 1996).

28. Healy et al., "Psychiatric Bed Utilisation," 779–90.

29. J. Feinman, "Rhyme, Reason and Depression: New Research Supports the Claim by Sylvia Plath's Doctor That an Inherited Condition Led to Her Suicide," *The Guardian*, February 16, 1993.

30. D. Healy and C. S. Whitaker, "Antidepressants and Suicide: Risk-Benefit Conundrums," *Journal of Psychiatry and Neuroscience* 28 (2003): 331–39.

31. J. Spijker, R. de Graaf, R. V. Bijl, A. T. F. Beekman, J. Ormel, and W. A. Nolen, "Duration of Major Depressive Episodes in the General Population: Results from the Netherlands Mental Health Survey and Incidence Study (NEMESIS)," *British Journal of Psychiatry* 181 (2002): 208–12.

32. Serotonin is also called 5-hydroxytryptamine, or 5HT.

33. G. Ashcroft, "The Receptor Enters Psychiatry," in Healy, *The Psychopharmacologists*, vol. 3, 189–200.

34. J. Axelrod, "The Discovery of Amine Reuptake," in Healy, *The Psychopharmacologists*, vol. 1, 29–50.

35. D. Eccleston, "The Receptor Enters Psychiatry (II)," in Healy, *The Psychopharmacologists*, vol. 3, 201–12.

36. J. J. Schildkraut, "The Catecholamine Hypothesis of Affective Disorders: A Review of Supporting Evidence," *American Journal of Psychiatry* 122 (1965): 519–22; J. J. Schildkraut, "The Catecholamine Hypothesis," in Healy, *The Psychopharmacologists*, vol. 3, 111–34.

37. Ashcroft, "The Receptor Enters Psychiatry," 189–200.

38. It is important to note what is *not* being said here. There are variations in serotonin levels and serotonergic receptors from person to person, and these may make us more or less sensitive to the effects of SSRIs and even to stress. SSRIs do act on serotonin, but there is no evidence of a serotonergic abnormality in depression.

39. One piece of evidence offered for lowered serotonin lies in the work of Pedro Delgado and colleagues, who gave recovered depressives a drink, which

lowers brain serotonin levels, among other things. This appeared to precipitate relapse. But many agents can trigger this kind of dysphoria, and even Delgado says that this only shows that serotonin may be necessary for the action of some antidepressants. See D. Healy, "The Case for an Individual Approach to the Treatment of Depression," *Journal of Clinical Psychiatry* 61, supplement 6 (2000): 24–28; P. Delgado, "Depression: The Case for a Monoamine Deficiency," *Journal of Clinical Psychiatry* 61, supplement 6 (2000), 7–11. P. L. Delgado, L. H. Price, H. L. Miller, G. R. Heninger, D. S. Charney, S. Woods, and W. Goodman, "Rapid Serotonin Depletion as a Provocative Challenge Test for Patients with Major Depression: Relevance to Antidepressant Action and the Neurobiology of Depression," *Psychopharmacology Bulletin* 27 (1991): 321–30.

40. Shepherd, "Psychopharmacology," 237–58; D. L. Davies and M. Shepherd, "Reserpine in the Treatment of Anxious Patients," *The Lancet* 269 (1955): 117–20.

41. Objections to a claim that reserpine is an antidepressant miss the point that the *designation* of a drug as an antidepressant is a business decision. Chlorpromazine is arguably much more antidepressant than Prozac, but the fact that it has never been licensed as, and therefore never called, an antidepressant owes everything to company perceptions of where they were likely to make money with it.

42. A. Pletscher, P. A. Shore, and B. B. Brodie, "Serotonin Release as a Possible Mechanism of Reserpine Action," *Science* 122 (1955): 374–75.

43. R. W. Wilkins, "Clinical Usage of Rauwolfia Alkaloids, Including Reserpine," *Annals New York Academy of Science* 59 (1954): 36–44. See D. Healy and M. Savage, "Reserpine Exhumed," *British Journal of Psychiatry* 172 (1998): 376–78.

44. D. C. Wallace, "Treatment of Hypertension: Hypotensive Drugs and Mental Changes," *The Lancet* 269 (1955): 116–17; F. H. Smirk and E. G. McQueen, "Comparison of Rescinamine and Reserpine as Hypotensive Agents," *The Lancet* 269 (1955): 115–16.

45. F. J. Ayd, "Drug Induced Depression—Fact or Fallacy," *New York State Journal of Medicine* (1958): 354–56.

46. R. W. P. Achor, N. O. Hanson, and R. W. Gifford, "Hypertension Treated with Rauwolfia Serpentina (Whole Root) and with Reserpine: Controlled Study Disclosing Occasional Severe Depression," *JAMA* 159 (1955): 841–45.

47. R. L. Faucett, E. M. Litin, and R. W. P. Achor, "Neuropharmacologic Action of Rauwolfia Compounds and Its Psychodynamic Implications," *AMA Archives of Neurology and Psychiatry* 77 (1957): 513–18.

48. G. J. Sarwer-Foner and W. Ogle, "Psychosis and Enhanced Anxiety Produced by Reserpine and Chlorpromazine," *Canadian Medical Association Journal* 74 (1955): 526–32.

49. H. Steck, "Le syndrome extrapyramidal et diencéphalique au cours des

traitements au Largactil et Serpasil," *Annales Medico-Psychologiques* (Paris) 112 (1954): 737–44; H.-J. Haase, "The Role of Drug-Induced Extrapyramidal Syndromes," in N. S. Kline (ed.), *Psychopharmacology Frontiers* (Boston: Little, Brown, 1958), 197–208.

50. See Healy and Savage, "Reserpine Exhumed," 376–78.

51. *Diagnostic and Statistical Manual*, 4th ed. (DSM-IV), text revision (Washington, D.C.: American Psychiatric Association Press, 2000).

52. For a consideration and definition of akathisia, see D. G. Cunningham-Owens, *A Guide to the Extrapyramidal Side-Effects of Antipsychotic Drugs* (Cambridge: Cambridge University Press, 1999).

53. A. Carlsson and D. T. Wong, "Correction: A Note on the Discovery of Selective Serotonin Reuptake Inhibitors," *Life Sciences* 61 (1997): 1203.

54. D. T. Wong, F. P. Bymaster, and E. A. Engleman, "Prozac (Fluoxetine, Lilly 110140), the First Selective Serotonin Reuptake Inhibitor and an Antidepressant Drug: Twenty Years since Its First Publication," *Life Sciences* 57 (1995): 411–41.

55. P. Kielholz, *Diagnose und Therapie der Depressionen fur Praktiker* (Munich: J. F. Lehmanns, 1971).

56. Arvid Carlsson was awarded a Nobel Prize in 2000.

57. A. Carlsson, "The Rise of Neuropsychopharmacology: Impact on Basic and Clinical Neuroscience," in Healy, *The Psychopharmacologists*, vol. 1, 51–80.

58. The articles first demonstrating these biochemical properties are by A. Carlsson, H. Corrodi, K. Fuxe, and T. Hokfelt, "Effects of Some Antidepressant Drugs in the Depletion of Intraneuronal Brain 5-Hydroxytryptamine Stores Caused by 4-Methyl-Alpha-Ethyl-Tyramine" and "Effects of Some Antidepressant Drugs on the Depletion of Intraneuronal Brain Catecholamine Stores Caused by 4-Alpha-Dimethyl-Meta-Tyramine," *European Journal of Pharmacology* 5 (1969): 357–66 and 367–73.

59. The zimelidine story and details of the drug can be found in A. Carlsson, C.-G. Gottfries, G. Holmberg, K. Modigh, T. Svensson, and S.-O. Ogren, *Acta Psychiatrica Scandinavia* 63, supplement 290 (1981): 1–475.

60. See L. Iversen, "Neuroscience and Drug Development," in Healy, *The Psychopharmacologists*, vol. 2, 325–50.

61. I owe some of these details to Sven Ove Ogren of Astra.

62. With figures like this, it is difficult to disentangle true development monies from marketing and other costs.

63. Omeprazole was marketed as Prilosec in North America and Losec in most European countries.

64. S. A. Montgomery, R. McAulay, S. J. Rani, D. Roy, and D. B. Montgomery, "A Double Blind Comparison of Zimelidine and Amitriptyline in Endogenous Depression," *Acta Psychiatrica Scandinavia* 63, supplement 290 (1981): 314–27.

65. E. Hellbom, M. Humble, and M. Larsson, "Antihistamines, SSRIs and Panic Disorder" (paper presented at the Twenty-sixth Annual Meeting of the Scandinavian Society for Psychopharmacology, 1999).

66. Through the 1970s, many companies developed SSRIs. For some this was simply an academic exercise to produce a behavioral probe. Serotonin was not the fashionable neurotransmitter. Ciba-Geigy, for instance, produced a series of the most potent SSRIs ever synthesized, but none were developed. Some of these SSRIs, including Prozac, in toxicological testing on dogs caused the appearance of vesicles in the lipid layers of the brain. No one was certain what this meant at the time. Some companies abandoned the development of their SSRI at this point, where others persisted. There appears to be no clear connection between this phenomenon in dogs and any comparable phenomenon in humans. See R. Pindar, "Approaching Rationality," in Healy, *The Psychopharmacologists*, vol. 2, 581–605. However, drugs active on the serotonin system do appear, perhaps in susceptible individuals only, to produce extensive pruning of nerve endings. This has been described clearly for Ecstasy and for some SSRIs. The scientific establishment often puts considerable effort into detecting problems with illicit substances, but little effort into seeing whether comparable changes may be happening with therapeutic drugs. See M. Kalia, J. P. O'Callaghan, D. B. Miller, and M. Kramer, "Comparative Study of Fluoxetine, Sibutramine, Sertraline and Dexfenfluramine on the Morphology of Serotonergic Nerve Terminals Using Serotonin Immunohistochemistry," *Brain Research* 858 (2000): 92–105.

67. On indalpine, see Comité Lyonnais de Recherches Thérapeutiques en Psychiatrie (CLRTP), "The Birth of Psychopharmacotherapy: Explorations in a New World, 1952–1968," in Healy, *The Psychopharmacologists*, vol. 3, 1–54; and P. Simon, "Twenty-first Century Drug Development," in Healy, *The Psychopharmacologists*, vol. 3, 523–42.

68. G. Naylor and B. Martin, "A Double-Blind Trial Out-Patient Trial of Indalpine vs. Mianserin," *British Journal of Psychiatry* 147 (1985): 306–9.

69. CLRTP, "Birth of Psychopharmacotherapy," 1–54.

70. Healy, *Creation of Psychopharmacology*, chap. 4.

71. The drug's manufacturer, Hoechst, knew of fourteen patients who died while taking the drug; one was the daughter of a politician. Author's conversation with P. Stonier, former medical director, Hoechst UK.

72. On the mianserin and other "hysterias," see R. Pinder, "Approaching Rationality," in Healy, *The Psychopharmacologists*, vol. 2, 581–605. See also R. Pinder, "The Benefits and Risks of Antidepressant Drugs," *Human Psychopharmacology* (1987): 73–86.

73. The company later brought out mirtazapine (Remeron), a closely related molecule, which, at the time of writing, has not achieved the same level of sales as mianserin.

74. Pinder, "Approaching Rationality," 581–605.

75. Fluovoxamine was developed from tripelennamine by Hendrik Welle and Volkert Classens in 1973.

76. J. S. Wakelin, "The Role of Serotonin in Depression and Suicide: Do Serotonin Reuptake Inhibitors Provide a Key?" in M. Gastpar and J. S. Wakelin (eds.), *Selective Serotonin Reuptake Inhibitors: Novel or Commonplace Agents* (Basel: Karger, 1988), 70–83.

77. P. Pichot, "The Discovery of Chlorpromazine and the Place of Psychopharmacology in the History of Psychiatry," in Healy, *The Psychopharmacologists*, vol. 1, 1–21.

78. CLRTP, "Birth of Psychopharmacotherapy," 1–54.

79. G. Beaumont and D. Healy, "The Place of Clomipramine in the Development of Psychopharmacology," *Journal of Psychopharmacology* 7 (1993): 383–93. See Healy, *Antidepressant Era*, chap. 6.

80. J. Rapoport, "Children, Phenomenology and Psychopharmacology," in Healy, *The Psychopharmacologists*, vol. 3, 333–56.

81. This doesn't necessarily mean that there is anything wrong with the serotonin system in OCD: see D. Healy, "What Do 5HT Reuptake Inhibitors Do in Obsessive-Compulsive Disorder," *Human Psychopharmacology* 6 (1991): 325–28.

82. J. L. Rapoport, *The Boy Who Couldn't Stop Washing* (New York: E. P. Dutton, 1989).

83. Luvox has other brand names in Europe, including Faverin in the United Kingdom.

84. V. Pedersen and K. Bøgesø, "Drug Hunting," in Healy, *The Psychopharmacologists*, vol. 2, 561–80.

85. A. Solomon, "Personal History: Anatomy of Melancholy," *New Yorker*, January 12, 1998, 47–61. This later became a book: A. Solomon, *The NoonDay Demon* (New York: Scribner, 2001).

86. A. Solomon, address to American Psychiatric Association (Chicago, May 2000).

87. S. Berfield, "A CEO and His Son," *Business Week*, May 27, 2002, 72–80.

88. D. Kirkpatrick, "Inside the Happiness Business," *New Yorker*, May 15, 2000, 36–43.

89. Zoloft is the trade name for sertraline in most of the world; in the United Kingdom, it trades as Lustral.

90. W. Welch, "Discovery and Preclinical Development of the Serotonin Reuptake Inhibitor Sertraline," *Advances in Medicinal Chemistry* 3 (1995): 113–48.

91. For example, less likely to lead to suicidality.

92. S. Woolley, "Science and Savvy," *Forbes*, January 11, 1999, 122–27.

93. On femoxetine, see J. Buus-Lassen, E. Petersen, B. Kjellberg, and S. Olsson, "Comparative Studies of a New 5HT (Serotonin) Uptake Inhibitor and Tricyclic Thymoleptics," *European Journal of Pharmacology* 32 (1975): 108–15; on

paroxetine, see J. Buus-Lassen, "Introduction to the Development of Paroxetine, a Novel Antidepressant," *Acta Psychiatrica Scandinavia* 80, supplement 350 (1989): 13. The entire supplement is given over to development work on paroxetine.

94. In the early 1980s, I was working on serotonin uptake, which appeared to be low in depression—one of the few things that could be shown to be abnormal. This brought me into contact with Beecham and paroxetine. See D. Healy and B. E. Leonard, "Monoamine Transport in Depression: Kinetics and Dynamics," *Journal of Affective Disorders* 12 (1987): 91–105.

95. Danish Universities Antidepressant Group, "Paroxetine: A Selective Serotonin Reuptake Inhibitor Showing Better Tolerance but Weaker Antidepressant Effect Than Clomipramine in a Controlled Multicenter Study," *Journal of Affective Disorders* 18 (1990): 289–99.

96. Around 1990, when the acronym was first coined, company marketers had in mind a model in which billiard or snooker balls being potted cleanly into pockets stood for the process of neurotransmission. This image would later recur in direct-to-consumer TV advertisements for modern medicines put out by the Pharmaceutical Manufacturers of America. The first use of this model to describe neurotransmission may have been in a London Weekend Television (LWT) series of programs called *How to Stay Alive,* aired in 1979. These details come from a conversation with Thelma Rumsey, a science researcher for LWT and later BBC, April 2002.

97. Edward Shorter, however, has pointed out that Roussel was advertising trazodone (Desyrel in North America and Molipaxin in the United Kingdom) as a selective serotonin inhibitor in 1982.

98. See Healy, *Antidepressant Era,* chap. 6.

99. D. Healy, "Have Drug Companies Hyped Social Anxiety Disorders to Increase Sales? Yes. Marketing Hinders the Discovery of Long-Term Solutions" and David Sheehan, "Response," *Western Journal of Medicine* 175 (2001): 364–65.

100. C. Medawar, "The Antidepressant Web," *International Journal of Risk and Safety in Medicine* 10 (1997): 75–125.

101. The issue of physical dependence to all SSRIs was raised most clearly in Britain by Charles Medawar, who had been an active player in the benzodiazepine dependence story. Medawar wrote to the Royal College of Psychiatrists, the Committee of Safety for Medicines in Britain, and others, noting the similarities in the emergence of a dependence problem with the SSRIs to the way the story had unfolded in the case of the benzodiazepines. His letters and their replies are laid out in fascinating detail on his Web site, www.socialaudit.org.uk. Minutes from Medicine Control Agency's meeting, Thursday, March 26, 1998, item 7.3.3, at http://www.socialaudit.org.uk/5003-2.htm#RESTRICTED.

102. At the time, Lilly lobbied British regulators to have the term *with-*

drawal syndrome changed to *discontinuation syndrome*—but this suggestion was not taken up. Minutes from Medicine Control Agency meetings 1997, available on http://www.socialaudit.org.uk/5003-2.htm.

103. J. F. Rosenbaum, M. Fava, S. L. Hoog, R. C. Ashcroft, and W. Krebs, "Selective Serotonin Reuptake Inhibitor Discontinuation Syndrome: A Randomised Clinical Study," *Biological Psychiatry* 44 (1998): 77–87. See also www.socialaudit.org.uk.

104. Among the insider takes on this, I have heard it said that the dependence story began to play at a time when Prozac was at real risk of being overtaken by Paxil and/or Zoloft.

105. Perhaps because they are so easy to get hold of legitimately.

106. L. Slater, *Prozac Diary* (Harmondsworth, Middlesex: Penguin Books, 1998).

107. D. Healy and R. Tranter, "Pharmacologic Stress Diathesis Syndromes," *Journal of Psychopharmacology* 13 (1999): 287–90, with commentaries by H. Ashton, A. Young and N. Ferrier, R. Baldessarini, A. Viguera and L. Tondo, L. Hollister, P. Haddad and I. Anderson, and P. Tyrer (291–98) and reply by Healy and Tranter, "In the Shadow of the Benzodiazepines" (299). See also Healy, *Creation of Psychopharmacology*; and D. Healy, *Psychiatric Drugs Explained*, 3d ed. (Edinburgh: Churchill-Livingstone, 2001), chap. 8.

108. J. Glenmullen, *Prozac Backlash* (New York: Simon and Schuster, 2000).

109. D. Healy, deposition and trial transcript in *Tobin vs. SmithKline* (2001); available on www.healyprozac.com/Trials. At a public debate in the Institute of Psychiatry in London (July 2003), before approximately 150 people, the editor of the *British Journal of Psychiatry*, Peter Tyrer, said that he had written to the company circa 1981 telling them of his concerns that their drug might be causing dependence. See also D. Healy, "SSRIs and Withdrawal/Dependence" (briefing paper presented to the British regulatory agency, the Medical and Healthcare Products Regulatory Agency, June 20, 2003), posted on http://www.socialaudit.co.uk; and deposition of B. Beard in *In re Paxil litigation*, CV-01-07937MRP (CWx), U.S. District Court, Central District of California, October 8, 2003, exhibit 7 and p. 297 *et seq.*

110. Many of the details here come from depositions in the Fentress/Wesbecker trials (see Chapter 2), taken by Paul Smith and Nancy Zettler from Irwin Slater, January 28 and 29, 1994; Ray Fuller, April 14 and 15, 1994; and David Wong, January 12 and April 13, 1994.

111. D. T. Wong, J. S. Horng, F. P. Bymaster, K. L. Hauser, and B. B. Molloy, "A Selective Inhibitor of Serotonin Uptake: Lilly 110140 3-(p-trifluoromethylphenoxy)-N-methyl-3-phenylpropylamine," *Life Sciences* 15 (1974): 471–79.

112. Its failure, and that of other SSRIs, on this test, along with the fact that older antidepressants do not cause marked akathisia, retrospectively suggests

that the reserpine test may in fact be a screening test for akathisia rather than for antidepressant activity.

113. A. Mundy, *Dispensing with the Truth: The Victims, the Drug Companies, and the Dramatic Story behind the Battle over Fen-Phen* (New York: St. Martin's Press, 2001). See M. Lemonick, "How Mood Drugs Work . . . and Fail," *Time*, Sept. 29, 1997, 75–82.

114. A. Coppen, "Biological Psychiatry in Britain," in Healy, *The Psychopharmacologists*, vol. 1, 265–86.

115. These are typically called extrapyramidal side effects; see Healy, *Psychiatric Drugs Explained*.

116. H. Y. Meltzer, "A Career in Biological Psychiatry," in Healy, *The Psychopharmacologists*, vol. 1, 483–508.

117. C. Beasley, exhibit 7 in deposition of Charles Beasley in *Fentress et al. vs. Shea Communications and Eli Lilly and Company* (1994), docket no. 90-CI-06033, Jefferson Circuit Court (hereafter *Fentress vs. Eli Lilly*). Adolph Pfefferbaum had six out of fifteen patients improve. Joyce Small found three out of eleven much improved. James Claghorn reported two out of seven improved and two out of seven much worse.

118. Fluoxetine Project Team Meeting Minutes, July 23, 1979; exhibit in *Fentress vs. Eli Lilly*. Available on www.healyprozac.com/CriticalDocs.

119. Deposition of Irwin Slater in *Fentress vs. Eli Lilly*.

120. Beasley, exhibit 7 in deposition of Charles Beasley. On Fabre, see J. Abraham and J. Sheppard, *The Therapeutic Nightmare* (London: Earthscan, 2000), 84.

121. See www.interbrand.com/papers_review.asp?sp_id=39.

122. A. Feuerstein, "Meet the Street: How to Name a Blockbuster Drug" (2001), at www.meetthestreet.com.

123. Deposition of Richard Wood in *Fentress vs. Eli Lilly*. This issue is picked up further in Chapter 10.

124. J. Wernicke, S. R. Dunlop, B. Dornseif, and R. Zerbe, "Fluoxetine Is Effective in the Treatment of Depression at Low Fixed Doses" (abstract prepared for Fifteenth Collegium Internationale Neuropsychopharmacologium [CINP] Congress, Puerto Rico, 1986), exhibit in *Fentress vs. Eli Lilly*.

125. Exhibit in *Fentress vs. Eli Lilly*. Quotes and abstract in PZ1135, 678–81 (1994).

126. S. A. Montgomery, D. James, M. de Ruiter, et al., "Weekly Oral Fluoxetine Treatment of Major Depressive Disorder, a Controlled Trial" (paper presented at Fifteenth CINP Congress, Puerto Rico, 1986).

127. See M. Fink, "A Clinician Researcher and ECDEU," in T. Ban, D. Healy, and E. Shorter (eds.), *The Triumph of Psychopharmacology* (Budapest: Animula, 2000). See also Healy, *Creation of Psychopharmacology*, chap. 6.

128. S. Stecklow and L. Johannes, "Questions Arise on New Drug Testing:

Drug Makers Relied on Clinical Researchers Who Now Await Trial," *Wall Street Journal*, August 15, 1997; K. Eichenwald and G. Kolata, "Drug Trials Hide Conflict for Doctors," *New York Times*, May 16, 1999, 1, 28, 29; "A Doctor's Drug Studies Turn into Fraud," *New York Times*, May 17, 1999, 1, 16, 17; S. Boseley, "Trial and Error Puts Patients at Risk," *The Guardian*, July 27, 1999, 8.

129. P. Leber, "Managing Uncertainty," in Healy, *The Psychopharmacologists*, vol. 2, 607–22.

130. FDA's Psychopharmacologic Drugs Advisory Committee, twenty-eighth meeting, October 10, 1985. The hearing this day was on Prozac (1985). The transcript is available on www.healyprozac.com/PDAC.

131. Ibid.

132. Ibid.

133. T. De Ciccio, Minutes of the "In-House Meeting on Fluoxetine" of the U.S. Food and Drug Administration, Washington, D.C., November 13, 1984. Obtained through Freedom of Information Act, available from author.

134. T. J. Moore, "Hard to Swallow," *The Washingtonian* 33 (1997): 68–71 and following.

135. FDA's Psychopharmacological Drugs Advisory Committee, thirty-third meeting, November 19, 1990. This hearing was given over to Zoloft. Transcript available at www.healyprozac.com/PDAC.

136. Ibid.

137. Ibid., 90–91.

138. M. Fink, "The Early Clinical Drug Evaluation Unit," in Ban, Healy, and Shorter, *Triumph of Psychopharmacology*, 441–62.

139. Minutes, Eli Lilly Pharmaceutical Product Strategy Meeting, April 6, 1983; exhibit in *Fentress vs. Eli Lilly*. Available from author.

140. Ibid.

141. I. M. Anderson and B. M. Tomenson, "The Efficacy of Selective Serotonin Reuptake Inhibitors in Depression: A Meta-Analysis of Studies against Tricyclic Antidepressants," *Journal of Psychopharmacology* 8 (1994): 238–49.

142. I. M. Anderson and B. M. Tomenson, "Treatment Discontinuation with Selective Serotonin Reuptake Inhibitors Compared to Tricyclic Antidepressants: A Meta-Analysis," *British Medical Journal* 310 (1995): 1433–38.

143. S. M. Gilbody and F. Song, "Publication Bias and the Integrity of Psychiatry Research," *Psychological Medicine* 30 (2000): 253–58; N. Freemantle, J. Mason, T. Phillips, and I. M. Anderson, "Predictive Value of Pharmacological Activity for the Relative Efficacy of Antidepressant Drugs: Meta-Regression Analysis," *British Journal of Psychiatry* 177 (2000): 292–302.

144. J. Donoghue, "Antidepressant Use in Primary Care," in A. Dawson and A. Tylee (eds.), *Depression: Social and Economic Timebomb* (London: BMJ Books, 2001), 151–56; J. Donoghue and D. M. Taylor, "Suboptimal Use of Antidepressants in the Treatment of Depression," *CNS Drugs* 5 (2000): 365–83.

145. May 25, 1984, communication to Lilly US from Lilly Bad Homburg by B. v. Keitz, containing a translation of an unofficially received medical comment on the fluoxetine application to the German regulators. Available at www.healyprozac.com/Trials/CriticalDocs.

NOTES TO CHAPTER I

1. The case described here was first described as Case A in W. Creaney, I. Murray, and D. Healy, "Antidepressant Induced Suicidal Ideation," *Human Psychopharmacology* 6 (1991): 329–32.

2. All quotes refer to extracts from this Mr. A's contemporary notes.

3. Several years later, he appeared able to tolerate venlafaxine, which is also a serotonin reuptake inhibitor. However, he was also on a thioridazine, which theoretically could block some of his SSRI problems.

4. M. H. Teicher, C. Glod, and J. O. Cole, "Emergence of Intense Suicidal Preoccupation during Fluoxetine Treatment," *American Journal of Psychiatry* 147 (1990): 207–10.

5. H. M. van Praag, "Biological Suicide Research: Outcome and Limitations," *Biological Psychiatry* 21 (1986): 1305–23.

6. D. Healy, "The Structure of Psychopharmacological Revolutions," *Psychiatric Developments* 5 (1987): 349–76.

7. Teicher, Glod, and Cole, "Emergence of Intense Suicidal Preoccupation during Fluoxetine Treatment," 207–10.

8. J. O. Cole, "The Evaluation of Psychotropic Drugs," in D. Healy (ed.), *The Psychopharmacologists*, vol. 1 (London: Arnold, 1996), 239–64.

9. M. H. Teicher, C. Glod, and J. O. Cole, "Suicidal Preoccupation during Fluoxetine Treatment," *American Journal of Psychiatry* 147 (1990): 1380–81.

10. Cole, "Evaluation of Psychotropic Drugs," 239–64.

11. Exhibit 83, Fluoxetine Project Team meeting minutes no. 79-2, July 23, 1979, in *Forsyth et al. vs. Eli Lilly and Company* (1999), civil no. 95-00185ACK, U.S. District Court for the District of Hawaii (hereafter *Forsyth vs. Eli Lilly*). These Eli Lilly minutes are available at www.healyprozac.com/Trials/CriticalDocs.

12. The case reported here was first reported as Case B in Creaney, Murray, and Healy, "Antidepressant Induced Suicidal Ideation," 329–32.

13. Flupenthixol is used in low doses in Europe and Canada as an antidepressant; it is not available in the United States. Parstelin is a combination of tranylcypromine and stelazine. Alprazolam trades as Xanax, thioridazine as Mellaril, viloxazine as Vivalan, and maprotiline as Ludiomil.

14. Interviews of this sort were a regular feature of psychiatric practice until the 1960s. They have since been implicated in the generation of memories of abuse that never happened. They are essentially a form of hypnosis.

15. Correspondence to author from Eli Lilly (1991).

16. Creaney, Murray, and Healy, "Antidepressant Induced Suicidal Ideation," 329–32.

17. M. Fava and J. F. Rosenbaum, "Suicidality and Fluoxetine: Is There a Relationship?" *Journal of Clinical Psychiatry* 52 (1991): 108–11.

18. Memo from David Graham, FDA, Sept. 11, 1990; obtained under the Freedom of Information (FOI) Act from FDA; available on www.healyprozac.com/Trials/CriticalDocs.

19. American College of Neuropsychopharmacology (ACNP), "Suicidal Behavior and Psychotropic Medication," *Neuropsychopharmacology* 8 (1992): 177–83.

20. M. H. Teicher, C. A. Glod, and J. O. Cole, "Antidepressant Drugs and the Emergence of Suicidal Tendencies," *Drug Safety* 8 (1993): 186–212.

21. See D. Healy, "A Failure to Warn," Guest Editorial, *International Journal of Risk and Safety in Medicine* 12 (1999): 151–56.

22. W. C. Wirshing, T. van Putten, J. Rosenberg, S. Marder, D. Ames, and T. Hicks-Gray, "Fluoxetine, Akathisia and Suicidality: Is There a Causal Connection?" *Archives of General Psychiatry* 49 (1992): 580–81.

23. Memo from P. Leber to T. Laughren, "Re: Akathesia and Fluoxetine," July 15, 1992; obtained from FDA under the Freedom of Information Act.

24. R. A. King, M. A. Riddle, P. B. Chappell, M. T. Hardin, G. M. Anderson, P. Lombroso, and L. Scahill, "Emergence of Self-Destructive Phenomena in Children and Adolescents during Fluoxetine Treatment," *Journal of American Academy of Child and Adolescent Psychiatry* 30 (1991): 171–76.

25. They are also significant in that more recent evidence suggests children may be at even greater risk of these problems than adults, leading British regulators to caution against the use of Paxil in children in June 2003.

26. A. J. Rothschild and C. A. Locke, "Re-Exposure to Fluoxetine after Serious Suicide Attempts by Three Patients: The Role of Akathisia," *Journal of Clinical Psychiatry* 52 (1991): 491–93.

27. There were further cases—K. Dasgupta, "Additional Case of Suicidal Ideations Associated with Fluoxetine," *American Journal of Psychiatry* 147 (1990): 1570; P. Masand, S. Gupta, and M. Dwan, "Suicidal Ideation Related to Fluoxetine Treatment," *New England Journal of Medicine* 324 (1991): 420; C. Hoover, "Additional Cases of Suicidal Ideation Associated with Fluoxetine," *American Journal of Psychiatry* 147 (1990): 1570–71.

28. D. Healy, W. Creaney, and I. Murray, "Antidepressant Induced Suicidal Ideation," Abstracts of Annual British Association for Pharmacology (BAP) Meeting, *Journal of Psychopharmacology* 6 (1992): 120.

29. C. M. Beasley, B. E. Dornseif, J. C. Bosomworth, M. E. Sayler, A. H. Rampey, J. H. Heiligenstein, V. L. Thompson, D. J. Murphy, and D. N. Massica, "Fluoxetine and Suicide: A Meta-Analysis of Controlled Trials of Treatment for Depression," *British Medical Journal* 303 (1991): 685–92.

30. For Lilly's figures, see P. Stark, C. D. Hardison, "A Review of Multi-centre Controlled Studies of Fluoxetine versus Imipramine and Placebo in Out-patients with Major Depressive Disorder," *Journal of Clinical Psychiatry* 46 (1985): 53–58. For an update, see W. M. Patterson, "Fluoxetine-Induced Sexual Dysfunction," *Journal of Clinical Psychiatry* 54 (1993): 71.

31. D. Healy and W. Creaney, "Antidepressant Induced Suicidal Ideation," *British Medical Journal* 303 (1991): 1058–59.

32. C. Beasley, letter, *British Medical Journal* 303 (1991): 1059.

33. Memo from Dr. J. Wernicke, July 2, 1986, in which he states that "the suicide factor on the HAMD does not provide an accurate predictor, thus we do not advocate it be used in place of the investigator's judgment"; exhibit 69 in *Forsyth vs. Eli Lilly*. See also exhibit 28 in the deposition of L. Fludzinski in *Fentress et al. vs. Shea Communications and Eli Lilly and Company* (1994), case no. 90-CI-06033, Jefferson Circuit Court (hereafter *Fentress vs. Eli Lilly*).

34. I. Oswald, *British Medical Journal* 303 (1991): 1058.

35. J. Abraham and J. Sheppard, *The Therapeutic Nightmare: The Battle over the World's Most Controversial Sleeping Pill* (London: Earthscan, 1999).

36. See ibid.; and "The Halcion Nightmare," in D. Hooper, *Reputations under Fire* (London: Little, Brown, 2000). The Halcion story is relevant to the Prozac story. Putting the two together could lead to a more company-hostile interpretation of what happened in the Prozac story than that offered here.

37. *Dispatches,* a current affairs program on Channel 4 in the United Kingdom, date filed December 19, 1990.

38. R. Behar, "The Thriving Cult of Greed and Power. Ruined Lives. Lost Fortunes. Federal Crimes. Scientology Poses as a Religion but Is Really a Ruthless Global Scam—and Aiming for the Mainstream," *Time,* May 6, 1991, 32–39.

39. Chasing the background to this book, almost ten years after the *Time* article, I came across a stand-alone Church of Scientology publication: *A Story That Time Couldn't Tell.* This claims that *Time* and Lilly had board members in common and that Lilly was threatening to remove its account from J. Walter Thompson, a subsidiary of the public relations company WPP, if Hill and Knowlton, another subsidiary of WPP, didn't drop their Scientology account. After the *Time* article, they did. These details are on record in a legal suit: *Church of Scientology vs. Eli Lilly and Company and Hill and Knowlton Inc.,* 848 F.Supp. 1018, U.S. District Court, Civil Action no. 92–1892, March 21, 1994.

40. J. F. Rosenbaum, "Clinical Trial by Media: The Prozac Story," in H. I. Schwartz (ed.), *Psychiatric Practice under Fire: The Influence of Government, the Media and Special Interests on Somatic Therapies* (Washington, D.C.: American Psychiatric Association Press, 1994), 3–27.

41. T. W. Burton, "Anti-Depression Drug of Eli Lilly Loses Sales after Attack by Sect," *Wall Street Journal,* April 19, 1991, 1 and thereafter.

42. Quote from letter from Melvin Sabshin, April 19, 1991, from the American Psychiatric Association Archives, Box 35, Folder 486 "Prozac."

43. Transcript of Food and Drug Administration, Psychopharmacological Drugs Advisory Committee, Thirty-fourth Meeting, Sept. 20, 1991. Available on www.healyprozac.com/PDAC.

44. See P. Breggin, *Talking Back to Prozac* (New York: St. Martin's Press, 1994).

45. Food and Drug Administration, Psychopharmacological Drugs Advisory Committee, Thirty-fourth Meeting, Sept. 20, 1991. Transcript available on www.healyprozac.com/PDAC.

46. Memo from David Graham, FDA, Sept. 11, 1990; obtained under Freedom of Information Act.

47. See G. Enas deposition in *Fentress vs. Eli Lilly;* exhibit 1 in *Fentress vs. Eli Lilly,* notes taken by James Kotsanos at an FDA meeting to discuss Fluoxetine Rechallenge Protocol, May 13, 1991; and Catherine Mesner, deposition in *Fentress vs. Eli Lilly.*

48. Transcript of Food and Drug Administration, Psychopharmacological Drugs Advisory Committee, Thirty-fourth Meeting, Sept. 20, 1991. Available on www.healyprozac.com/PDAC. See also FDA minutes of meeting on Prozac, May 13, 1991, taken by Paul David: The division had required that the firm submit protocols to determine whether a relationship exists between taking Prozac and suicidal ideation. Lilly submitted two draft protocols. See corresponding minutes from Lilly side taken by J. Kotsanos, Wheadon exhibit 9 in *Fentress vs. Eli Lilly.* See also memo from L. Thompson to colleagues, July 18, 1990, on this issue, and draft protocol for rechallenge study submitted to FDA on March 29, 1991, Wheadon exhibit 10 in *Fentress vs. Eli Lilly.*

49. Transcript of Food and Drug Administration, Psychopharmacological Drugs Advisory Committee, Thirty-fourth Meeting, Sept. 20, 1991. Available on www.healyprozac.com/PDAC.

50. Deposition of Martin Teicher in *Greer vs. Eli Lilly* (1996), October 29 and 30, 1996, case 91-1790 JGP.

51. Martin Teicher volunteered some information about this pressure in an interview with the author on March 30, 2000.

52. Food and Drug Administration, Psychopharmacological Drugs Advisory Committee, Thirty-fourth Meeting, Sept. 20, 1991.

53. Teicher claims he had been told that the session was informal and that no slides or prepared data were permitted. The issue of handouts was not covered by the organizer Carl Salzman from Massachusetts Mental Hospital. From author's interview with Martin Teicher, March 2000.

54. I have these details from Teicher and one other witness. Teicher also claims that at this meeting he was told that continuing in this position would ruin his career.

55. ACNP, "Suicidal Behavior and Psychotropic Medication," 177–83.

56. J. J. Mann and S. Kapur, "The Emergence of Suicidal Ideation and Behavior during Antidepressant Pharmacotherapy," *Archives of General Psychiatry* 48 (1991): 1027–33.

57. Deposition of D. Healy in *Miller vs. Pfizer Inc.* (2000), case no. 99-2326 KHV, U.S. District Court for the District of Kansas, March 27 and 28, 2000.

58. Teicher, Glod, and Cole, "Antidepressant Drugs and the Emergence of Suicidal Tendencies," 186–212.

NOTES TO CHAPTER 2

1. J. Cornwell, *The Power to Harm: Mind, Medicine and Murder on Trial* (New York: Viking, 1996).

2. L. Coleman, deposition in *Fentress et al. vs. Shea Communications and Eli Lilly and Company* (1994), civil case no. 90-CI-06033, Jefferson Circuit Court, Sept. 9, 1993 (hereafter *Fentress vs. Eli Lilly*).

3. Brenda Camp, trial testimony in *Fentress vs. Eli Lilly*, Oct. 31, 1994.

4. James Wesbecker, trial testimony in *Fentress vs. Eli Lilly*, Nov. 18, 1994.

5. J. Glenmullen, *Prozac Backlash* (New York: Simon and Schuster, 2000).

6. Ibid. But in addition, the discovery of the antidepressants came from imipramine's capacity to make patients psychotic—see D. Healy, *The Antidepressant Era* (Cambridge, Mass.: Harvard University Press, 1997), chap. 2.

7. Letter of Paul Smith to other plaintiffs' counsel, April 27, 1983, on file as exhibit in *Winkler vs. Eli Lilly MDL* (1997), Indianapolis, case no. C95-732C filed in 274th Judicial District of Comal County, Texas.

8. By convention, the case is named after the first plaintiff, listed alphabetically.

9. This section depends heavily on author's interview with Nancy Zettler (July 2001), who has subsequently reviewed the section for accuracy.

10. There is also a set of documents from the Halcion cases and the trial of Ian Oswald. See J. Abraham and J. Sheppard, *The Therapeutic Nightmare* (London: Earthscan, 1999).

11. The depositions included Max Talbott, June 4, 1992, and January 13, 1994; David Wheadon, June 9 and 10, 1992; Catherine Mesner, Aug. 17 and Oct. 15, 1993; David Wong, Jan. 12 and April 13, 1994; Paul Stark, March 5, 29, and 30, 1994; John Heiligenstein, April 27, 28, and 29, 1994; Richard Wood, May 12, 1994; Robert Zerbe, May 13 and Aug. 9, 1994; Charles Beasley, May 17 and 18, 1994; Dorothy Dobbs, July 11, 1994; Leigh Thompson, July 20, 21, and 22, 1994; Hans Weber, Sept. 10, 1994; Nick Schulze-Solce, Sept. 16, 1994.

12. C. Mesner, deposition in *Fentress vs. Eli Lilly*, Aug. 17, 1993.

13. J. Heiligenstein, deposition in *Fentress vs. Eli Lilly*, April 27 and 28, 1994.

14. C. Mesner, deposition in *Fentress vs. Eli Lilly*, Aug. 17, 1993.

15. Including the following cases: *Biffle vs. Eli Lilly*, 91-02496-A; *Welch vs. Eli Lilly*, 93-04911-A; *Crossett vs. Eli Lilly*, 92-14775-E; *Reves vs. Eli Lilly*, A-921,405-C; *Saines vs. Eli Lilly*, SC 008331; *Huslig vs. Eli Lilly*, 94-C-192; *Kung vs. Eli Lilly*, 93-8792-D.

16. Teicher and Zettler agree on his discomfort with the approach to the regulatory and company documents the attorneys wanted him to consider. Author's interviews with Martin Teicher, March 2000, and with Nancy Zettler, July 2001.

17. P. Breggin, *Toxic Psychiatry: Why Therapy, Empathy and Love Must Replace the Drugs, Electroshock and Biochemical Theories of the "New Psychiatry"* (New York: St. Martin's Press, 1991).

18. P. Breggin, *Talking Back to Prozac: What Doctors Aren't Telling You about Today's Most Controversial Drug* (New York: St. Martin's Press, 1994).

19. J. Cornwell, *Power to Harm*; D. Kurschner, "Interview with Randall Tobias," *Business Ethics* 9 (1995): 31–34; R. Stodghill II, "Lilly Rides a Mood Elevator," *Business Week*, Nov. 11, 1996, 63–64.

20. The details here come from Cornwell, *Power to Harm*; and the trial transcript in *Fentress et al. vs. Shea Communications and Eli Lilly and Company* (1994), civil case no. 90-CI-06033, Jefferson Circuit Court.

21. Cross examination of Dr. P. Breggin by Mr. J. Freeman in *Fentress vs. Eli Lilly*, Oct. 19, 1994. Transcript of cross examination available at www.healyprozac.com/Trials, p. 114 *et seq.*, Oct. 19.

22. Trial testimony from Nancy Lord in *Fentress vs. Eli Lilly*, Oct. 24, 1994. Transcript of testimony available on www.healyprozac.com/Trials, p. 46, Oct. 24.

23. Ibid., p. 49.

24. Ibid., p. 54.

25. Ibid., p. 52.

26. Further testimony of Dr. Nancy Lord in *Fentress vs. Eli Lilly*, Oct. 24, 1994.

27. N. Schulz-Solce, trial testimony in *Fentress vs. Eli Lilly*, from deposition, Sept. 16, 1994. Transcript of deposition available at www.healyprozac.com/Trials, p. 185. See also Chapter 9, below, for relevant figures on suicidal acts.

28. In Cornwell, *Power to Harm*, 284. See also J. Chetley, *Problem Drugs* (London: Health Action International, 1995), 141–52.

29. The sidebar conversations between the judge and lawyers are available on www.healyprozac.com, under "The Trials: *Fentress v. Eli Lilly*." It should be noted that no one has accused any lawyer or officer of the court here of lying.

30. In *Fentress vs. Eli Lilly*, Jury Instructions, Dec. 9, 1994.

31. In Cornwell, *Power to Harm*, 286. The entire summing up is available as part of the *Fentress* trial transcript on www.healyprozac.com/Trials.

32. From author's interview with Nancy Zettler, May 15, 2000.

33. All three quotes in Cornwell, *Power to Harm,* 286 and 287.

34. John Cornwell later suggested to me that the settlement figure was of the order of $500 million; my other contacts suggest no more than $20 million.

35. In Cornwell, *Power to Harm,* 299.

36. This quote comes from case 926 S.W.2d 449, *Hon. John W. Potter, Judge, Jefferson Circuit Court vs. Eli Lilly and Company,* hearing, May 23, 1996.

37. John Potter on BBC TV's *File on Four,* Tuesday, May 30, 2000.

38. D. Healy, "The Fluoxetine and Suicide Controversy," *CNS Drugs* 1 (1994): 223–31.

39. J. Nakielny, with reply from D. Healy, "The Fluoxetine and Suicide Controversy, *CNS Drugs* 2 (1994): 252–54.

40. A. J. Bond, "Drug Induced Behavioural Disinhibition: Incidence, Mechanisms and Therapeutic Implications," *CNS Drugs* 9 (1998): 41–57; C. M. Beasley, "Suicidality with Fluoxetine," *CNS Drugs* 9 (1998): 513–14.

41. Comments from Alyson Bond, personal communication with the author (1999).

42. J. O. Cole, "The Evaluation of Psychotropic Drugs," in D. Healy (ed.), *The Psychopharmacologists,* vol. 1 (London: Arnold, 1996), 239–64.

43. I found out through a further interview in March 2000 that he had no awareness of my involvement with Prozac and suicide cases.

44. The David King review is in the author's files.

45. S. Jick, A. D. Dean, and H. Jick, "Antidepressants and Suicide," *British Medical Journal* 310 (1995): 215–18.

46. Mianserin and flupenthixol were not available in the United States.

47. G. Isacsson, P. Holmgren, D. Wasserman, and U. Bergman, "Use of Antidepressants among People Committing Suicide in Sweden," *British Medical Journal* 308 (1994): 506–9.

48. D. Healy, C. Langmaak, and M. Savage, "Suicide in the Course of the Treatment of Depression," *Journal of Psychopharmacology* 13 (1999): 9499.

49. J. Feinman, "Rhyme, Reason and Depression: New Research Supports the Claim by Sylvia Plath's Doctor That an Inherited Condition Led to Her Suicide," *The Guardian,* February 16, 1993. There are a great number of theories about Plath's nervous problems, including PMS and manic-depressive illness. Treatment may have caused her suicide though, whatever was wrong with her, or even if nothing had been wrong with her.

50. For an example of this kind of work, see G. C. Harborne, F. L. Watson, D. Healy, and L. Groves, "The Effects of Sub-Anaesthetic Doses of Ketamine on Memory, Cognitive Performance and Subjective Experience in Healthy Volunteers," *Journal of Psychopharmacology* 10 (1996): 134–40.

51. The results were, however, presented at the 1998 annual general meet-

ing of the British Association for Psychopharmacology in Cambridge, UK, in July.

52. D. Healy and G. Farquhar, "The Immediate Effects of Droperidol," *Human Psychopharmacology* 13 (1998): 113–20.

53. R. Bentall, *Madness Explained* (London: Allen Lane, 2003); R. Bentall and E. Else, "Power to the Patients!" *New Scientist* 179, Aug. 30, 2003, 40–43.

54. G. Jones-Edwards, "An Eye-Opener," *OpenMind* (1998): 17–19.

55. Merton Sandler, personal communication, September 1998. Some of this was presented at an ECNP meeting and published in D. Healy, "The Case for an Individual Approach to the Treatment of Depression," *Journal of Clinical Psychiatry* 61, supplement 6 (2000): 24–28.

56. K. S. Kendler, "A Medical Student's Experience with Akathisia," *American Journal of Psychiatry* 133 (1977): 454–55.

57. D. J. King, M. Burke, and R. A. Lucas, "Antipsychotic Drug-Induced Dysphoria," *British Journal of Psychiatry* 167 (1995): 480–82; see also G. Lynch, J. F. Green, and D. J. King, "Antipsychotic Drug Induced Dysphoria," *British Journal of Psychiatry* 169 (1996): 524.

58. See V. Pedersen and K. Bøgesø, "Drug Hunting," in D. Healy, *The Psychopharmacologists,* vol. 2 (London: Arnold, 1998), 561–80.

59. D. Healy and D. Nutt, "British Association for Psychopharmacology Consensus on Childhood and Learning Disabilities Psychopharmacology," *Journal of Psychopharmacology* 11 (1997): 291–94. The principles at the heart of this statement were drawn from the lessons of the Osheroff case—see Healy, *Antidepressant Era,* chap. 7.

60. Abraham and Sheppard, *Therapeutic Nightmare.*

61. Cornwell, *Power to Harm.*

NOTES TO CHAPTER 3

1. M. Lurie, "The Enigma of Isoniazid," in D. Healy (ed.), *The Psychopharmacologists,* vol. 2. (London: Arnold, 1996), 119–34.

2. D. Healy, *The Psychopharmacologists* (London: Chapman and Hall, 1996).

3. Tony Rothschild later ended up as an expert witness for Lilly in *Cassidy and Cassidy vs. Eli Lilly and Company,* civil action no. CA-00821, U.S. District Court for the Western District of Pennsylvania, where he argued that his study with Carol Locke could not be used as evidence that Prozac causes suicide induction.

4. Based on depositions of Susan Forsyth, Feb. 29, 1996; Riggs Roberts, March 4, 1996; Deborah Mihalek, March 6, 1996; Thomas Brady, March 6, 1996; Randolph Neal, March 8, 1996; Ann Blanchard, Aug. 15, 1996; Mark Barrett, Aug. 15, 1996; Kathleen Iannitello, Aug. 15, 1996; Barbara Comstock, Aug. 16,

1996; William Forsyth Jr., Aug. 19, 1996; and Jennifer Capelouto, Sept. 18, 1996. These depositions were taken in *Forsyth et al. vs. Eli Lilly and Company* (1996), civil case no. 95-00185ACK, U.S. District Court for the District of Hawaii (hereafter *Forsyth vs. Eli Lilly*).

5. Xanax is alprazolam, which, in common with other benzodiazepines, can cause depression.

6. Quotes in the following are taken from D. Healy deposition in *Forsyth vs. Eli Lilly*, July 11, 1997.

7. D. Healy, "The Fluoxetine and Suicide Controversy," *CNS Drugs* 1 (1994): 223–31.

8. C. Hoover, "Additional Cases of Suicidal Ideation Associated with Fluoxetine," *American Journal of Psychiatry* 147 (1990): 1570–71.

9. These reviews are all available on the Web site www.healyprozac.com/EditorsDilemma.

10. With a review like this, the author will often know who the reviewer is from aspects of writing style, arguments, or even the font used. Being polite to this person when next you meet is part of the game.

11. D. Healy, C. Langmaak, and M. Savage, "Suicide in the Course of the Treatment of Depression," *Journal of Psychopharmacology* 13 (1999): 94–99.

12. S. Jick, A. D. Dean, and H. Jick, "Antidepressants and Suicide," *British Medical Journal* 310 (1995): 215–18.

13. S. Guze and E. Robins, "Suicide and Primary Affective Disorder: A Study of Ninety-five Cases," *British Journal of Psychiatry* 117 (1970): 437–38.

14. H. M. Inskip, E. C. Harris, and B. Barraclough, "Lifetime Risk of Suicide for Affective Disorder, Alcoholism and Schizophrenia," *British Journal of Psychiatry* 172 (1998): 35–37.

15. A. P. Boardman, A. H. Grimbaldeston, C. Handley, P. W. Jones, and S. Willmott, "The North Staffordshire Suicide Study: A Case-Control Study of Suicide in One Health District," *Psychological Medicine* 29 (1999): 27–33.

16. Data presented at British Association for Psychopharmacology Annual Meeting, Harrogate, July 1999; A. Boardman and D. Healy, "Modeling Suicide Risk in Affective Disorders," *European Psychiatry* 16 (2001): 400–405.

17. E. van Weel-Baumgarten, W. van Den Bosch, H. van Den Hoogen, and F. G. Zitman, "Ten Year Follow Up of Depression after Diagnosis in General Practice," *British Journal of General Practice* 48 (1998): 1643–46.

18. O. Hagnell, J. Lanke, and B. Rorsman, "Suicide Rates in the Lundby Study: Mental Illness as a Risk Factor for Suicide," *Neuropsychobiology* 7 (1981): 248–53.

19. G. E. Simon and M. Von Korff, "Suicide Mortality among Patients Treated for Depression in an Insured Population," *American Journal of Epidemiology* 147 (1998): 155–60.

20. H. Jick, M. Ulcickas, and A. Dean, "Comparison of Frequencies of Suicidal Tendencies among Patients Receiving Fluoxetine, Lofepramine, Mianserin or Trazodone," *Pharmacotherapy* 12 (1992): 451–54.

21. D. Healy, "The Antidepressant Drama," in M. Weissman (ed.), *Treatment of Depression: Bridging the Twenty-first Century*, Proceedings of the American Psychopathological Association Meeting, March 1999 (Washington, D.C.: American Psychiatric Association Press, 2000), 7–34.

NOTES TO CHAPTER 4

1. J. Abraham and J. Sheppard, *The Therapeutic Nightmare: The Battle over the World's Most Controversial Sleeping Pill* (London: Earthscan, 1999); and D. Hooper, "The Halcion Nightmare," in *Reputations under Fire* (London: Little, Brown), 2000.

2. Because norepinephrine is called noradrenaline in Europe, reboxetine began as an NARI. The company realized this acronym wouldn't work in America. The compromise was NRI, which involved having to redo European marketing material. Given the state of antidepressant "science" in the late 1990s, getting details such as this right probably count for more in the long run than getting the science right. Instead of going down the depression route with an NRI, Lilly has followed an attention deficit/hyperactivity disorder (ADHD) route with atomoxetine, which has a similar action to reboxetine.

3. P. Melloni, G. Carniel, A. Della Toree, A. Bonsignori, M. Buonamici, O. Pozzi, S. Raccardi, and A. C. Rossi, "Potential Antidepressant Agents: A-Aryloxy-benzyl Derivatives of Ethanolamine and Morpholine," *European Journal of Medical Chemistry and Therapeutics* 19 (1984): 235–42.

4. Details based on interview with Adriana Dubini, who was closely involved with the development of the drug from the start, in August 1998. Supplementary details from interview with Max Lagnado, September 1998.

5. Max Lagnado was a primary-care physician who had several months before switched into the pharmaceutical industry. He subsequently moved to PR companies and communication agencies, quickly building up a reputation as creative—perhaps too creative for what is a very conservative industry.

6. I. Oswald, "The Hypnotic Business," in D. Healy (ed.), *The Psychopharmacologists*, vol. 3 (London: Arnold, 2000), 459–78.

7. A. Dubini, M. Bosc, and V. Polin, "Do Noradrenaline and Serotonin Differentially Affect Social Motivation and Behaviour?" *European Neuropsychopharmacology* 7 (1997): 49–56.

8. P. Pichot, "The Discovery of Chlorpromazine and the Place of Psychopharmacology in the History of Psychiatry," in D. Healy (ed.), *The Psychopharmacologists*, vol. 1 (London: Arnold, 1996), 1–21.

9. S. Garattini, "Experimental and Clinical Activity of Antidepressant Drugs," in D. Healy and D. Doogan (eds.), *Psychotropic Drug Development: Social, Economic and Pharmacological Aspects* (London: Chapman and Hall, 1996), 1–12.

10. Traded as Zispin in Britain.

11. D. P. Wheatley, M. van Moffaert, L. Timmerman, and C. M. Kremer, "Mirtazapine: Efficacy and Tolerability in Comparison with Fluoxetine in Patients with Moderate to Severe Major Depressive Disorder," *Journal of Clinical Psychiatry* 59 (1998): 306–12. See R. Pinder, "Approaching Rationality?" in D. Healy (ed.), *The Psychopharmacologists*, vol. 2 (London: Arnold, 1998), 581–604.

12. M. Bosc, A. Dubini, and V. Polin, "Development and Validation of a Social Functioning Scale, the Social Adaptation Self-evaluation Scale," *European Neuropsychopharmacology* 7, supplement 1 (1997): 57–70.

13. M. M. Weissman, G. L. Klerman, E. S. Paykel, B. Prusoff, and B. Hanson, "Treatment Effects on the Social Adjustment of Depressed Patients," *Archives of General Psychiatry* 30 (1974): 771–78.

14. G. L. Klerman, M. M. Weissman, B. Rounsaville, and E. S. Chevron, *Interpersonal Therapy of Depression* (New York: Basic Books, 1984).

15. D. Healy, *The Antidepressant Era* (Cambridge, Mass.: Harvard University Press, 1997), chap. 7.

16. M. M. Weissman, "Gerald Klerman and Psychopharmacotherapy," in Healy, *The Psychopharmacologists*, vol. 2, 521–42.

17. M. M. Weissman, "Beyond Symptoms: Social Functioning and the New Antidepressants," *Journal of Psychopharmacology* 11 (1997): 4 (supplement), 5–8.

18. See the following for content: D. Healy and T. M. McMonagle, "Enhancement of Social Functioning as a Therapeutic Principle in the Treatment of Depression," *Journal of Psychopharmacology* 11 (1997): supplement, 25–31; D. Healy, "Reboxetine, Fluoxetine and Social Functioning as an Outcome Measure in Antidepressant Trials: Implications," *Primary Care Psychiatry* 4 (1998): 81–89; D. Healy and H. Healy, "The Clinical Pharmacological Profile of Reboxetine: Does It Involve the Putative Neurobiological Substrates of Wellbeing?" *Journal of Affect Disorders* 51 (1998): 313–22; D. Healy, "The Case for an Individual Approach to the Treatment of Depression," *Journal of Clinical Psychiatry* 61, supplement 6 (2000): 24–28.

19. Examples of the message are in Healy, "The Case for an Individual Approach to the Treatment of Depression," 24–28; Healy, "Reboxetine, Fluoxetine and Social Functioning as an Outcome Measure in Antidepressant Trials," 81–89.

20. P&U was taken over by Pfizer in 2002 to become the largest pharmaceutical company.

21. Oswald, "Hypnotic Business," 459–77.

22. S. A. Glantz, L. A. Bero, P. Hanauer, D. E. Barnes, *The Cigarette Papers*

(Berkeley: University of California Press, 1996). See D. Kessler, *A Question of Intent* (New York: Public Affairs, 2001). For a consideration of the impact of this on pharmaceutical cases, see Oswald, "Hypnotic Business," 459–77.

23. See Healy, *Antidepressant Era,* chap. 6; D. Healy, "The Psychopharmacological Era: Notes toward a History," *Journal of Psychopharmacology* 4 (1990): 152–67; D. Healy, "The Marketing of 5HT: Anxiety or Depression," *British Journal of Psychiatry* 158 (1991): 737–42; D. Healy, "Psychopharmacology in the New Medical State," in Healy and Doogan, *Psychotropic Drug Development,* 15–39.

24. T. A. Sheldon and G. D. Smith, "Consensus Conferences as Drug Promotion," *Lancet* 341 (1993): 100–102.

25. L. A. Bero, A. Galbraith, and D. Rennie, "The Publication of Sponsored Symposiums in Medical Journals," *New England Journal of Medicine* 327 (1992): 1135–40.

26. The Institute for International Research (IIR) describes itself as the world's largest independent conference company and a leader in the provision of business information. See www.iir-conferences.com.

27. From a brochure for a London meeting on "Creating Targeted Patient Education Campaigns," organized by IIR, October 29–30, 1996.

28. P. Breggin, *Toxic Psychiatry* (New York: St. Martin's Press, 1991); R. Whitaker, *Mad in America* (Cambridge, Mass.: Perseus, 2002).

29. On the development of patient organizations in the OCD field, see J. Rapoport, "Phenomenology, Psychopharmacology and Child Psychiatry," in Healy, *The Psychopharmacologists,* vol. 3, 333–56.

30. One of the best histories of a patient organization and its power to lobby for a treatment can be found in H. Kushner, *A Cursing Brain: Gilles de la Tourette and His Syndrome* (Cambridge, Mass.: Harvard University Press, 1998).

31. Even though largely a group of individuals who accept the NAMI model that mental illnesses are brain illnesses, DA was at this time still aware of and offered resistance to the continuing pressure toward pathologizing and medicalizing emotional distress, and favored a more "commonsense" and human response. DA at this point received over 25 percent of its funding from industry.

32. And may directly conflict with their charitable status, if they are a charity.

33. My information on these patient group–related issues all comes from sources it seems better at present to leave nameless.

34. D. L. Shuey, T. W. Sadler, and J. M. Lauder, "Serotonin as a Regulator of Craniofacial Morphogenesis: Site Specific Malformations Following Exposure to Serotonin Reuptake Inhibitors," *Teratology* 46 (1992): 367–78. Other data suggest babies are more likely to be born prematurely or underweight, and that these babies may show withdrawal from SSRIs.

35. Thus D. Healy, "Antidepressant Psychopharmacotherapy at the Cross-roads," *International Journal of Psychiatry in Clinical Practice* 3, supplement 2 (1999): 9–16, sits beside S. Kasper, "Bridging the Gap between Psychopharmacology and Clinical Symptoms," *International Journal of Psychiatry in Clinical Practice* 3, supplement 2 (1999): 17–20. In this case a recognizably "Healy" article, complete with Healy references still, appearing under another name, sits beside a recognizably Healy article. Articles on www.healyprozac.com/GhostlyData.

36. This is a practice not confined to pharmaceutical company productions. In academia, it is probably more common in big centers such as Ivy League universities or their equivalent in Europe, where more books are produced and there are more trainees who can be encouraged for the sake of their careers to help out. The example I base this characterization on came from the Institute of Psychiatry.

37. For details on venlafaxine and related agents, see Chapter 9. The e-mail came from CMED, a communication agency based in Toronto, on Jan. 1, 2001. Available on www.healyprozac.com/GhostlyData/CMED.pdf. The meeting was being held in Laguna Beach, California.

38. M. E. Thase, A. R. Entsuah, and R. L. Rudolph, "Remission Rates during Treatment with Venlafaxine or SSRIs," *British Journal of Psychiatry* 178 (2001): 234–41.

39. "Conflict of Interest and the British Journal of Psychiatry," *British Journal of Psychiatry* 180 (2002): 82–83.

40. Editorial. "Just How Tainted Has Medicine Become?" *Lancet* 359 (2002): 1167. See also responses in "How Tainted Is Medicine?" *Lancet* 359 (2002): 1775–76. It is important to note that there may be absolutely no problem here—the critical issue is the potential for discrepancy between what is written and the raw data. This point is developed further in chapter 9.

41. This was scheduled to appear as D. Healy et al., "The Prevalence and Outcome of Partial Remission in Depression," *Journal of Psychiatry and Neuroscience* (2001). It appears under the same title as being by R. Tranter, C. O'-Donovan, P. Chandarama, and S. Kennedy, in *Journal of Psychiatry and Neuroscience* 27 (2002): 241–47. I removed my name. All drafts of the article are available at www.healyprozac.com/GhostlyData.

42. In this instance, the final author or authorization was a senior academic from the Centre of Addiction and Mental Health at the University of Toronto.

43. S. Okie, "A Stand for Scientific Independence," *Washington Post*, August 5, 2001, A1.

44. A. Mundy, *Dispensing with the Truth* (New York: St. Martin's Press, 2001); see also S. Rampton and J. Stauber, "Trust Us, We're Experts!" (New York: Tarcher, Putnam, 2001), chap. 8.

45. R. M. Hirschfeld, M. Keller, M. Bourgeois, D. S. Baldwin, D. Healy, M. Humble, S. Kasper, and S. Montgomery, "Focus on Social Functioning in Depression," *International Journal of Psychiatry in Clinical Practice* 2 (1998): 241–43; and R. M. Hirschfeld, S. A. Montgomery, M. Keller, S. Kasper, A. Schatzberg, H. J. Moller, D. Healy, D. Baldwin, M. Humble, M. Versiani, R. Montenegro, and M. L. Bourgeois, "Social Functioning in Depression," *Journal of Clinical Psychiatry* 61 (2000): 268–75.

46. I. Marks, "Marketing the Evidence," in Healy, *The Psychopharmacologists,* vol. 2, 543–60; Oswald, "Hypnotic Business," 459–77.

47. N. Pearce, "Adverse Reactions, Social Responses: A Tale of Two Asthma Mortality Epidemics," in P. Davis (ed.), *Contested Ground: Public Purpose and Private Interest in the Regulation of Prescription Drugs* (Oxford: Oxford University Press, 1996), 57–74.

48. Current Medical Directions (CMD) Web site, http://www.cmdconnect.com, 2002. The specific wording cited here has since been removed but appears in D. Healy and D. Cattell, "The Interface between Authorship, Industry and Science in the Domain of Therapeutics," *British Journal of Psychiatry* 182 (2003): 23.

49. The entire series of articles can be seen on www.healyprozac.com/GhostlyData/Zoloftpublications.htm.

50. Healy and Cattell, "Interface between Authorship, Industry and Science in the Domain of Therapeutics," 22–27.

51. CMD Web site, http://www.cmdconnect.com, 2002. The specific wording cited here has since been removed but appears in Healy and Cattell, "Interface between Authorship, Industry and Science in the Domain of Therapeutics," 23.

52. Exhibit in *Motus vs. Pfizer Inc.,* case no. CV00-298AHM (SHx), U.S. District Court, Central District of California, and in *Miller vs. Pfizer Inc.,* case no. 99-2236KHV, U.S. District Court for the District of Kansas.

53. Letter from Roger Lane of Pfizer to Ulrik Malt, February 16, 1994; in author's files. This letter was part of *Motus vs. Pfizer Inc.,* case no. CV00-298AHM (SHx), Bates pages 015980–016037, and exhibits 51–53 in "Plaintiff's Opposition to Defendant Pfizer's Motion to Exclude the Testimony of Dr. David Healy." Lane himself discounts the Beasley study in other settings; his (and Pfizer's) view of the study's faults is available from the author and as exhibit 27 in "Plaintiff's Motion to Strike Pfizer's Exhibit 7 to Its Motion to Exclude the Testimony of Dr. David Healy," *Motus vs. Pfizer.*

54. U. F. Malt, O. H. Robak, H.-B. Madsbu, O. Bakke, and M. Loeb, "The Norwegian Naturalistic Treatment Study of Depression in General Practice (NORDEP). I: Randomized Double Blind Study," *British Medical Journal* 318 (1999): 1180–84.

55. Pfizer Expert Report, "Sertraline Hydrochloride for Obsessive Compulsive Disorder in Paediatric Patients," approved Oct. 20, 1997. Available on www.healyprozac.com/GhostlyData/expertreport.htm.

56. Psychopharmacology means never having to go without a pen.

57. I owe this phrase from 1998 to Edward Shorter, the author of *A History of Psychiatry* (New York: John Wiley and Sons, 1996).

58. D. A. Kessler, "Drug Promotion and Scientific Exchange," *New England Journal of Medicine* 325 (1991): 201–3.

59. See O. Vinar, "A Psychopharmacology That Nearly Was," in Healy, *The Psychopharmacologists,* vol. 3, 55–79.

60. D. Rennie, "Fair Conduct and Fair Reporting of Clinical Trials," *JAMA* 282, 1 (1999): 766–1768.

61. The program for the Collegium Internationale Neuropsychopharmacologium (CINP) meeting in Brussels in July 2000 had twenty-three symposia/workshops supported by unrestricted educational grants out of a total of fifty-eight symposia/workshops on the main program in addition to twenty-five satellite symposia.

62. A. Bass, "Drug Companies Enrich Brown Professor," *Boston Globe,* October 4, 1999, Metro section, A1.

63. G. J. Hankey and J. W. Eikelboom, "Homocysteine and Vascular Disease," *Lancet* 354 (1999): 407–13; C. Bolander-Gouaille, *Focus on Homocysteine* (Paris: Springer, 2000).

64. D. F. Klein, "Reaction Patterns to Psychotropic Drugs and the Discovery of Panic Disorder," in Healy, *The Psychopharmacologists,* vol. 1, 329–52; Marks, "Marketing the Evidence," 543–60.

65. Greg Birnbaum and Douglas Montero, "Shrinks for Sale. Analyze This: Docs Get Drug Co. $$," *New York Sunday Post,* Feb. 28, 1999, 2–3 plus front cover. See also Loren Mosher's Dec. 4, 1998, letter of resignation from the American Psychiatric Association, on the Web at www.oikos.org/mosher.htm, for the details that follow.

66. Borison was chairman of the Department of Psychiatry and professor in the Department of Pharmacology at the Medical College of Georgia, and chief of neuropsychopharmacology at Augusta VA Medical Center, Georgia.

67. S. Stecklow and L. Johannes, "Questions Arise on New Drug Testing: Drug Makers Relied on Clinical Researchers Who Now Await Trial," *Wall Street Journal,* Aug. 15, 1997; K. Eichenwald and G. Kolata, "Drug Trials Hide Conflict for Doctors," *New York Times,* May 16, 1999, 1, 28, 29; "A Doctor's Drug Studies Turn into Fraud," *New York Times,* May 17, 1999, 1, 16, 17; S. Boseley, "Trial and Error Puts Patients at Risk," *The Guardian,* July 27, 1999, 8.

68. See M. Fink, "A Clinician Researcher and ECDEU: 1959–1980," in T. Ban, D. Healy, and E. Shorter (eds.), *The Triumph of Psychopharmacology* (Budapest: Animula, 2000), 82–96.

69. D. Healy, "The Assessment of Outcomes in Depression: The Place for Measures of Social Functioning," *Reviews in Contemporary Psychopharmacology* 11 (2000): 295–301.

70. The first discussion of quality of life in medicine came in 1966, in an article on renal dialysis, see J. R. Elkington, "Medicine and the Quality of Life," *Annals of Internal Medicine* 64 (1996): 711–14.

71. BGA is the Bundesgesundheitsamt, translated as Federal Health Department—the German equivalent of the FDA.

72. H. Weber, deposition in *Fentress et al. vs. Shea Communications and Eli Lilly and Company* (1994), case no. 90-CI-06033, Jefferson Circuit Court, September, exhibit 1, memo from J. Schenk and H. Weber to E. Ashbrook and C. Hardison, June 26, 1984.

73. H. Weber, deposition in *Fentress vs. Eli Lilly*, exhibit 3, unofficial copy of the medical comments on the fluoxetine application to the BGA, sent by Barbara von Keitz to colleagues in London and Indianapolis, May 25, 1984.

74. Healy, "Assessment of Outcomes in Depression," 295–301.

75. This was written in 1995–1996.

76. T. S. Eliot, "Burnt Norton," in *Four Quartets* (London: Faber and Faber, 1944).

NOTES TO CHAPTER 5

1. Details of the two companies can be found on the Web at www.justice-seekers.com and www.baumhedlundlaw.com.

2. Fluoxetine Project Team Meeting Minutes, July 1978, exhibit 30 in *Forsyth et al. vs. Eli Lilly and Company* (1999), civil case no. 95-00185ACK, U.S. District Court for the District of Hawaii (hereafter *Forsyth vs. Eli Lilly*). All documents available at www.healyprozac.com/Trials/CriticalDocs.

3. Fluoxetine Project Team Meeting Minutes, July 23, 1979, in *Forsyth vs. Eli Lilly*.

4. March 6, 1992 German package insert (translation), exhibit 5 to May 17, 1994 deposition of Charles Beasley in *Fentress et al. vs. Shea Communications and Eli Lilly and Company* (1994), case no. 90-CI-06033, Jefferson Circuit Court (hereafter *Fentress vs. Eli Lilly*). For translation, see text below, at note 39.

5. Memo by Dr. J. Wernicke, July 2, 1986. Exhibit 69 in *Forsyth vs. Eli Lilly*.

6. D. Healy and W. Creaney, "Antidepressant Induced Suicidal Ideation," *British Medical Journal* 303 (1991): 1058–59.

7. C. Beasley, letter to *British Medical Journal* 303 (1991): 1059.

8. J. Heiligenstein, memorandum to L. Thompson, Sept. 14, 1990, exhibit 110 in *Forsyth vs. Eli Lilly*.

9. October 3, 1986, memorandum from J. Wernicke, "Fluoxetine Suicides and Suicide Attempts," exhibit 73 in *Fentress vs. Eli Lilly*.

10. Unless otherwise stated, these documents were also exhibits in the *Fentress* case or in depositions associated with that case. Further details of each of these exhibits can be obtained on the company Web sites (www.justiceseekers.com and www.baumhedlundlaw.com) or from the legal offices of Nancy Zettler, Two North LaSalle Street #1600, Chicago, Illinois, 60602.

11. J. Heiligenstein, memo to Dr. L. Thompson, Sept. 14, 1990, plaintiff's exhibit 110 in *Forsyth vs. Eli Lilly*.

12. E. Daniels, memo to Leigh Thompson, coaching for a television appearance, April 15, 1991, plaintiffs' exhibit 123 in *Forsyth vs. Eli Lilly*. See also deposition of Leigh Thompson in *Fentress vs. Eli Lilly*, July 20, 1994.

13. June 1990 letter to Lilly by concerned physician ("Some of these cases appear to be in patients taking Prozac for reasons other than depression"), exhibit 102 in *Forsyth vs. Eli Lilly*.

14. Internal FDA memo, Oct. 23, 1986, exhibit 74 in *Forsyth vs. Eli Lilly*.

15. Leigh Thompson memo, February 7, 1990, exhibit 98 in *Forsyth vs. Eli Lilly*.

16. Letter from Eli Lilly to FDA, March 26, 1990, exhibit 102 in *Forsyth vs. Eli Lilly*.

17. T. P. Laughren, J. Levine, J. G. Levine, and W. L. Thompson, "Premarketing Safety Evaluation of Psychotropic Drugs," in R. F. Prien and D. S. Robinson (eds.), *Clinical Evaluation of Psychotropic Drugs* (New York: Raven Press, 1994), 185–215.

18. L. Thompson, memo regarding call from Paul Leber, July 18, 1990, exhibit 104 in *Forsyth vs. Eli Lilly*.

19. Lilly memos between Max Talbott (formerly of the FDA) and Leigh Thompson, Sept. 12, 1990, exhibit 109 in *Forsyth vs. Eli Lilly*.

20. Memo from Claude Bouchy to Leigh Thompson, Nov. 13, 1990, exhibit 117 in *Forsyth vs. Eli Lilly*.

21. Memo from Claude Bouchy to Leigh Thompson, Nov. 14, 1990, exhibit 118 in *Forsyth vs. Eli Lilly*.

22. *Forsyth vs. Eli Lilly*, trial transcript, March 9 to March 12, 1999.

23. Rhonda Hawkins caught the phenomenon best when I later commented on his transformation to her. "Yep," she said, "he cleans up real good."

24. M. G. Warshaw and M. B. Keller, "The Relationship between Fluoxetine Use and Suicidal Behavior in 654 Subjects with Anxiety Disorders," *Journal of Clinical Psychiatry* 57 (1996): 158–66.

25. D. S. Baldwin, N. A. Fineberg, and S. Montgomery, "Fluoxetine, Fluvoxamine and Extra-Pyramidal Tract Disorders," *International Clinical Psychopharmacology* 6 (1991): 51–58.

26. D. Healy, *Psychiatric Drugs Explained* (London: Mosby Yearbooks Ltd., 1993; 2d ed., 1996).

27. D. Healy, *The Psychopharmacologists,* vols. 1–3 (London: Arnold, 1996, 1998, 2000).

28. P. Leber, "Managing Uncertainty," in Healy, *The Psychopharmacologists,* vol. 2, 607–22.

29. Deposition of Randolph Neal in *Forsyth vs. Eli Lilly,* March 8, 1996.

30. What follows is from *Forsyth* trial transcript, March 12, 1999.

31. Inderal is propranolol, a beta-blocker that Rothschild and Locke reported eased Prozac-induced akathisia. See A. Rothschild and C. Locke, "Re-exposure to Fluoxetine after Serious Suicide Attempts by Three Patients," *Journal of Clinical Psychiatry* 52 (1991): 491–93.

32. G. Tollefson, "Fluoxetine and Suicidal Ideation," *American Journal of Psychiatry* 147 (1990): 1691–92; M. Teicher, C A. Glod, and J. O. Cole, "Dr. Teicher and Associates Reply," *American Journal of Psychiatry* 147 (1990): 1692–93.

33. *Forsyth vs. Eli Lilly,* trial transcript, March 23, 1999.

34. Ibid.

35. R. M. Lane, "SSRI-Induced Extrapyramidal Side Effects and Akathisia: Implications for Treatment," *Journal of Psychopharmacology* 12 (1998): 192–214.

36. Personal communication from A. Vickery, March 1999. Whatever the reason for the Lane article, senior pharmaceutical company contacts whom I have asked about this article have suggested it is unlikely it could have come out without senior figures in Pfizer knowing about it.

37. *Forsyth vs. Eli Lilly,* trial transcript, closing statements, March 30, 1999.

38. Evidentiary hearings to determine allegations of juror misconduct, Honolulu, Hawaii, transcript, July 1, 1999, civil case no. 95-00185 ACK.

39. March 6, 1992, German package insert (translation), exhibit 5 to May 17, 1994, deposition of Charles Beasley in *Fentress vs. Eli Lilly.*

40. Appeal Brief, *Forsyth vs. Eli Lilly,* April 20, 2000, case no. CV00-00401 ACK-LEK.

NOTES TO CHAPTER 6

1. C. M. Beasley, B. E. Dornseif, J. C. Bosomworth, M. E. Sayler, A. H. Rampey, J. H. Heiligenstein, V. L. Thompson, D. J. Murphy, and D. N. Massica, "Fluoxetine and Suicide: A Meta-Analysis of Controlled Trials of Treatment for Depression," *British Medical Journal* 303 (1991): 685–92.

2. Deposition of Charles Beasley, May 17 and 18, 1994, in *Fentress et al. vs. Shea Communications and Eli Lilly and Company* (1994), case no. 90-CI-06033, Jefferson Circuit Court (hereafter *Fentress vs. Eli Lilly*).

3. *Physician's Desk Reference* (Montvale, N.J.: Medical Economics Inc., 1991), entry on Prozac.

4. See Chapter 5; and testimony of Nancy Lord in *Fentress vs. Eli Lilly*, Chapter 2.

5. Food and Drug Administration, Psychopharmacologic Drugs Advisory Committee, Twenty-eighth Meeting, Thursday, Oct. 10, 1985. Transcript available at www.healyprozac.com/PDAC.

6. Deposition of Catherine Mesner, August 17, 1993, in *Fentress vs. Eli Lilly*.

7. Deposition of John Heiligenstein, April 27 and 28, 1994, in *Fentress vs. Eli Lilly*.

8. Deposition of Charles Beasley, May 17 and 18, 1994, in *Fentress vs. Eli Lilly*.

9. Memorandum from Richard Huddleston to Hans Weber, December 7, 1990, exhibit 35 in the deposition of W. Leigh Thompson in *Fentress vs. Eli Lilly*, July 20, 1994.

10. Deposition of Wilma Harrison, March 14, 2000, in *Miller vs. Pfizer Inc.*, case no. 99-2236 KHV, U.S. District Court for the District of Kansas.

11. Depositions of J. Heiligenstein and C. Mesner in *Fentress vs. Eli Lilly* (1994).

12. Deposition of John Heiligenstein, April 27 and 28, 1994, in *Fentress vs. Eli Lilly*.

13. Deposition of Charles Beasley, May 17 and 18, 1994, in *Fentress vs. Eli Lilly*.

14. Quote from anonymous *BMJ* referee for the Beasley paper, exhibit 3 in deposition of Greg Enas in *Fentress vs. Eli Lilly*, Sept. 16, 1994.

15. Further quote from *BMJ* reviewer, exhibit 3 in deposition of Greg Enas, in *Fentress vs. Eli Lilly*.

16. *Forsyth et al. vs. Eli Lilly and Company* (1999), civil case no. 95-00185ACK, U.S. District Court for the District of Hawaii (hereafter *Forsyth vs. Eli Lilly*), trial transcript, March 12, 1999.

17. M. Fava and J. F. Rosenbaum, "Suicidality and Fluoxetine: Is There a Relationship?" *Journal of Clinical Psychiatry* 52 (1991): 108–11. See D. Healy, Guest Editorial, "A Failure to Warn," *International Journal of Risk and Safety in Medicine* 12 (1999): 151–56.

18. M. G. Warshaw and M. B. Keller, "The Relationship between Fluoxetine Use and Suicidal Behavior in 654 Subjects with Anxiety Disorders," *Journal of Clinical Psychiatry* 57 (1996): 158–66.

19. A. C. Leon, M. B. Keller, M. G. Warshaw, T. I. Mueller, D. A. Solomon, W. Coryell, et al., "Prospective Study of Fluoxetine Treatment and Suicidal Behavior in Affectively Ill Subjects," *American Journal of Psychiatry* 156 (1999): 195–201.

20. M. N. G. Dukes and B. Schwartz, *Responsibility for Drug-Induced Injury* (Amsterdam: Elsevier, 1988).

21. Letter to the author from Graham Dukes, October 13, 1998.

22. J. Rosenbaum, Eli Lilly and Company, personal communication, June 12, 1991. Cited in "Clinical Trial by Media: The Prozac Story," in H. I. Schwartz (ed.), *Psychiatric Practice under Fire* (Washington, D.C.: American Psychiatric Press, 1994), 3–28.

23. See D. Wilkinson, "Loss of Anxiety and Increased Aggression in a Fifteen-Year-Old Boy Taking Fluoxetine," *Journal of Psychopharmacology* 13 (1999): 420; reply by D. Healy, *Journal of Psychopharmacology* 13 (1999): 421.

24. Given that none of the studies in the Beasley paper was designed to answer the question, it is debatable whether publication bias has anything to do with what happened to this article. The sheer embarrassment of recognizing this may have played a part in Richard Smith's inability to accept any papers drawing attention to the issue.

25. Correspondence from Richard Smith, April 12 (for first sentence) and April 19 (for the rest), 1999. This correspondence from Richard Smith is included here because, as will be clear from the rest of the book, Richard Smith and the *BMJ* are on the side of the angels. Their "failures" in the Prozac case therefore serve doubly to illustrate the extent of confusions in the field, and the problems with bringing hazards to light. The full correspondence is on www.healyprozac.com/EditorsDilemma.

26. R. Smith, "An Amnesty for Unpublished Trials" and R. Smith, "Doctor's Information: Excessive, Crummy and Bent," *British Medical Journal* 315 (1997): 611 and 622.

27. All correspondence available on www.healyprozac.com/EditorsDilemma/British%20Medical%20Journal.pdf.

28. Starting from the 1960s, the *Guardian* had risen to become Britain's leading liberal broadsheet. While the *Times* and *Sunday Times* were better known internationally, they had been replaced as the leading papers for investigative journalism, certainly for issues like this.

29. J. Diamond, "In Praise of Prozac," *Times*, June 5, 2000.

30. S. Boseley, "Prozac: Can It Make You Kill?" *Guardian*, October 30, 1999, "Weekend" section.

31. S. O'Neill, "Coroner Calls for Warning Note on Prozac Packets," *Daily Telegraph*, November 3, 1999.

32. Details of this case were confirmed by Craig Clark's doctor in a follow-up telephone conversation with the author, January 2000.

33. G. Monbiot, "Getting Your Science from Charlatans," *The Guardian*, March 16, 2000, "Comment and Analysis" section, 24. For support for this view from the opposite side of political divide, see R. Bate, *What Risk? Science, Politics and Public Health.* (London: Butterworth-Heinemann, 1997).

34. As I understand it, Lilly gave the Hastings Center $25,000 per year. See contributions from C. Elliott, D. Healy, P. Kramer, J. Edwards, and D. DeGrazia, *Hastings Center Report* 30 (March 2000).

35. D. Healy, Guest Editorial, "A Failure to Warn," *International Journal of Risk and Safety in Medicine* 12 (1999): 151–56. Quote from letter to the author from Graham Dukes, January 8, 2000.

36. Memo from C. Bouchy to L. Thompson, "Re: Adverse Drug Event Reporting—Suicide Fluoxetine," Nov. 13, 1990, exhibit 117 in *Forsyth vs. Eli Lilly.*

37. Memo from Claude Bouchy to Leigh Thompson, Nov. 14, 1990, exhibit 118 in *Forsyth vs. Eli Lilly.*

38. Memo from L. Thompson to C. Bouchy, Nov. 14, 1990, exhibit 118 in *Forsyth vs. Eli Lilly.*

39. Unpublished editorial sent to the *British Medical Journal*; see www.healyprozac.com/EditorsDilemma/British%20Medical%20Journal.pdf.

40. Letter from Richard Smith to the author, Dec. 20, 1999.

41. Letter from the author to Richard Smith, Jan. 6, 2000.

42. Letter from Richard Smith to the author, Jan. 14, 2000.

43. T. Lemmens and B. Freedman, "Ethics Review for Sale? Conflict of Interest and Commercial Research Review Boards," *Milbank Quarterly* 78 (2000): 547–84.

44. D. Healy, "Clinical Trials and Legal Jeopardy," *Bulletin of Medical Ethics* 153 (1999): 13–18.

45. Memo from B. von Keitz and H. Weber to J. Wernicke, "Fluoxetine Suicides and Suicide Attempts, October 1986," exhibit 19 in the deposition of Joachim Wernicke in *Fentress vs. Eli Lilly.* See Brickler exhibit 1 at www.healyprozac.com, in the "Critical Documents" section.

46. S. Kasper, "The Place of Milnacipran in the Treatment of Depression," *Human Psychopharmacology* 12 (1997): supplement 135–41.

47. D. Baldwin, "The Treatment of Recurrent Brief Depression" (paper presented at the European College of Neuropsychopharmacology Meeting, London, Sept. 24, 1999). There is, however, another study—R. J. Verkes, R. C. Van der Mast, M. W. Hengeveld, J. P. Tuyl, A. H. Zwinderman, and G. M. Van Viemper, "Reduction by Paroxetine of Suicidal Behavior in Patients with Repeated Suicide Attempts but Not Major Depression," *American Journal of Psychiatry* 155 (1998): 543–47. This appears to show a reduction in suicide attempts on paroxetine compared to placebo; but with forty-five patients on paroxetine of whom thirty-five drop out, and forty-five on placebo of whom thirty-seven drop out, it is difficult to know what the results mean.

48. Communications from R. Baldessarini by e-mails during 1999–2000.

49. A. Khan, H. A. Warner, W. A. Brown, "Symptom Reduction and Suicide Risk in Patients Treated with Placebo in Antidepressant Clinical Trials: Analysis of the FDA Database," *Archives of General Psychiatry* 57 (2000): 311–17.

50. FDA Adverse Events Reporting System (AERS), Freedom of Information Act report, June 2, 1999, 407.

51. UK Prozac sales figures, source Dinlink Compufile Ltd.

52. After the book was finished, a study appeared that directly supported these observations: S. Donovan, A. Clayton, M. Beeharry, S. Jones, C. Kirk, K. Waters, D. Gardner, J. Faulding, and R. Madely, "Deliberate Self-Harm and Antidepressant Drugs: Investigation of a Possible Link," *British Journal of Psychiatry* 177 (2000): 551–56.

53. Statement from local Lilly representative in my office in November 1999, witnessed by Drs. Tony Roberts and Dave Wilkinson.

54. *Day by Day: A Guide to Your First Three Weeks of Treatment,* brochure distributed by Eli Lilly representatives during the 1990s in the United Kingdom. No publication date or details.

NOTES TO CHAPTER 7

1. Deposition of John Heiligenstein, April 27, 1997, in *Fentress et al. vs. Shea Communications and Eli Lilly and Company* (1994), case no. 90-CI-06033, Jefferson Circuit Court (hereafter *Fentress vs. Eli Lilly*).

2. D. Healy, "The Case for an Individual Approach to the Treatment of Depression," *Journal of Clinical Psychiatry* 61, supplement 6 (1999): 24–28; D. Healy, "Reboxetine, Fluoxetine and Social Functioning as an Outcome Measure in Antidepressant Trials: Implications," *Primary Care Psychiatry* 4 (1998): 81–89.

3. R. Hoehn-Saric, J. R. Lipsey, and D. R. McLeod, "Apathy and Indifference in Patients on Fluvoxamine and Fluoxetine," *Journal of Clinical Psychopharmacology* 10 (1990): 343–45.

4. For instance, E. J. Garland and E. A. Baerg, "Amotivational Syndrome Associated with Selective Serotonin Reuptake Inhibitors in Children and Adolescents," *Journal of Child and Adolescent Psychopharmacology* 11 (2001): 181–86.

5. L. Slater, *Prozac Diary* (New York: Random House, 1998).

6. APA Online release no. 99–19, April 28, 1999, statement by APA President Rodrigo Munoz, at www.psych.org/news_stand/nr_990428.html.

7. £400 at that point was approximately $600—$75 per week of the study.

8. Further details of this study can be found in D. Healy, "Emergence of Antidepressant Induced Suicidality," *Primary Care Psychiatry* 6 (2000): 23–28. Details were also presented at the Annual Royal College of Psychiatrists meeting in Edinburgh in July 2000, the BAP meeting in Cambridge in July 2000, and the ECNP meeting in Munich in September 2000.

9. P. R. Joyce, R. T. Mulder, and C. R. Cloninger, "Temperament Predicts Clomipramine and Desipramine Response in Major Depression," *Journal of Affective Disorders* 30 (1994): 35–46.

10. K. Fitzgerald and D. Healy, "Dystonias and Dyskinesias of the Jaw Associated with the Use of SSRIs," *Human Psychopharmacology* 10 (1995): 215–20.

11. It was only clear at the end of the study that up to 50 percent were affected.

12. I. M. Anderson and B. M. Tomenson, "Treatment Discontinuation with Selective Serotonin Reuptake Inhibitors Compared to Tricyclic Antidepressants: A Meta-Analysis," *British Medical Journal* 310 (1995): 1433–38.

13. Results presented at the Royal College of Psychiatrists annual meeting in Edinburgh, July 2000; the BAP annual meeting in Cambridge, July 2000; and the ECNP meeting in Munich, September 2000.

14. R. Tranter, H. Healy, D. Cattell, and D. Healy, "Functional Effects of Agents Differentially Selective to Serotonergic or Noradrenergic Systems," *Psychological Medicine* 32 (2002): 517–24.

15. A peer-reviewed version of this section can be found in Healy, "Emergence of Antidepressant Induced Suicidality." The full study is in R. Tranter, H. Healy, D. Cattell, and D. Healy, "Functional Effects of Agents Differentially Selective to Serotonergic or Noradrenergic Systems," *Psychological Medicine* 32 (2002): 517–24.

16. See J. Glenmullen, *Prozac Backlash* (New York: Simon and Schuster, 2000), for more details on this issue.

17. For the best description of encounters between critics and the industry, see J. Braithwaite, *Corporate Crime in the Pharmaceutical Industry* (London: Routledge and Kegan Paul, 1986).

18. *Medieval* is being used here to refer to Scholastic views of the devil. Prior theologies had seen good and evil as opposite powers in the universe (good guys and bad guys), but Thomas Aquinas introduced the idea of evil as an absence of good—a void.

19. A. Solomon, "Anatomy of Melancholy," *New Yorker*, January 12, 1998, 47–61.

20. B. Saletu, J. Grunberger, and L. Linzmayer, "On the Central Effects of Serotonin Reuptake Inhibitors: Quantitative EEG and Psychometric Studies with Sertraline and Imipramine," *Journal of Neural Transmission* 67 (1986): 241–66; J. Grunberger and B. Saletu, "Determination of Pharmacodynamics of Psychotropic Drugs by Psychometric Analysis," *Progress in Neuropsychopharmacology* 4 (1980): 417–34.

21. S. J. Warrington, J. Dana-Haeri, and A. J. Sinclair, "Cardiovascular and Psychomotor Effects of Repeated Doses of Paroxetine: A Comparison with Amitriptyline and Placebo in Healthy Men," *Acta Psychiatrica Scandinavia* 80, supplement 350 (1989): 42–44.

22. These figures have all been calculated conservatively and are favorable for Lilly and Pfizer.

23. These calculations and the details behind them were presented at the Royal College of Psychiatrists Meeting in Edinburgh in July 2000 and the BAP Meeting in Cambridge in July 2000; see D. Healy, "Antidepressant Associated Suicidality," *Journal of Psychopharmacology* 14, abstract PC23 (2000).

24. Deposition of W. Leigh Thompson, July 20, 1994, in *Fentress vs. Eli Lilly.*

25. The full correspondence with the MCA, stretching over almost two years, is on www.socialaudit.org.uk and on www.healyprozac.com.

NOTES TO CHAPTER 8

1. Deposition of D. Healy, Boston, March 29, 2000, p. 341, in *Miller vs. Pfizer Inc.* (2000), case no. 99-2236 KHV, U.S. District Court of Kansas. Unfortunately, further details of this study remain unavailable due to a confidentiality order.

2. Deposition of D. Healy, Boston, March 29, 2000, in *Miller vs. Pfizer.*

3. In the case of the FDA, the details were faxed directly to David Graham and Tom Laughren.

4. The full correspondence is available on www.socialaudit.org.uk and on www.healyprozac.com/MCA.

5. D. Healy, trial testimony, Cheyenne, May 22, 2001, in *Tobin vs. SmithKline Beecham Pharmaceutical,* civil case no. 00-CV-0025 BEA. The entire correspondence between the author and the UK regulators is available on www.socialaudit.org.uk and on www.healyprozac.com/MCA.

6. D. Healy and D. Nutt, "British Association for Psychopharmacology Consensus on Childhood and Learning Disabilities Psychopharmacology," *Journal of Psychopharmacology* 11 (1997): 291–94.

7. R. Fisher and S. Fisher, "Antidepressants for Children: Is Scientific Support Necessary?" *Journal of Nervous and Mental Disease* 184 (1996): 99–102. Accompanying commentaries from Leon Eisenberg and Edmund Pellegrino (pp. 103–8) make this set of contributions a benchmark for what was happening preadult antidepressant prescribing in the 1990s. See also P. J. Ambrosini, "A Review of Pharmacotherapy of Major Depression in Children and Adolescents," *Psychiatric Services* 51 (2000): 627–33.

8. G. J. Emslie, A. J. Rush, W. A. Weinberg, R. A. Kowatch, R. W. Hughes, T. Carmody, and J. Funkelman, "A Double-Blind, Randomized, Placebo-Controlled Trial of Fluoxetine in Children and Adolescents with Depression," *Archives of General Psychiatry* 54 (1997): 1031–37.

9. N. Shute, T. Locy, and D. Pasternak, "The Perils of Pills: The Psychiatric Medication of Children Is Dangerously Haphazard," *U.S. News and World Report,* March 6, 2000, 44–50.

10. Deposition of Douglas Geenens, Dec. 16, 1999, in *Miller vs. Pfizer.*

11. Deposition of Matthew Miller's grandmother Jane, Dec. 29, 1999, in *Miller vs. Pfizer.*

12. Deposition of Hilary Burton, Feb. 15, 2000, in *Miller vs. Pfizer.*

13. May 27, 1999, was the date of the homicide-suicide.

14. Expert report of Parke Dietz (1999), in *Miller vs. Pfizer Inc.,* case no. 99-CV-2326 KHV. See transcript of November 20, 2001, hearing in Kansas City at p. 420 (full transcript available from the author). Dietz had some years before

offered the view that Anita Hill might be suffering from an erotomanic fantasy for Clarence Thomas and that her delusional beliefs led to the claims against him; see S. Kutchins and S. Klerk, *Making Us Crazy* (New York: Simon and Schuster, 1998).

15. Pfizer clinical trial database, subject to confidentiality order, December 1991.

16. Exhibit 40 in *Miller vs. Pfizer* at p. 23 (transcript). See www.healyprozac .com/Trials/expertreport.htm. The publications stemming from these trials, however, refer to only one suicidal act, other than obliquely; one article on the side effects of sertraline refers to the fact that no other side effects occurred in more than 10 percent of subjects.

17. Exhibit 40 in *Miller vs. Pfizer* at pp. 17, 18, and 20.

18. A subsequent trial on paroxetine in children—M. B. Keller, N. D. Ryan, M. Strober, et al., "Efficacy of Paroxetine in the Treatment of Adolescent Major Depression: A Randomised Controlled Trial," *Journal of the American Academy of Child and Adolescent Psychiatry* 40 (2001): 762–72—also reported rates of suicidal acts much higher on paroxetine than on placebo. The authors dismissed this finding by saying that in their opinion these acts in May 2001 were not caused by the drug.

19. Communications from Allison Sesnon, the program maker for *20/20*, by e-mail and telephone in during April and May 2001.

20. C. Poitras, "Prozac Defence Brings Acquittal," *Hartford Courant*, February 25, 2000.

21. The details in this case remain confidential, but I was involved as an expert witness.

22. J. Swiatek, "Lilly's Legal Tactics Disarmed Legions of Prozac Lawyers," *Indianapolis Star*, April 23, 2000, A1 and 18–19; April 24, 2000, A1 and A8.

23. Glenmullen, *Prozac Backlash*.

24. M. H. Teicher, D. A. Klein, S. L. Andersen, and P. Wallace, "Development of an Animal Model of Fluoxetine Akathisia," *Progress in Neuropsychopharmacology and Biological Psychiatry* 19 (1995): 1305–19.

25. J. M. Young, T. J. Barberich, and M. H. Teicher, U.S. Patent number 5,708,035, January 13, 1998.

26. Martin Teicher subsequently went on to work on an isomer of Ritalin for Sepracor.

27. All of these reviews are available on www.healyprozac.com/GhostlyData/prozacbacklash.pdf.

28. Based on an April 2000 telephone conversation with Leah Garnett, the author of the *Boston Globe* article. John Cornwell had originally planned to call *The Power to Harm* "The Prozac Trials." His publisher objected. Cornwell felt that a number of hostile reviews of his book had been strategically placed, and he was threatened with legal action. Cornwell also wrote *Hitler's Pope*, a book

that implicated the Catholic Church in the Holocaust, if only by failing to do anything; this book blocked efforts to beatify Pius XII. This did not make Cornwell popular in the Vatican, but overall, in his estimation, the Vatican was much less of a problem to deal with than a pharmaceutical company can be. (From author's conversation with John Cornwell, June 2002.)

29. I am indebted to Kitty Moore, then of Guilford University Press, for copies of this material from *Newsday.*

30. Letter from Robert Schwadron to Jamie Talan at *Newsday,* April 6, 2000.

31. L. R. Garnett, "Prozac Revisited: As Drug Is Remade, Concerns about Suicides Surface," *Boston Globe,* May 7, 2000, 1+.

32. Young, Barberich, and Teicher, U.S. Patent number 5,708,035, January 13, 1998, at p. 10.

33. Ibid., p. 12.

34. G. Tollefson, Letter, "Article on Prozac Ignored Overwhelming Evidence," *Boston Sunday Globe,* May 21, 2000.

35. This building is striking partly because it is now derelict, and at night shows as a darkened and jagged stump on the skyline.

36. "Pharmacologist" was how Dr. McNeil's lawyer, Lawrence Finn, designated him; see deposition of D. Healy, Sept. 25, 2000, in *Berman vs. Dr. David McNeil, Dr. Daryl Pure and Eli Lilly and Company,* case no. 93 L 7223, Circuit Court of Cook County, Illinois (hereafter *Berman vs. McNeil, Pure and Eli Lilly*).

37. Deposition of Darryl Pure, April 18 and June 11, 1998, in *Berman vs. McNeil, Pure and Eli Lilly.*

38. Deposition David McNeil, April 22, 1998, in *Berman vs. McNeil, Pure and Eli Lilly.*

39. G. W. Murgatroyd, K. A. Barth, A. Vickery, and R. K. Chang, Independent action to set aside judgment for fraud on court, *Forsyth* appeal brief (2000), case 95-00185 ACK, U.S. District Court of Hawaii.

40. *Pumphrey vs. K. O. Thompson Tool Co.,* Ninth Circuit Court, 62 F.3d 1128 (1995).

41. The cardiac profile of psychotropic drugs has been a problem since 1996, when sertindole, an antipsychotic that Abbott hoped to market in the United States, was shown to produce the cardiac abnormality later found in R-fluoxetine. No one knew whether this was a real problem, but it was enough to stall sertindole's licensing. The company that benefited from this was Lilly, whose antipsychotic olanzapine in consequence enjoyed a free run. This story illustrates that the power of regulation at present lies before a drug is licensed. For details, see D. Healy, *The Creation of Psychopharmacology* (Cambridge, Mass.: Harvard University Press, 2001). As Prozac, which almost necessarily has the same cardiac profile as R-fluoxetine, doesn't cause many cardiac problems, the question arises whether Lilly were using this anomaly to get rid of R-fluoxetine.

42. R. Pierson, "Sepracor Falls as Lilly Pulls Plug on Version of Prozac," *Reuters*, October 19, 2000.

43. On February 7, 2004, nineteen-year-old Traci Johnson, a healthy volunteer on a Lilly duloxetine study, committed suicide. See: www.indystar.com/articles/2/12004-8092-092.html, accessed 15/02/04 "Student's suicide cries out to FDA for drug warnings," by Ruth Hollady.

44. Exhibit 10 in deposition of J. Potvin, Oct. 10, 1993, in *Fentress et al. vs. Shea Communications and Eli Lilly and Company* (1994), case no. 90-CI-06033, Jefferson Circuit Court (hereafter *Fentress vs. Eli Lilly*).

45. L. Fludzinski, deposition in *Fentress vs. Eli Lilly*, Oct. 28, 1993.

46. D. B. Montgomery, A. Roberts, M. Green, T. Bullock, D. Baldwin, and S. A. Montgomery, "Lack of Efficacy of Fluoxetine in Recurrent Brief Depression and Suicidal Attempts," *European Archives of Psychiatry and Clinical Neuroscience* 244 (1994): 211–15.

47. Exhibit 4 in the deposition of L. Thompson in *Fentress vs. Eli Lilly*, July 20, 1994.

48. Exhibit 21 in the deposition of Joachim Wernicke in *Fentress vs. Eli Lilly*, Aug. 25, 1994. The significance level in favor of placebo is cited as $p = 0.006$.

49. D. Baldwin, "The Treatment of Recurrent Brief Depression" (paper presented at ECNP meeting, London, Sept. 24, 1999).

50. D. Healy, Cheyenne, May 23, 2001, testimony in *Tobin vs. SmithKline Beecham*.

51. Details from David Baldwin, an investigator on the study, in a number of conversations with the author ca. 1999.

52. SmithKline later supported another study in this patient group by R. J. Verkes, R. C. Van der Mast, M. W. Hengeveld, J. P. Tuyl, A. H. Zwinderman, and G. M. Van Viempen, "Reduction by Paroxetine of Suicidal Behaviour in Patients with Reported Suicide Attempts but Not Major Depression," *American Journal of Psychiatry* 155 (1998): 543–47, who reported that Paxil reduced suicide rates compared to placebo. However, all but nineteen out of ninety-one patients entered into the trial dropped out, making the study meaningless without a proper analysis of the reasons for dropout.

53. Exhibit 28 in the deposition of L. Fludzinski in *Fentress vs. Eli Lilly*, Oct. 28, 1993.

54. Exhibit 16 in the deposition of A. Webber in *Fentress vs. Eli Lilly*, Dec. 16, 1993.

55. S. A. Montgomery, D. L. Dunner, and G. Dunbar, "Reduction of Suicidal Thoughts with Paroxetine in Comparison to Reference Antidepressants and Placebo," *European Neuropsychopharmacology* 5, (1995): 5–13.

56. J. J. Lopez-Ibor, "Reduced Suicidality on Paroxetine," *European Psychiatry* 1, supplement 8 (1993): 17s–19s.

57. Letter from Andrea Smith Lilly in April 2000 to Sara [*sic*] Boseley of the *Guardian* newspaper, copied by S. Boseley to the author.

58. Deposition of Daniel Casey in *Miller vs. Pfizer*, April 6, 2000, 69.

59. Deposition of J. Mann in *Miller vs. Pfizer*, March 29, 2000, 65.

60. Deposition of R. Lane in *Miller vs. Pfizer*, July 21, 1999, 96; deposition of D. Wheadon in *Tobin vs. SmithKline*, Oct. 18, 2000, 44; deposition of C. Beasley, Nov. 8, 2000, 10, in *Espinoza vs. Eli Lilly and Company*, case no. 2:99-CV-393, U.S. District Court of Vermont.

61. I have these details from George Beaumont and several others.

62. This conversation was witnessed by Claus Langmaack. It was recorded in note form immediately afterward. Obviously, such conversations are open to misinterpretation, and it cannot be excluded that Dr. Nemeroff was simply concerned about my welfare.

63. "Speaking on behalf of Lilly, Charles Nemeroff . . . was quick to discredit the anecdotal testimony of alleged Prozac victims. Asserting that anecdotal reports fail to establish cause and effect, Nemeroff said that double-blind, placebo controlled trials were necessary to prove such a link. Criticizing studies of Prozac's adverse effects that were based on anecdotal evidence with small numbers of patients, Nemeroff said that Teicher's study has launched 'a maelstrom of activity' in the lay press. Teicher's conclusions were based on six patients who had 'multiple complicating factors,' including alcohol abuse, multiple personalities and 'other factors known to be associated with suicidality,' Nemeroff maintained. He also emphasized that 'suicidality is part and parcel of this disease [depression]' and therefore it is difficult to attribute suicidal behavior to the drug." *Health News Daily*, September 23, 1991.

64. As of the summer of 2001, C. Nemeroff listed himself on conflict-of-interest statements as a major equity shareholder in Lilly, Bristol-Myers Squibb, Forrest, Organon, SmithKline Beecham, Astra-Zeneca, Pfizer, Janssen, Wyeth-Ayerst, and Merck. In addition, he has grant/research support and other financial and material support from the same companies. He is also a paid consultant for, on the speakers bureau for, and receives direct payments for talks from the same companies. Nemeroff said that, under current conflict-of-interest guidelines, being a major equity shareholder means owning $10,000 worth of stock or more, and that he had got a few shares from Eli Lilly some years before and when he found that they had increased in value to over $10,000, he declared this. (My recollection of his explanation of what being a major equity shareholder meant is open to error, but the listing of his links to companies was prepared by him and not me).

65. *T.E.N.* 2, 9 (Sept. 2000).

66. Some years later, a range of Nemeroff's conflicts of interest featured in the *New York Times*: Melody Petersen, "Undisclosed Financial Ties Prompt Reproval of Doctor," August 3, 2003.

67. G. D. Tollefson and J. F. Rosenbaum, "Selective Serotonin Reuptake Inhibitors," in A. F. Schatzberg and C. B. Nemeroff (eds.), *The American Psychiatric Press Textbook of Psychopharmacology* (Washington, D.C.: APA Press, 1998), 219–37.

68. Declaration in support of plaintiff's opposition to defendant's motion for partial summary judgment on plaintiff's inadequate-warning claims, in *Motus vs. Pfizer Inc.* (October 30, 2000), CV00-298AHM (SHx), U.S. District Court, Central District of California.

69. According to Martin Teicher, as related to the author (March 2000), there was, for example, a phone call to Joe Coyle as head of the department of psychiatry and other efforts to get Teicher to drop these matters, for the sake of his career and the public good.

70. D. Cauchon, "FDA Advisers Tied to Industry," *USA Today*, September 25, 2000, 1; and D. Cauchon, "Number of Drug Experts Available Is Limited," 10.

71. In Cauchon, "Number of Drug Experts Available Is Limited," 10.

72. J. Calvert and L. Johnston, "How Safe Is the Meningitis Vaccine?" *Sunday Express*, August 6, 2000, 1, 2, 8, 9, and 32; M. Bright and T. McVeigh, "Meningitis Advisers Funded by Drug Firms," *The Observer*, Sept. 3, 2000, 10; S. Boseley, column in *The Guardian*, Sept. 5, 2000, G2.

73. The entire correspondence is available on www.socialaudit.org.uk and www.healyprozac.com/MCA.

74. Letter to the author from Dr. K. Jones, Medicines Control Agency, Aug. 23, 2000.

75. F. J. Mackay, N. R. Dunn, M. R. Martin, G. L. Pearce, S. N. Freemantle, and R. D. Mann, "Newer Antidepressants: A Comparison of Tolerability in General Practice," *British Journal of General Practice* 49 (1999): 892–96.

76. E. A. Ashleigh and F. A. Fesler, "Fluoxetine and Suicidal Preoccupation," *American Journal of Psychiatry* 149 (1992): 1750.

77. S. Donovan, A. Clayton, M. Beeharry, S. Jones, C. Kirk, K. Waters, D. Gardner, J. Faulding, and R. Madely, "Deliberate Self-Harm and Antidepressant Drugs: Investigation of a Possible Link," *British Journal of Psychiatry* 177 (2000): 551–56.

78. S. Donovan, M. J. Kelleher, J. Lambourn, and R. Foster, "The Occurrence of Suicide Following the Prescription of Antidepressant Drugs," *Archives of Suicide Research* 5 (1999): 181–92.

79. Letter to the author from Dr. K. Jones, Medicines Control Agency, Aug. 23, 2000.

80. Correspondence, April 2001, from Tania Evers of New South Wales Legal Aid, lawyer for David Hawkins, acquitted of a murder charge in May 2001, who had been on Zoloft.

81. Deposition of Dr. Suhany, Feb. 20, 2001, in *Tobin vs. SmithKline* (2001).

82. Most of this book antedates the events of November 30, 2000.

83. Formerly the Clarke Institute.

84. D. Healy, *The Creation of Psychopharmacology* (Cambridge, Mass.: Harvard University Press, 2002).

85. It was not a talk about SSRIs and suicide.

86. D. Healy, "Conflicting Interests in Toronto: The Anatomy of a Controversy at the Interface of Academia and Industry," *Perspectives in Biology and Medicine* 45 (2002): 253–63.

87. All correspondence regarding these issues is available on www.healyprozac.com/AcademicFreedom.

88. M. L. Barer, K. M. McGrail, K. Cardiff, L. Wood, and C. J. Green (eds.), *Tales from the Other Drug Wars* (Vancouver: The Centre for Health Services and Policy Research, 2000).

89. J. Thompson, P. Baird, and J. Downie, *The Olivieri Report* (Toronto: James Lorimer & Co., 2001); J. L. Turk (ed.), *The Corporate Campus: Commercialization and the Dangers to Canada's Colleges and Universities* (Toronto: James Lorimer & Co, 2000).

90. A. McIlroy, "Prozac Critic Sees U. of T. Job Revoked," *Globe and Mail,* April 16, 2000, 1.

91. Deposition of Martin Teicher, October 29 and 30, 1996, in *Greer vs. Eli Lilly,* case 91-1790 JGP.

92. One of the witnesses in favor of Teicher had been Jerrold Rosenbaum.

93. S. A. Montgomery and G. C. Dunbar, "Paroxetine Is Better Than Placebo in Relapse Prevention and the Prophylaxis of Recurrent Depression," *International Clinical Psychopharmacology* 8 (1993): 189–95.

94. Comment on the Cheng report in the expert report of K. Tardiff, April 3, 2001, in *Tobin vs. SmithKline Beecham.*

95. Deposition of Ian Hudson, December 15, 2000, in *Tobin vs. SmithKline Beecham*, 30–33.

96. Healy, "Conflicting Interests in Toronto," 253–63.

NOTES TO CHAPTER 9

1. L. Meyler, *Side Effects of Drugs* (New York: Elsevier, 1952).

2. D. Healy, *The Creation of Psychopharmacology* (Cambridge, Mass.: Harvard University Press, 2002).

3. See D. Healy, *The Antidepressant Era* (Cambridge, Mass.: Harvard University Press, 1997), chap. 1.

4. T. Stephens and R. Brynner, *Dark Remedy: The Impact of Thalidomide and Its Revival as a Vital Medicine* (New York: Perseus Publishing, 2001).

5. See M. N. G. Dukes and B. Swartz, *Responsibility for Drug-Induced Injury* (New York: Elsevier, 1988).

6. P. Temin, *Taking Your Medicine: Drug Regulation in the United States* (Cambridge, Mass.: Harvard University Press, 1980).

7. L. Lasagna, "Back to the Future: Evaluation and Drug Development, 1948–1998," in D. Healy, *The Psychopharmacologists*, vol. 2 (London: Arnold, 1998), 135–66.

8. M. Fink, "A Clinician-Researcher and ECDEU: 1959–1980," in T. Ban, D. Healy, and E. Shorter (eds.), *The Triumph of Psychopharmacology* (Budapest: Animula, 2000), 82–92; D. Healy, *The Creation of Psychopharmacology* (Cambridge, Mass.: Harvard University Press, 2002).

9. See D. Healy, "Evidence Biased Psychiatry," *Psychiatric Bulletin* 25 (2001): 290–91; D. Healy, "The Dilemmas of New and Fashionable Treatments," *Advances in Psychiatric Therapy* 7 (2001): 322–27; Healy, *Antidepressant Era*, chap. 3; Healy, *Creation of Psychopharmacology*, chap. 7.

10. See A. S. Evans, *Causation and Disease* (New York: Plenum Medical Book Co., 1993); M. Susser, *Criteria of Judgement in Causal Thinking in the Health Sciences: Concepts and Strategies in Epidemiology* (New York: Oxford University Press, 1973). Koch's efforts gave rise to what are called Koch's postulates.

11. N. Tomes, *The Gospel of Germs* (Cambridge, Mass.: Harvard University Press, 1998).

12. P. Mazumdar, *Species and Specificity* (Cambridge: Cambridge University Press, 1995).

13. Ibid.; L. Altman, *Who Goes First? The Story of Self-Experimentation in Medicine* (New York: Random House, 1987). The passions in the SSRI ivory tower may stem in part from the fact that many key players have suicides or suicidal acts in their backgrounds.

14. A. B. Hill, "Reflections on the Controlled Trial," *Annals of the Rheumatic Diseases* 25 (1966): 107–13.

15. Healy, "Dilemmas of New and Fashionable Treatments," 322–27.

16. F. E. Karc and L. Lasagna, "Towards the Operational: Identification of Adverse Drug Reactions," *Clinical Pharmacology and Therapeutics* 21 (1977): 247–53; A. Kazdin, *Single-Case Research Designs* (New York: Oxford University Press, 1982); H. Jick, M. Ulcickas, and A. Dean, "Comparison of Frequencies of Suicidal Tendencies among Patients Receiving Fluoxetine, Lofepramine, Mianserin or Trazodone," *Pharmacotherapy* 12 (1992): 451–54; M. Stevens, "Deliberate Drug Rechallenge," *Human Toxicology* 2 (1983): 573–77; M. Girard, "Conclusiveness of Rechallenge in the Interpretation of Adverse Drug Reactions," *British Journal of Clinical Pharmacology* 23 (1987): 73–79; C. Beasley, "Fluoxetine and Suicide," *British Medical Journal* 303 (1991): 1200. See also C. Beasley, Draft Rechallenge Protocol by Dr. Charles Beasley (1990), in testimony of Dr. G. Tollefson, March 24, 1999, in *Forsyth et al. vs. Eli Lilly and Company* (1999), civil case no. 95-00185ACK, U.S. District Court for the District of Hawaii (hereafter *Forsyth vs. Eli Lilly*); T. P. Laughren, J. Levine, J. G. Levine, and W. L. Thompson, "Premarketing Safety Evaluation of Psychotropic Drugs," in R. F. Prien and D. S. Robinson (eds.), *Clinical Evaluation of Psychotropic Drugs* (New York: Raven

Press, 1994), 185–215; M. N. G. Dukes and B. Swartz, *Responsibility for Drug-Induced Injury* (Amsterdam: Elsevier Press, 1988); *Federal Judicial Center Reference Manual on Scientific Evidence* (Washington, D.C., 1994), 160–61.

17. Dukes and Swartz, *Responsibility for Drug-Induced Injury.*

18. Stephens and Brynner, *Dark Remedy.*

19. Ibid.

20. A. B. Hill, "The Environment and Disease: Association or Causation," *Proceedings of Royal Society of Medicine* 58 (1966): 295–300.

21. S. A. Glantz, L. A. Bero, P. Hanauer, and D. E. Barnes, *The Cigarette Papers* (Berkeley: University of California Press, 1996). See also D. Kessler, *A Question of Intent* (New York: Public Affairs, 2001).

22. M. Green, *Bendectin and Birth Defects: The Challenges of Mass Toxic Substances Litigation* (Philadelphia: University of Pennsylvania Press, 1996).

23. M. Angell, *Science on Trial* (New York: Norton, 1997).

24. This point, it should be noted, does not apply to antidepressants, where even a relative risk of 0.5 may be compatible with antidepressants triggering suicide.

25. See Healy, *Antidepressant Era,* chap. 7; G. L. Klerman, "The Psychiatric Patient's Right to Effective Treatment: Implications of Osheroff versus Chestnut Lodge," *American Journal of Psychiatry* 147 (1990): 409–18; G. L. Klerman, "The Osheroff Debate: Finale," *American Journal of Psychiatry* 148 (1991): 387–88; A. A. Stone, "Law, the Science and Psychiatric Malpractice: A Response to Klerman's Indictment of Psychoanalytic Psychiatry," *American Journal of Psychiatry* 147 (1990): 419–27; A. A. Stone, "Dr. Stone Replies," *American Journal of Psychiatry* 148, (1991): 388–90.

26. D. Healy, July 11, 1999, deposition in *Forsyth vs. Eli Lilly*; and *Forsyth* trial transcript, March 9 and 10, 1999.

27. Green, *Bendectin and Birth Defects.* See *Daubert vs. Merrill Dow Pharmaceuticals, Inc.,* 727 F.Supp. 570, 572 (S.D. Cal. 1989).

28. *Frye vs. United States,* 293 F. 1013 (D.C. Cir. 1923).

29. *Miller vs. Pfizer Inc.,* case no. 99-2236KHV, U.S. District Court of Kansas.

30. R. M. Lane, "SSRI-Induced Extrapyramidal Side Effects and Akathisia: Implications for Treatment," *Journal of Psychopharmacology* 12 (1998): 192–214.

31. Glantz, Bero, Hanauer, and Barnes, *Cigarette Papers.*

32. K. H. Vratil, "Order to Show Cause," August 18, 2000, in *Miller vs. Pfizer.*

33. *Miller vs. Pfizer,* case no. 99-CV-2326KHV, transcript of proceedings, Nov. 19 and 20, 2001, Kansas City.

34. C. Elliott, "Caring about Risks: Are Severely Depressed Patients Competent to Consent to Research?" *Archives of General Psychiatry* 54 (1997): 113–16. See *American Journal of Bioethics.*

35. A. Khan, H. A. Warner, and W. A. Brown, "Symptom Reduction and

Suicide Risk in Patients Treated with Placebo in Antidepressant Clinical Trials," *Archives of General Psychiatry* 57 (2000): 311–17.

36. T. P. Laughren, "The Scientific and Ethical Basis for Placebo-Controlled Trials in Depression and Schizophrenia: An FDA Perspective," *European Psychiatry* 1 (2001): 418–23. A similar analysis, reaching similar conclusions, was undertaken by J. G. Storosum, B. J. van Zwieten, W. van den Brink, B. P. Gersons, and A. W. Broekman, "Suicide Rate in Placebo Controlled Studies of Major Depression," *American Journal of Psychiatry* 158 (2001): 1271–75.

37. Exhibit 1 from the deposition of G. Brickler, Dec. 1, 1993, in *Fentress et al. vs. Shea Communications and Eli Lilly and Company* (1994), case no. 90-CI-06033, Jefferson Circuit Court (hereafter *Fentress vs. Eli Lilly*). Available on www.healyprozac.com/Trials/CriticalDocs.

38. H. Lee, "Statistical Review on Sertraline," January 1991. This FDA review is available on www.healyprozac.com/Trials/CriticalDocs.

39. M. Brecher, FDA Review and Evaluation of Clinical Data Original NDA 20–031, Paroxetine Safety Review, June 19, 1991. See also exhibit 5 in the deposition of M. Brecher, March 13, 2003, in *In re Paxil litigation*, case no. CV-01-07937MRP (Cwx), U.S. District Court, Central District of California.

40. Memorandum from B. von Keitz and H. Weber to J. Wernicke, "Fluoxetine Suicides and Suicide Attempts" (1986), exhibit 19 in the deposition of J. Wernicke in *Fentress vs. Eli Lilly* (1994).

41. A. Khan, S. R. Khan, R. M. Leventhal, and W. A. Brown, "Symptom Reduction and Suicide Risk in Patients Treated with Placebo in Antidepressant Clinical Trials: A Replication Analysis of the Food and Drug Administration Database," *International Journal of Neuropsychopharmacology* 4 (2001): 113–18.

42. Khan, Warner, and Brown, "Symptom Reduction" (2000); Khan et al., "Symptom Reduction" (2001); B. Von Keitz, suicide report for the BGA, December 1986; deposition of G. Brickler, exhibit 1 in *Fentress vs. Eli Lilly*; also C. D. Hardison, "Summary of Suicide Attempt Rate," April 10, 1985, in deposition of E. Ashbrook, Dec. 9, 1993, exhibit 5 in *Fentress vs. Eli Lilly*. Venlafaxine data come from Thomas Moore, through an FDA Freedom of Information request to T. Moore, 2002.

43. See D. Healy, "Lines of Evidence on SSRIs and Risk of Suicide," *Psychotherapy and Psychosomatics* 72 (2002): 71–79. D. Healy and C. J. Whitaker, "Antidepressants and Suicide: Risk-Benefit Conundrums," *Journal of Psychiatry and Neuroscience* 28, 5 (2003): 331–39. Using an exact Mantel-Haenszel procedure, with a one-tailed test for significance, the odds ratio of a suicide on these new antidepressants as a group compared to placebo is 4.40 (95 percent Confidence Interval is $1.32 - \infty$; $p = 0.0125$). The odds ratio for a suicidal act on these antidepressants compared to placebo is 2.39 (95 percent Confidence Interval $1.655 - \infty$; $p \leq 0.0001$). The odds ratio for a completed suicide on an SSRI antidepressant (including venlafaxine) compared to placebo is 2.46 (95 percent

Confidence Interval 0.707 – infinity; p = 0.16), with an odds ratio for a suicidal act on SSRIs compared to placebo of 2.22 (95 percent Confidence Interval 1.47 – infinity; p ≤ 0.001).

44. In some of their dealings on these issues, FDA officials took phone calls from and otherwise made contact with company personnel outside normal official channels. See deposition of W. L. Thompson, July 20, 1994, in *Fentress vs. Eli Lilly* (available at www.healyprozac.com/Trials) and deposition of M. Brecher, March 13, 2003, in *In re Paxil litigation*.

45. S. A. Montgomery, D. L. Dunner, and G. Dunbar, "Reduction of Suicidal Thoughts with Paroxetine in Comparison to Reference Antidepressants and Placebo," *European Neuropsychopharmacology* 5 (1995): 5–13.

46. J. J. Lopez-Ibor, "Reduced Suicidality on Paroxetine," *European Psychiatry* 1, supplement 8 (1993): 17s–19s.

47. F. J. MacKay, N. R. Dunn, M. R. Martin, G. L. Pearce, S. N. Freemantle, and R. D. Mann, "Newer Antidepressants: A Comparison of Tolerability in General Practice," *British Journal of General Practice* 49 (1999): 892–96.

48. These figures have all been reviewed by many different colleagues. They are at present accepted for publication in one journal and being considered by two others.

49. See the data sheet for Prozac from the *Physician's Desk Reference* (Montvale, N.J.: Medical Economics Co. Inc., 2000).

50. SmithKline Beecham Corporation's memorandum in support of the motion to exclude or limit the testimony of plaintiff's experts Dr. Healy and Dr. Maltsberger, filed in *Tobin vs. SmithKline Beecham Pharmaceutical*, civil case no. 00—CV-025D, April 9, 2001; available at www.healyprozac.com/Trials. Order denying defendant SmithKline Beecham Corporation's motion to exclude or limit the testimony of plaintiff's experts, William C. Beaman, May 8, 2001. Order denying SmithKline Beecham Corporation's motion for judgment as a matter of law for a new trial, William C. Beaman, August 9, 2001. Concato and Davis, in their *Miller* report and later hearing in Kansas in November 2001, failed to take into consideration any of this evidence. The Miller case is now under appeal. Subsequent Daubert and Frye hearings in *Cassidy and Cassidy vs. Eli Lilly and Company* (civil action no. CA-00821, U.S. District Court for Western District of Pennsylvania), *Lown vs. Eli Lilly and Company* (civil action no. 3:01-3674-10, U.S. District Court for South Carolina), and *Berman vs. Dr. David McNeil, Dr. Daryl Pure and Eli Lilly and Company* (case no. 93 L 7223, Circuit Court of Cook County, Illinois) have considered a fuller array of evidence and have supported the plaintiffs.

51. P. Stark and C. D. Hardison, "A Review of Multicentre Controlled Studies of Fluoxetine versus Imipramine and Placebo in Outpatients with Major Depressive Disorder," *Journal of Clinical Psychiatry* 46 (1985): 53–58; W. M. Patterson, "Fluoxetine-Induced Sexual Dysfunction," *Journal of Clinical Psychiatry* 54 (1993): 71.

52. It is unconventional to use the name Prozac, instead of the generic fluoxetine, throughout a book like this, but I have chosen to stick with Prozac, as one of the important hinges of this whole story appears to be the patenting system, which makes Prozac out of fluoxetine.

53. Memo from Leigh Thompson to Allan Weinstein, Feb. 7, 1990, exhibit 98 in *Forsyth vs. Eli Lilly.*

54. There is no problem with patents per se. Alternative systems have been in place before and could be devised that would minimize the kind of problem outlined here.

55. T. Lemmens and B. Freedman, "Ethics Review for Sale? Conflict of Interest and Commercial Research Review Boards," *Milbank Quarterly* 78 (2000): 547–84.

56. When corresponding with Lilly about suicide data for their antipsychotic Zyprexa, which is listed as unavailable by Khan and colleagues in another article on suicidality on psychotropic drugs (A. Khan, S. R. Khan, R. M. Leventhal, and W. A. Brian, "Symptom Reduction and Suicide Risk among Patients Treated with Placebo in Antipsychotic Trials: An Analysis of the Food and Drug Administration Database," *American Journal of Psychiatry* 158 [2001]: 1449–54), I was informed by the company that the material was unavailable. Letter to the author from A. Simpson, Nov. 29, 2001.

57. Memo from J. Schenk (Bad Hamburg, Germany) to S. Bandak (London), "Benefit/Risk Considerations," March 29, 1985, exhibit 58 in *Forsyth vs. Eli Lilly,* 18 and 22.

58. Deposition of David Wheadon, June 9, 1994, and deposition of Joachim Wernicke, August 25, 1994, in *Fentress vs. Eli Lilly.*

59. Details in discovery papers in *Nyugen vs. SmithKline Beecham Corporation,* case no. CV791998, Superior Court, Santa Clara County, California.

60. Depositions of Nick Schulz-Solce, Sept, 16, 1994, and Hans Weber, Sept. 10, 1994, in *Fentress vs. Eli Lilly.*

61. Deposition of W. Leigh Thompson, July 20, 21, and 22, 1994, in *Fentress vs. Eli Lilly.*

62. Deposition of Richard Wood, May 12, 1994, in *Fentress vs. Eli Lilly.*

63. Letter to Max Talbott of Lilly from Robert Temple of FDA, Sept. 9, 1987, in a series of correspondences that followed eighty-eight submissions from Lilly about Prozac starting in September 6, 1983; exhibit 40 in deposition of W. L. Thompson, July 20, in *Fentress vs. Eli Lilly.*

64. Letter from Max Talbott to FDA, *Fentress* exhibit 40.

65. Trial testimony of Joachim Wernicke in *Fentress vs. Eli Lilly:* Nov. 10, 1994, pp. 173–90; Nov. 11, 1994, pp. 29–140; Nov. 14, 1994, pp. 5–167.

66. Letter from Max Talbott to the FDA, Dec. 4, 1987, exhibit 10 in deposition of N. Schulz-Solce, Sept. 16, 1994, in *Fentress vs. Eli Lilly.*

67. Memo from Richard Kapit of the FDA, Dec. 8, 1987, to file NDA 18-936, exhibit 11 in deposition of N. Schulz-Solce, Sept. 16, 1994, in *Fentress vs. Eli Lilly.*

68. Deposition of W. Leigh Thompson, July 22, 1994, in *Fentress vs. Eli Lilly.*

69. Joachim Wernicke, trial testimony, Nov. 10–14, 1994, in *Fentress vs. Eli Lilly.*

70. At   www.justiceseekers.com/Newsletter.cfm?category=SSRIWrong-fulDeathCase . . . ; accessed April 17, 2003.

71. This estimate is based on tobacco litigation precedents.

NOTES TO CHAPTER 10

1. H. K. Beecher, "Ethics and Clinical Research," *New England Journal of Medicine* 74 (1966): 1354–60. For a history of this article, see D. Rothman, *Strangers at the Bedside: A History of How Law and Bioethics Transformed Medical Decision Making* (New York: Basic Books, 1991).

2. J. D. Moreno, *Undue Risk: Secret State Experiments on Humans* (New York: Routledge, 2001).

3. D. Healy, *The Creation of Psychopharmacology* (Cambridge, Mass.: Harvard University Press, 2002), chap. 4.

4. T. Lehrer, "Werner von Braun," from *That Was the Year That Was,* recorded July 1965 on the Reprise Label.

5. Deposition of Catherine Mesner, August 17, 1993, in *Fentress et al. vs. Shea Communications and Eli Lilly and Company* (1994), case 90-CI-06033, Jefferson Circuit Court (hereafter *Fentress vs. Eli Lilly*).

6. Deposition of Richard Wood, May 12, 1994, in *Fentress vs. Eli Lilly.*

7. D. Healy, *The Antidepressant Era* (Cambridge, Mass.: Harvard University Press, 1997), chap. 1.

8. Harold Shipman was a general practitioner from Manchester in England, jailed in March 2000 on fifteen counts of murder, mostly of elderly women, who is thought, over a twenty-year career, to have killed more than 200 and up to 260 of his patients—the greatest serial killer of all time.

9. See L. Cook, "Pharmacology, Behavior and Chlorpromazine," in D. Healy, *The Psychopharmacologists,* vol. 2 (London: Arnold, 1998), 17–38.

10. L. Hollister, "From Hypertension to Psychopharmacology—A Serendipitous Career," in Healy, *The Psychopharmacologists,* vol. 2, 215–36; M. Fink, "Neglected Disciplines in Psychopharmacology," in D. Healy, *The Psychopharmacologists,* vol. 3 (London: Arnold, 2000), 431–58.

11. H. Weber, deposition in *Fentress vs. Eli Lilly,* Sept. 10, 1994, exhibit 3, unofficial copy of the medical comments on the fluoxetine application to the BGA, sent by Barbara von Keitz to colleagues in London and Indianapolis, May 25, 1984.

12. See L. Cook, "Psychopharmacology, Chlorpromazine and Behaviour," in Healy, *The Psychopharmacologists,* vol. 2, 17–38.

13. L. Buckingham and S. Busfield, "Game, Set and Unmatched," *The*

Guardian, March 26, 1999, 26; Editorial, "The Options Drug," *The Guardian*, March 26, 1999, 21.

14. S. A. Glantz, L. A. Bero, P. Hanauer, and D. E. Barnes, *The Cigarette Papers* (Berkeley: University of California Press, 1996).

15. D. Hooper, *Reputations under Fire* (London: Little, Brown, 2000), 194.

16. See D. Kessler, *A Question of Intent* (New York: Public Affairs, 2001).

17. Deposition of C. Beasley in *Espinoza vs. Eli Lilly and Co.* (2000), case no. 2:99-CV-393, U.S. District Court, District of Vermont, p. 10; deposition of M. Brumfield in *Motus vs. Pfizer Inc.* (2000), case no. CV00-298AHM (SHx), U.S. District Court, Central District of California, Oct. 12, p. 21; deposition of D. Casey in *Miller vs. Pfizer Inc.* (2000), case no. 99-2236 KHV, U.S. District Court for the District of Kansas, April 6, p. 69; deposition of R. Lane in *Miller vs. Pfizer* (1999), July 21, p. 96; deposition of J. Mann in *Miller vs. Pfizer* (2000), March 9, p. 65; deposition of D. Wheadon in *Tobin vs. SmithKline Beecham Pharmaceutical* (2000), civil case no. 00-CV-025D, U.S. District Court for the District of Wyoming, Oct. 18, p. 44.

18. The trial protocol and Suicide Ideation Scale are available on www.healyprozac.com/Trials/CriticalDocs, and from the author.

19. S. A. Montgomery, D. James, M. de Ruiter, et al., "Weekly Oral Fluoxetine Treatment of Major Depressive Disorder, a Controlled Trial" (paper presented at the Fifteenth CINP Congress, Puerto Rico, June 1986).

20. Part of the problem here is the publication has vanished and hence it is not possible, based on a knowledge of the dose used, to say whether this compound would have been safer. Other Montgomery reference lists in Montgomery articles continue, however, to list this study. I can also personally attest to awareness of this study in the 1980s. This situation has close parallels to the tobacco research situation.

21. J. Wernicke, S. R. Dunlop, D. Dornseif, and R. Zerbe, "Fluoxetine Is Effective in the Treatment of Depression at Low Fixed Doses" (abstract prepared for the Fifteenth CINP Congress, Puerto Rico, June 1986), exhibit in *Fentress vs. Eli Lilly*. J. F. Wernicke et al., "Low Dose Fluoxetine Therapy for Depression," *Psychopharmacology Bulletin* 24 (1988): 183–88.

22. Deposition of Richard Wood (CEO, Lilly, 1990) in *Fentress vs. Eli Lilly*, May 12, 1994.

23. The related documentation is available in *Forsyth et al. vs. Eli Lilly and Company* appeal, CV00-00407 ACK-LEK.

24. Janet Reno, cited in *The Guardian*, Sept. 23, 1999.

25. E. K. Ong and S. A. Glantz, "Tobacco Industry Efforts Subverting International Agency for Research on Cancer's Second-Hand Smoke Study," *Lancet* 355 (2000): 1253–59.

26. Editorial, "Resisting Smoke and Spin," *Lancet* 355 (2000): 1197.

27. J. Quick, director of World Health Organization (WHO) Essential

Drugs and Medicines policy, quoted in *Bulletin of World Health Organization*, Press Bulletin 9, Dec. 17, 2001.

28. At present, it is estimated that the United States constitutes 70 percent of the world's market in pharmaceuticals.

29. Mimi Hall, "'You Have to Get Help': Frightening Experience Now a Tool to Help Others," *USA Today*, May 7, 1999.

30. O. James, "The Happiness Gap," *The Guardian*, Sept. 15, 1997, G2–G4.

31. J. Clarke, "Happy Eaters," *Observer Weekend Magazine*, Jan. 30, 2000, 34; see Jane Clarke, *Body Foods for Life* (London: Weidenfield Nicolson, 1998).

32. P. Kramer, *Listening to Prozac* (New York: Viking Penguin, 1993).

33. Not only do such statements deflect but they are used as a defense by corporate lawyers, e.g., it is well known that antidepressants do not work for two or three weeks and therefore they could not have caused this problem, which happened in the first week of treatment.

34. See I. Kawachi and P. Conrad, "Medicalization and the Pharmacological Treatment of Blood Pressure," in P. Davis (ed.), *Contested Ground: Public Purpose and Private Interest in the Regulation of Prescription Drugs* (New York: Oxford University Press, 1996), 26–41.

35. See S. J. Jachuk, H. Brierley, S. Jachuk, and P. M. Wilcox, "The Effect of Hypotensive Drugs on the Quality of Life," *Journal of the Royal College of General Practitioners* 32 (1982): 103–5.

36. Healy, *Creation of Psychopharmacology*.

37. In J. Cornwell, *The Power to Harm: Mind, Medicine, and Murder on Trial* (New York: Viking, 1996), 286.

38. The phrase was apparently a favorite of German Chancellor Helmut Kohl, who became enmeshed in a series of scandals once he lost his grip on power.

39. This appears on the back of British packets, at least.

40. J. Glenmullen, *Prozac Backlash* (New York: Simon and Schuster, 2000).

41. This is an unsustainable position. If a problem emerges on reducing the dose of a drug or within days of halting it, this is dependence rather than a new illness. If the problem clears up quickly on going back on the drug, this is dependence rather than a new illness, which would take time to respond to treatment. If new symptoms appear on discontinuation, this again is dependence rather than a new illness.

42. D. Healy, expert testimony in *Tobin vs. SmithKline*, esp. 11:49 a.m., May 23, 2001: "In terms of the arguments Mr. Preuss made yesterday about Mr. Schell and the fact he didn't adhere to treatment the way he should have done, one of the extraordinarily interesting things about the healthy volunteer data in Harlow was that they have a group of studies there where totally healthy volunteers, people like members of the court here, go on this drug for very brief periods of time, a week or two at the most, and after only two weeks on the drug

SmithKline Beecham recognized that they're having physical dependence on this drug so when the drug is halted there are withdrawal syndromes." Available at www.healyprozac.com/Trials. See D. Healy, "SSRIs and Withdrawal/Dependence," briefing paper, June 20, 2003, presented to the British regulatory agency, the Medical and Healthcare Products Regulatory Agency, and posted on www.socialaudit.org.uk; deposition of Barry Brand in *In re Paxil litigation*, CV-01-07927 MRP (CWx), Oct. 8, 2003, exhibit 7 and pp. 297 *et seq.*; and the depositions of Martin Brecher (March 13, 2003), Paul Leber (May 20, 2003), Thomas Kline (August 298, 2003), and Alan Metz (Nov. 21, 2003) in *In re Paxil litigation*.

43. S. A. Montgomery and G. C. Dunbar, "Paroxetine Is Better Than Placebo in Relapse Prevention and the Prophylaxis of Recurrent Depression," *International Clinical Psychopharmacology* 8 (1993): 189–95; S. A. Montgomery, D. P. Doogan, and R. Burnside, "The Influence of Different Relapse Criteria on the Assessment of Long-Term Efficacy of Sertraline," *International Clinical Psychopharmacology* 6, supplement 2 (1991): 37–46. Dr. Montgomery was the editor of this journal at the time.

44. C. Medawar, A. Herxheimer, A. Bell, and S. Jofre, "Paroxetine, Panorama and User Reporting of ADRS: Consumer Intelligence Matters in Clinical Practice and Post-Marketing Drug Surveillance," *International Journal of Risk and Safety in Medicine* 15 (2002): 161–69; and C. Medawar and A. Herxheimer, "A Comparison of Adverse Drug Reaction Reports from Professionals and Users, Relating to Risk of Dependence and Suicidal Behaviour with Paroxetine," *International Journal of Risk and Safety in Medicine* 16 (2003): 5–19.

45. The action was filed by Karen Barth of Baum, Hedlund, Guildford, Aristei and Schiavo, *In re Paxil litigation*, CV-01-07937 MRP (CWx).

46. Revised wording for Paxil requested by the FDA, Dec. 14, 2001, as appears in product information material in *Physician's Desk Reference*, January 2002.

47. D. Healy, "A Dance to the Music of the Century," *Psychiatric Bulletin* 24 (2000): 1–3.

48. P. V. Rosenau and C. Thoer, "The Liberalization of Access to Medication in the United States and Europe," in Davis, *Contested Ground*, 194–206. See G. Cowley, "Right Off the Shelf," *Newsweek*, July 10, 2000, 50–51.

49. J. Abraham and J. Sheppard, *The Therapeutic Nightmare* (London: Earthscan, 2000).

50. For a comprehensive discussion of the changing climate on the university campus, see J. L. Turk (ed.), *The Corporate Campus: Commercialization and the Dangers to Canada's Colleges and Universities* (Toronto: James Lorimer & Co., 2002).

51. This wonderful phrase, which would have made a marvelous title for this book, comes in the first instance from a piece by Peter Medawar, used more

recently in a paper given by Charles Medawar, "A Conspiracy of Goodwill," at the British Association for Science, London, Sept. 5, 2000.

52. N. Pearce, "Adverse Reactions, Social Responses: A Tale of Two Asthma Mortality Epidemics," in Davis, *Contested Ground*, 57–75.

53. A first action against Barr pharmaceuticals, makers of generic fluoxetine, has in fact been lodged: *Radke vs. Barr Pharmaceuticals Inc.*, CV03-3654P.

54. "Spirit of the Age: Malignant Sadness Is the World's Great Hidden Burden," *The Economist*, Dec. 19, 1998, 123–29.

55. D. Healy, "The Marketing of 5HT: Anxiety or Depression," *British Journal of Psychiatry* 158 (1991): 737–42.

56. Marketed by Lundbeck as Cipralex in Europe and by Forrest as Lexapro in North America.

57. Text for a direct-to-consumer (DTC) advertisement for Paxil in the *Readers' Digest*, November and December 2001.

58. This phrase should be taken simply as a statement of fact rather than a judgment about causality.

59. See www.healyprozac.com/AcademicFreedom for more on the case.

NOTES TO THE EPILOGUE

1. See M. B. Keller, N. D. Ryan, M. Strober, R. G. Klein, S. P. Kutcher, B. Birmaker, O. R. Hagino, H. Kopleuicz, G. A. Carlsson, G. N. Clarke, G. J. Emslie, D. Feinberg, B. Geller, V. Kusumakar, G. Papatheodoru, W. H. Sack, M. Sweeney, K. D. Wagner, E. B. Weller, N. C. Winters, R. M. Oakes, and J. P. McCafferty, "Efficacy of Paroxetine in the Treatment of Adolescent Major Depression: A Randomised Controlled Trial," *Journal of the American Academy of Child and Adolescent Psychiatry* 40 (2001): 762–72.

2. From transcript of BBC *Panorama* program "The Secrets of Seroxat," October 13, 2002.

3. "Dear Doctor" letter from Glaxo-SmithKline in the United Kingdom, June 2003, and in Canada, July 2003.

4. S. Boseley, "Scientist in Rethink over Drug Link to Suicide," *The Guardian*, Oct. 1, 2003, 1. This article refers to Karen Wagner of the University of Texas.

5. D. Healy, *The Creation of Psychopharmacology* (Cambridge, Mass.: Harvard University Press, 2002).

6. D. Healy, "The Psychopharmacological Era: Notes toward a History," *Journal of Psychopharmacology* 4 (1990): 152–67. D. Healy, "The Marketing of 5HT: Anxiety or Depression," *British Journal of Psychiatry* 158 (1991): 737–42.

7. J. Spijker, R. de Graaf, R. V. Bijl, A. T. F. Beekman, J. Ormel, and W. A. Nolen, "Duration of Major Depressive Episodes in the General Population: Results from the Netherlands Mental Health Survey and Incidence Study

(NEMESIS)," *British Journal of Psychiatry* 181 (2002): 208–12; R. C. Kessler, P. Berglund, O. Demler, R. Jin, D. Koretz, K. R. Merikangas, A. D. Rush, E. E. Walters, and P. S. Wang, "The Epidemiology of Major Depressive Disorder: Results from the National Comorbidity Survey Replication," *JAMA* 289 (2003): 3095–3105.

8. Rachel Carson, *Silent Spring* (Boston: Houghton Mifflin, 1962).

Index

Abney v. Spring Shadows Glen, 129
abuse liability, 6, 29
academia, xiii, 209–11; interface with industry, xiv-xv, 15–16, 128, 191, 226,
   277–78, 286–88; silence of, 191, 275, 288
academic freedom, xiii, 209–12, 215–17,
   222–23, 279–81, 282–83
addiction. *See* dependence
Agent Orange, 234
agitation, 32, 43, 50–53, 72, 81–84, 182, 200,
   236. *See also* akathisia
akathisia, 14–15, 32, 43, 50–53, 81–84, 103;
   definition, 14–15; and suicide, 81–84,
   182–85, 200–201, 236–37
Alan L, 45–48, 89
alprazolam. *See* Xanax (alprazolam)
American College of Neuropsychopharmacology (ACNP), 50, 63, 160, 223
American Foundation for Suicide Prevention, 217
American Journal of Psychiatry, 116–17, 156
American Psychiatric Association (APA),
   42, 58–60, 86, 87, 120–22, 125, 175, 251
American Psychopathological Association
   (APPA), 125, 128
amitriptyline, 8, 38
Amytal interview, 47
anecdotal reports of suicidal effects, 56,
   77–78, 150, 208
Angell, Marcia, 233
antibiotics, 226, 267
antidepressants: action of, 16–17; causality,
   229–30; children and adolescents, 84,
   195–97; delayed effectiveness, 10; dependence, 26–29; development of early,
   7–11; development of SSRIs, 16–39;
   lethal in overdose, 21–22, 80; market for,
   8, 31; suicidal effects, 79–81; withdrawal
   suicides, 241
antidotes, 53, 131
antihistamines, 18, 20, 22, 30
antihypertensive drugs, 31, 267
anti-obesity agents, 31

antipsychiatry, 21–22, 111. *See also* "fringe
   groups"
antipsychotics, suicidal effects, 82–84
anxiety disorders, 26–29, 42, 53
anxiolytics, 4–7, 38, 281–82; dependence, 7,
   26–29; as lifestyle drugs, 7; marketing, 7,
   280–82
Archives of General Psychiatry, 116, 216
Ashcroft, George, 11, 205
AstraZeneca, 18–20, 87, 215
attorney-client privilege, 66, 69, 231
authors/authorship, 112–19. *See also* ghost
   writing
autoerotic asphyxiation, 197
Aviation Safety Board (U.S.), 276
Axelrod, Julius, 11
Ayd, Frank, 8

bacteria, 226–29; infections, 226
Baerlein, Rasky, 200
Baldessarini, Ross, 170
Baldwin, David, 170, 206
barbiturates, 4–5,
Barchas, Jack, 216
Barth, Karen, 129–30
Baum, Hedlund, 87, 129–30, 202, 271
Beaman, Judge William, 219, 244
Beasley, Charles, 55–58, 62, 67, 78, 150–54,
   209; meta-analysis of Lilly's data, 55–58,
   119, 131, 158, 204, 259
Beaumont, George, 23
Beecham Pharmaceuticals, 26
Beecher, Henry, 254–55
Bendectin, 232–33
benoxaprofen. *See* Oraflex (benoxaprofen,
   Opren)
Bentall, Richard, 82
benzodiazepines, 5–7; acceptance in Japan,
   6; as antidote to stimulating effects, 53,
   131; decline in use of, 6–7, 282; depend-
   ence, 6–7, 28–30, 266, 282; marketing of,
   5–7; similarity to SSRIs, 282
Berger, Frank, 4

Berman, "Corky," 86, 201–2
Berndtsson, Peder, 18
"better than well" response to medication, 13, 179, 185, 264
BGA (Bundesgesundheitsamt). *See* German regulators
Biffle, Martin, 66, 85
biobabble, 264
Birgenau, Robert, 223
"blame the disease, not the drug" defense, 59, 71, 132, 151–53, 224, 245,
Blowers, Hugh, 202
Boardman, Jed, 99
Bøgesø, Klaus, 24
Bond, Alyson, 78
Borison, Richard, 126
Bosc, Marc, 106
Boseley, Sarah, 160–61, 208
Boston Globe, 123, 200–201
Bouchy, Claude, 134, 165
Boy Who Couldn't Stop Washing, The (Rapoport), 24
brain function, restoring to normal, 11–12, 265–66
breach of contract, 223
breast implants, 232–33
Brecher, Martin, 213, 240
Breggin, Peter, 70–71, 137
Bristol-Myers Squibb, 7
British Association for Psychopharmacology, 54, 84, 137, 209
British Journal of Psychiatry, 113
British Medical Journal (BMJ), 55–58, 119, 150, 156–60, 165–69, 259–61
Brodie, Steve, 13
burnout, 275
buspirone (Buspar), 7
Buus-Lassen, Jorgen, 26
Bymaster, Frank, 30

Canadian Association for University Teachers (CAUT), 223
Carlsson, Arvid, 17–20
Casey, Daniel, 60–62, 209
Cassady, Tim, 78, 101
Castle Medical Center, 92
"Catecholamine Hypothesis of Depression" (Schildkraut), 12
cause and effect, 57, 97, 156, 227–33, 235–44. *See also* challenge, dechallenge, rechallenge (CDR); epidemiological studies; randomized controlled trials (RCTs)

Celexa (citalopram), 24–25, 239–40, 281
Centre for Addiction and Mental Health (CAMH), Healy affair, 215–17, 222, 283
challenge, dechallenge, rechallenge (CDR), 40–47, 51, 230–37. *See also* Prozac, CDR
Chamberlain Communications Group, 200
chemical imbalance. *See* brain function, restoring to normal; serotonin (5HT) levels
Chemie-Grünenthal, 224–25
childhood attention deficit disorder (CHADD) group, 111
children and adolescents, 265–69; antidepressants, 84–85, 195–97, 265–69; depression, 195–97; IQ testing, 269; OCD, 51–52; suicide, 195–97
chlorpheniramine, 18–19
Church of Scientology, 22, 55, 58–59, 138
Ciba-Geigy Pharmaceutical Company, 7, 8, 109
Cigarette Papers, 109
Cipramil, 24
citalopram. *See* Celexa
Citizens Commission on Human Rights (CCHR), 55
Clark, Craig, 162–63
"clinical immune-deficiency virus" (CIV), 286
clinical trials: children and adolescents, 195–97; design and management, 33–35, 105–7, 258, 266–69; failed, 35–36; legal jeopardy, 166–68
clinical trials data: access to, 277–79; analysis, 239–42; faked, 126; generalized to all individuals, 266; manipulation of, 37–38, 73–77, 150–52, 166–68, 236–42; reporting, 118–26, 159; used as evidence in lawsuits, 166
clomipramine, 17, 23–24
CMED, 113–14
Cohn, Jay, 35, 151
Cole, Jonathan, 42–45, 50–52, 78, 142, 165
Coleman, Lee, 64, 71
collateral estoppel, 253
Columbine High School, 24, 175
Committee for the Prevention and Treatment of Depression (CPTD), 8
communications agencies, 112–20
Concato, John, 238
conflict of interest, 60, 116, 203–12
conspiracies of goodwill, 297–98
consultants, 54–55, 70, 200, 211, 261, 272
Coppen, Alec, 31

Cornwell, John, 85
coroners, 161–63, 172
Corrodi, Hanns, 18
corruption 119–27; of medico-legal process, 241–51
Cox, John, 163
Coyle, Joe, 62
Creation of Psychopharmacology, The (Healy), 215
cultural side effects of SSRIs, 263–66
Current Medical Directions (CMD), 116–19
Cutthroat legal tactic, 157

Daniels, Mitch, 132, 198
data, proprietary, 119–27, 241–45; suppression of, 119–27, 241–45
Daubert hearings, 134, 236–37, 244
Davis, John, 238
Day by Day, 172
Defeat Depression (UK), 9–11, 251, 270
dependence, 26–29, 270–72. *See also* withdrawal, as cause of dependence
depression: about, 7–11; children and adolescents, 265–69; clinical cases, 40–53; diagnosis and treatment, 71, 100, 189, 265, 286; economic consequences, 70; education campaigns, 91, 110–12; hospitalized, 7–11, 32, 69, 98; marketing of, 10–11, 70; mild, 35, 100; monoamine theories of, 11–12; non-hospitalized, 35, 100; risk of suicide, 100, 154, 195–97, and serotonin levels, 11–12; and suicide, 99–101, 144, 152; unrecognized, 7–11; untreated, 200
Depression–Awareness, Recognition, and Treatment (DART) (U.S.), 9–11, 251, 270
Depression: What You Need to Know, 9
Depressive Alliance (DA), 111
Diagnostic and Statistical Manual of Mental Disorders (DSM-III), 8
Dianetics: The Modern Science of Mental Health (Hubbard), 58
diethylstilbestrol (DES), 74
Dietz, Parke, 197
diphenhydramine, 30
discontinuation syndromes. *See* dependence; withdrawal, as cause of dependence
discontinuation trials, 286
disinhibition, 174–75, 182–84
doctor-patient relationships, 10, 226, 254–55, 273–75

dose-response relationships, 136, 228, 231
dothiepin, 79–81
Dow Corning, 334
Downey, William, 129, 151–52, 158–62, 202, 213
drive-enhancing drugs, 48, 50, 171. *See also* norepinephrine system
droperidol, 143–45
drug-induced injury, 15, 29, 237, 323–24, 327, 333–34, 382
drugs, 326; development, 33, 35–36, 368, 383; efficacy overestimated, 193; generic, 395; inherent risk, 30; launched on market in groups, 350; licensing, 87; marketing, 32, 86, 268; regulation, 225–27; resistance to taking, 265; structural problem in system, 13; worse than condition, 224.
Drugs Safety Research Unit (DSRU), 243
DSM-III. See *Diagnostic and Statistical Manual of Mental Disorders*
Dubini, Adriana, 106
Dukes, Graham, 157, 165
duloxetine, 203
Dunner, David, 60, 205
Duphar Laboratories, 22

earnings, 123
eating disorders, 267–69
ecologists, 21
ECT (electroconvulsive therapy), 21, 58, 124, 195
education campaigns, 111–12, 194; marketing as, 9–10; by pharmaceutical companies, 8, 26, 109–11
Edwards, Gwen Jones, 83
Efexor, 113–15, 240
Eliashof, Byron, 143–45
Eli Lilly, 9, 16, 30–39, 49, 54–59, 112, 150–55, 244–51; defense of Prozac, 30–39, 54–59, 131–34, 150–56, 244–51; education campaigns, 9; favored access to FDA, 353; FDA hearings on Prozac, 60–62; Hastings Center support, withdrawal of, 164, 313; indemnification of psychiatrists, 202; lawsuits, 54–59, 87–97, 129–49, 282; Prozac-suicide link, awareness of, 132–34, 244–51; CDR study, 61; responsibility, 241–51; R-fluoxetine, 201–3; settlements, out of court, 198–99; S-fluoxetine, 260; and University of Toronto, 215
Elliott, Carl, 164

emotional blunting, 174–75, 182–84
Emslie, Graham, 196, 199
epidemiological studies, 155–56, 212, 231–23, 243; cause and effect, 231; indiTs, 229–30
ethics committees, 169, 254–55
European College of Neuropsychopharmacology, 170
evidence-biased medicine, 227
expert witnesses, 70, 87–90, 93–96, 100–101, 130–39, 217–19, 272; attempts to discredit, 87–90, 217–19; credentials, 233; indemnification, 202

Fabre, Louis, 32, 35, 151
Farmitalia Carlo Erba, 103
Faucett, Robert, 14
Fava, Maurizio, 49, 155, 212
Fawcett, Jan, 60
Federal Aviation Authority (FAA) (U.S.), 277
Federal Rules of Evidence, 236
Fentress v. Eli Lilly, 71–77, 85–86, 249–51
Ferrosan, 26
Fink, Max, 165, 169
Finz, Leonard, 65
Fisher, Seymour and Rhonda, 195
Fluctin, 39, 148
Fludzinski, Laura, 204–9
fluvoxamine. *See* Luvox
Food and Drug Administration (FDA) (U.S.), 33–37; Adverse Event Database, 171; breast implants, 233; clinical trials with placebo, 33–37, 238–42; conflict of interest waivers, 211; employees, 212–13; favored access, 248; Leber's reforms, 33–36; liaising with Lilly, 206–7, 247–51; 1991 hearings on antidepressants and suicide, 59–62, 150; Paxil, 220, 239–40, 282; and pharmaceutical company officers, 251; Prozac, 33–37, 59–62, 171, 247–51; regulations 1962, 225–27; role of, 272–77; thalidomide, 225; Zoloft, 36, 239–40. *See also* Leber, Paul; prescription-only drugs
Food and Drugs Act, 1962 amendments, 225–27
Forrest Laboratories, 25
Forsyth, Billy Jr., 90–93, 134
Forsyth, June, 90–93
Forsyth, Susan, 90–93

Forsyth, William, 90–93
Forsyth v. Eli Lilly, 87–102, 129–49, 235–36; appeal, 202; settlement, 282
"fringe groups," 21–22, 54–55, 58–60
Fuller, Ray, 30, 32, 67

Gandhi, on doing good, xvi
Garnett, Leah, 200
Geenens, Douglas, 196
Geigy, 7–8, 23–24
generalized anxiety disorder (GAD), 281
German regulators (Bundesgesundheitsamt), licensing of Prozac, 39, 128, 131, 134, 148, 248–50
ghost writing, 112–20, 259, 277
GlaxoSmithKline, 27–29, 124, 214, 220–22, 282–83, 284–85
Glenmullen, Joseph, 199–200
globalization, pharmaceutical companies, 266–69
Glod, Carol, 42
Goldbloom, David, 215–17
Goodwin, Fred, 1, 8
Gore, Tipper, 263
Graham David, 50, 148
Grain, Donna, 147
Granacher, Robert, 74
Greer v. Eli Lilly, 217–19
Greist, John, 199
Guardian, 160–61, 208, 263
Guillain-Barré Syndrome, 18
Gussack, Nina, 217–19
Guze, Samuel, 98

Haase, Hans, 14
Halcion, 103, 109, 277
Hall, Cindy, 88, 94, 129, 138–39
haloperidol, 32
Hamilton Depression Rating Scale (HAM-D), 105; item 3, 56–57, 131, 150, 207; item 17, 57
Harris, Eric, 175
Harrison, Wilma, 152
Hartman, Brynn, 96, 197
Hastings Center, 216
Hastings Center Reports, 164–65
Hawkins, David, 219
hazards: exposing, 224, 277–80; failure to recognize, 286; lack of warnings, 234; no incentive for competitor companies, 245; risk, in early phase of treatment, 10; warning, 224
health news, in mass media, 6

healthy volunteers, studies, 81–84, 174–93, 194, 209, 213; dependence, 270; suicidality, 180–93
Heiligenstein, John, 68, 132, 151–52, 154, 174
helicobacter pylori, 124
Henry, John, 22
Hill, Austin Bradford, 229
Hindmarch, Ian, 189, 194, 209, 213
Hippocratic Oath, de facto, 268
Hoechst Pharmaceutical Company, 21
Hoffman La Roche, 5–7; marketing of benzodiazepines, 5–7; overpricing, 7
Hoover, Cynthia, 95
Hubbard, L. Ron, 58
Hudson, Ian, 213, 221–22
Hurcombe, Caitlin, 2–3, 189
5-hydroxytryptamine (5HT). *See* Serotonin
hypertension, 31, 267

imipramine, 7, 35, 41, 48, 95
indalpine (Upstene), 20–22
independent research, 33, 122–26, 258–62; lack of funding for, 33, 261; tobacco, 258–62
Indianapolis Star, 198
industry, interface with academia, 156, 109–28, 191, 227, 256–59, 272–79, 286
informed consent, 254–55, 262, 277
Institute for International Research, 110
Institutional Review Boards (IRBs), 169, 191, 246, 254–55; privatization of, 169
Interbrand, 32
International Journal of Risk and Safety in Medicine, 157, 165
Interpersonal Psychotherapy (ITP), 106
iproniazid, 7
"I Saved Prozac," 203–4
isomers, 199

Jamison, Kay Redfield, 1–2, 11
Japan, benzodiazepines, 7; social phobia, 27–28
Jick, Hershel, 79–81, 101, 155, 171, 212
Jones, Keith, 213
Journal of the American Medical Association (JAMA), 116–19
Journal of Psychiatry & Neuroscience, 114
Journal of Psychopharmacology, 97–98
Joyce, Peter, 178
Judd, Lew, 9
juries, 75, 130–31, 146–48, 222

Kapit, Richard, 249–50
Kay, Judge Alan, 101, 130, 134, 144–45, 147–48
Kefauver, Estes, 225
Keller, Marty, 78, 135, 155, 210
Kentucky Supreme Court, 77
Kessler, David, 248
Khan, Arif, 238–42
Kielholz, Paul, 8–9, 16, 24, 80
Klein, Don, 8
Klerman, Gerald, 106
Kline, Nathan, 7–8, 13
Koch, Robert, postulates, 227–31
Kramer, Peter, 164, 180, 264
Kuhn, Roland, 7

labeling, 148, 207; of drugs, for hazards, 60, 273, 282–83
Lader, Malcolm, 6
Lagnado, Max, 104–5
Lambert, Pierre, 20
Lancet, 113, 120, 260
Lane, Roger, 119, 145, 209
Langmaack, Claus, 98
Laughren, Tom, 133, 239, 249–50
law firms, acting for tobacco and pharmaceutical companies, 259–61
lawsuits, 85–86, 155–56; contingent fees, 251–52, 272; costs of, 251–52
Leber, Paul, 33–36, 54, 60–61, 84, 133, 137, 213, 272; reform of regulatory rules, 33–34
Lee, Hilary, 240
legal immunity, pharmaceutical companies, 273
legal jeopardy, 165–69, 244–45; regulators, 22
legal liability, for off-patent drugs, 280; of patient groups, 112; of regulators, 57
Lenz, Siegfried, 225
Leon, A. C., 155, 160, 212
Leonard, Brian, 21–22, 205
Leschly, Jan, 259
Librium, 5–7
lifestyle drugs, 264–65
Listening to Prozac (Kramer), 180, 264
Loban, 31
Locke, Carol, 52, 200
lofepramine, 80, 104
Lopez-Ibor, Juan, 208, 220, 242
lorazepam, 81, 214
Lord, Nancy, 70, 72–73
Lundbeck Pharmaceutical Company, 24

Lundby study, 99
Lurie, Max, 87
Luvox, 22–24; OCD, 23; side effects, 22, 174; suicidal acts, 23, 243
LY–110140, 30–31. *See also* Prozac (fluoxetine, Fluctin, Loban, LY–82816, LY–110140)

Malt, Ulrik, 119
Maltsberger, Terry, 220
Manic-Depressive Illness (Jamison and Goodwin), 1–2
Mann, John, 63, 209, 220
Marketing: of depression, 8; of drugs, 36–37, 165; to physicians as education, 103–28
Marks, Don, 219
Marks, Isaac, 27, 116
Marshall, John, 162, 187
Matthews, Daryl, 142–43
McBride, William, 225
McNeil, David, 202
medical journals, editorial decisions, 116, 158; ghost writing, 112–20; pharmaceutical companies, 160, 260–62, 286; supplements, 112–16
medical writing agencies. *See* communications agencies
Medicines Control Agency (MCA) (U.K.), 103, 163; dual responsibilities, 276; correspondence with, 191, 194, 212–14; Halcion, 103; Paxil, 213, 220
Meltzer, Herbert, 32
meprobamate. *See* Miltown
Merck, marketing of depression, 8
Merrell-Dow Pharmaceutical Company, 236
Mesner, Catherine, 67, 69, 151, 256
meta-analysis of Lilly's data (Beasley), 55–58, 67, 97, 150–56, 158–59, 205–8
mianserin, 21–22, 34, 80, 106, 205; defense of, 21–22
Michels, Bob, 165, 312
Miller, Matthew, 136, 194–99
Miller v. Pfizer, 152–53, 194–99, 236–38
Miltown (meprobamate), 4
mirtazapine (Remeron), 80, 240
Molloy, Bryan, 30
monoamine oxidase inhibitors (MAOIs), 7, 48, 50–51
monoamine theories of depression, 112, 263–65

Montgomery, Stuart, 22, 33, 53, 60, 104, 136, 170, 205–8, 220, 242, 260
Mosher, Loren, 125
Murgatroyd, Skip, 129, 131

Nakielny, Joanna, 77
National Alliance for the Mentally Ill (NAMI), 111
National Depressive and Manic-Depressive Association, 60
"nature's Prozac," 263
Neal, Randolph, 92, 139–41
Nemeroff, Charles, 60, 209–12, 213
neurotransmission/neurotransmitter systems, 168
New England Journal of Medicine, 116, 254
Newsday, 200
New Yorker, 25
New York Sunday Post, 125
New York Times, 126
nisoxetine, 30
nomifensine, 21
norepinephrine levels, 11, 16
norepinephrine reuptake inhibitors (NRIs), 11, 16, 103–5, 127, 178
norepinephrine system, 11, 16, 103–5, 127
Norman, Doug, 149, 203
nortriptyline, 30
Nutt, David, 97–98

obsessive-compulsive disorder (OCD), 23–24, 40, 51–52, 111
Olivieri, Nancy, 216, 277
opinion leaders, 21, 118, 122
Oraflex (benoxaprofen, Opren), 73–75
Organon, 21, 105, 204; defense of mianserin, 21–22
Osheroff, Rafael, 234
Oswald, Ian, 57–58, 103, 109, 259; fear for personal safety, 109
overdose, of older antidepressants, safety in, 22
over the counter drugs, 273–75

Panorama, 57, 137, 284–85
paroxetine. *See* Paxil
Patel, Dr., 214, 220
patents on drugs, 244–46; expiry of, 267, 280; profitability, 18
patients, 266–68; compliance, 10, 26, 181, 273–75; education, 1102; globalization of treatment, 266–68; harmed by treat-

ment, 267–69; patients' rights, 255; personality differences, 178–82; support groups, 110–12; testimonials, 59–62, 111, 128; welfare, 277–79

Paxil: agitation, 194; clinical trials, 206, 208, 220, 249–53, 270; compared with coffee, 25, 188; dependence, 26–29, 194, 220, 270, 282; development, 26–29; dropout, 206, 282; labeling, 282; lawsuits, 220–24; marketing, 27, 282; reporting, 192; social phobia, 27, 107; suicidal acts, 239–43; suicidal effects, cases of, 214; suicidal effects, discussion of, 221–23, 239–43; violent acts, 214, 221; withdrawal, 220, 282. *See also* SmithKline Beecham

Paykel, Eugene, 53, 106

Payne, Reginald, 96

peer review, 97–98, 116

personality changes on SSRIs, 174–80, 201

Pfizer: Central Research Assists Marketing program (CRAM), 26; defense of Zoloft, 245–51; and Eli Lilly, 222, 303; funding of research, 116–19; ghost writing, 116–19; healthy volunteer studies, 194, 212–13; lawsuits, 136, 196–97, 236–41; marketing, 25–27; patient education program, RHYTHMS, 27; physician education program, PRIME–MD, 27

pharmaceutical companies: and academia, interface with, 15–16, 191; authorship, 112–20, 259, 277; blockbuster drugs, 245, 277; business practices, 164, 224–31, 260; clinical trials, 33–35, 266–69; communications agencies, 112–20; compared with tobacco industry, 109, 259–62; contract with society, 272–81; control of scientific agenda, 123–24; critics, 89, 111, 188; data, proprietary, 277–79; data reporting, 126, 166–69, 191, 244–46; Daubert ruling, 236–39; defense of products, 157, 203–9, 244–46; executive compensation, 259; funding of medical research, 33–35, 123–27, 176, 215–17, 256–58, 269; genetic technologies, 258; globalization, 266–68; lawsuits, 22, 227–39, 269; legal immunity, 273; management, 259–62; marketing, 35–39, 103–28, 244–46; meetings of medical associations, funding, 120–23; patient groups, 110–12; and physicians, 256–58, 259–62; prescription-only arrangements, 273–75; profits, 245,

258–62; and regulators, 33–34, 60–61, 225–26, 249–52, 272–76; and researchers, 34–35, 112–28, 259–62, 286; satellite symposia, 120–23; shareholders, 210–11, 256–62; sponsorship of delegates, 120–23; sorcerer's apprentice, 8

Pharmaceutical Research and Manufacturers of America, 114

Pharmacia & Upjohn: creation of, 169; marketing of reboxetine, 103–9; SASS, 1179, 174–82

pharmacovigilantes, 22, 286

physicians, 363–68, 385–88; as consumer watchdogs, 87, 385–86; duty to warn of hazards, 120, 133, 139, 219, 244–45, 257, 302, 305, 321, 323–25, 367, 387; education, 43–44, 47, 71, 380; liability and indemnification, 238, 251, 294; and pharmaceutical companies, 71, 75, 365, 368, 378–79, 386; prescribing wrong drug, 267; reluctance of patients to sue, 225, 244; tobacco, 386; treatment of depression, 359; treatment of suicide, 166

Pinder, Roger, 21–22, 205, 275

Placebo: and children, 195–97; in clinical trials, 33–39, 55, 71, 81, 170, 220, 239–43; washout suicides misreported, 170, 239–43; ethics, 242–43; and suicide, 239–43

Plath, Sylvia, 10, 80

poop-out, 29

post-marketing surveillance, 156, 172, 242–43; independent, 276

post-traumatic stress disorder, 281

Potter, Judge John, 66, 73–77, 146

Power to Harm, The (Cornwell), 85

prescription-only drugs, 148, 222, 225–27, 256–59, 273–77

Primary Care Psychiatry, 190

Protocol 27 study, 35, 257

Prozac (fluoxetine, Fluctin, Loban, LY–82816, LY–110140), 30–39; agitation, 32, 40–54, 64–65, 201, 205; behavioral effects, 31–33; CDR, 40–50, 52–53, 61, 235–36; children and adolescents, 195–96; clinical trials, 34–39, 55–58, 72–73, 150–55, 205–7, 240–42, 258–59; dependence, 270–71; depression cases, 40–53; development, 30–39; dosage, 33, 37, 53, 136, 260; drugs to minimize stimulating effects, 32, 41, 52, 72, 131, 142, 148, 202, 214; generic, legal liability, 280;

Prozac (*Continued*)
    lawsuits, 58–59, 65–77, 85–86, 93–97,
        100–102, 129–49, 200–202, 282; licensing,
        34–39, 127–28, 148–49, 244–51; market-
        ing, 38–39, 264; "most researched drug
        in history," 59, 67, 132, 145; the "new
        Valium," 100, 189; over-the-counter ac-
        cess, 273; package insert, 143–45,
        172–73, 208; patent, 198–203, 280; qual-
        ity of life scales, 127–28; relative risk,
        99–100, 243; safety in overdose, 38; sex-
        ual dysfunction, 56–57, 244; suicidal
        acts, cases of, 2–3, 40–41, 42–54, 90–93,
        201–4; suicidal acts, discussion, 58, 73,
        77–80, 95–97, 131–36, 150–56, 161–62,
        169–72, 182–88; violent acts, 64–65, 88,
        96, 198; warnings, 77, 131, 143–44, 148,
        161, 172–73, 201; weight loss, 38–39
Prozac Backlash (Glenmullen), 199–200
Prozac Diary (Slater), 175
Prozac Survivors Support Group, 89
psychiatric disorders, classification of, 8
psychoanalysis, 264, 279
psychobabble, 264
Psychopharmacologists, The (Healy), 89,
    137
psychosocial setting, of patients, 226
psychotherapy, 84, 106, 274–75; history,
    279–80; lack of warnings, 234–35; recov-
    ered memory, 129, 235
psychotic disorders, 32, 69
public accountability, of psychiatry, 126,
    275–76
public perception: of antidepressants as
    addictive, 28–29, 270–72, 282; of benefits
    of treatment, 267–69, 279; of link be-
    tween serotonin levels and depression,
    263–66
Putnam, Monica, 66
python, dancing with a, 277

quality of life, 38, 126–28, 174–76, 267
Quick, Jonathan, 262

randomized controlled trials (RCTs) data:
    misuse of, 229–30, 238; to prove cause
    and effect, 67, 94–95, 156, 220–22,
    229–31; reliance on, by physicians, 275;
    results generalized to all populations,
    266–68; role in regulation of drugs,
    276–78
Rapoport, Judith, 23–24
rating scales, 268–69

raw data, 114–16, 117–19, 208, 239–42; ac-
    cess by independent experts, 245–46,
    277–80
reboxetine, 103–9, 126–28, 174–82; cardiac
    side effects, 104–5
Recognizing the Depressed Patient (Ayd), 8
recovered memory, 129, 235
Redux, 31
regulation of drugs, 225–26, 272; no guar-
    antee of protection, 273–76
regulators: access to research data, 191–92,
    212, 258; and pharmaceutical compa-
    nies/industry, 132–34, 212–13; role of,
    33–34, 60–61, 249–52, 272
Remeron. *See* mirtazapine
remoxipride, 18
Reno, Janet, 260
research subjects, 83, 254–55; compensa-
    tion, 177; legal jeopardy, 166–69; social
    contract, 262
reserpine, 136; side effects, 15; suicidal
    acts, 156
R-fluoxetine (dexfluoxetine), 199–203, 260
Rhône-Poulenc, 20; chlorpromazine, 13
Richardson-Merrell, 231
Rickels, Karl, 35
Ring, Leonard, 65–66
risk: efforts to minimize, 266–69; relative,
    268; relative, of adverse effects, 235–38;
    of suicidal acts, 237; tyranny of, 269
risk *vs.* benefit of treatment, 21, 224–27,
    247–51; direct and indirect, 185–87
Ritalin, 84–85, 111, 196
Roberts, Riggs, 92
Roberts, Tony, 179–82
Robins, Eli, 98
Rosenbaum, Jerrold, 49, 59, 200
Rosenthal Peter, 283
Rothschild, Anthony, 52–53, 89, 101, 200
Royal College of Psychiatrists, 28, 163, 251
Ruben, Harvey, 199

Sabshin, Melvin, 59
Saletu, Berndt, 189
Sandler, Merton, 83
Sarwer-Foner, Gerald, 14
satellite symposia, 112–16, 120–23
scales, weighing, 268–69
Schatzberg, Alan, 210
Schell, Donald, 214, 220. See also *Tobin v.
    SmithKline Beecham*
Schildkraut, Joseph, 12, 17
Schwadron, Robert, 200

Science on Trial (Angell), 233
Scientologists. *See* Church of Scientology
See, Andy, 94–97, 130, 130–45, 154–55
selectivity, definition, 27
separation of powers, judiciary and government, 282–83
Sepracor, 62, 146, 199–203, 260
serotonin (5HT) levels: and anxiety, 282; and depression, 112, 167, 263–68; and suicide, 25
serotonin hypothesis of depression, 112, 167
Seroxat, 27. *See* Paxil
sertraline. *See* Zoloft
Serzone, 239–40
settlements, out of court: Dow Corning, 233; Lilly, 76–77, 85–86, 197, 202, 282; SmithKline Beecham, 253
S-fluoxetine, 260
shareholders, 2092, 256, 259–62
share options, 259
Shepherd, Michael, 8, 13
Shipman, Harold, 257
Shlensky, Ron, 94, 141
Shook, Hardy and Bacon, 94, 109, 259
shyness, 27
Silent Spring, 288
Simon, Gregory, 100
Singer, James, 32
Slater, Irwin, 32
Slater, Lauren, 175
Smith, Paul, 66–79, 85–86, 139; breach of fiduciary trust, 85–86, 139
Smith, Richard, 158–60, 165–69, 261
SmithKline Beecham: appeal of Tobin verdict, 253; defense of Paxil, 206–7, 220–22, 235–38; guilty verdict, 222; healthy volunteer studies, 189, 194; settlements out of court, 253. *See also* GlaxoSmithKline; Paxil
Social Adaptation Scale (SAS), 106
Social Adaptation Self Evaluation Scale (SASS), 105–7, 127–28, 174, 181
social anxiety disorder. *See* social phobia
social functioning, 106–8, *See also* quality of life
social phobia, 27–28, 111, 281
Solomon, Andrew, 25, 188
Solomon, Howard, 25
Space shuttle fallacy, 241
Spilker, Bert, 114
SSRIs (selective serotonin reuptake inhibitors), action of, 169, 103; benefits *vs.*

harm, 267; brain stressors, 29; children and adolescents, 194–98, 266–69; clinical trials, 37–39, 239–41, 266–69; compared with placebo, 178; cultural side effects, 263–65; dependence, 28–30, 270–72, 282; development, 16–39; in early stages of treatment, 101, 274–75; future of, 280–82; healthy volunteers, 188–93; licensing, 276; marketing, 37–39, 104, 124; OCD, 23–24, 195; patient compliance, 38; in pregnancy, 112; quality of life scales, 126–28; risk of suicide, 239–44; safety in overdose, 37; side effects, 175, 188; suicidal acts, 19, 23, 40–47, 119, 169–72, 239–43; warnings, lack of, 172–73
Steck, Hans, 14
St. John's Wort, 275
Suhany, Mark, 214
suicidality and suicide: and akathisia, 135, 63, 81–83, 142–44, 166–67, 171, 201–3, 240–41; in early stages of treatment, 24, 80, 119, 241; healthy volunteers, 182–85; measurement, 61, 256; in persons left untreated, 99–100, 171–72; in persons not depressed, 62, 152–53; public perception, 270; rates of, 132, 171–72, 190, 239–43; reporting, lack of, 150–52, 206; risk of, 98–100, 190–93, 239–43; stopped when treatment discontinued, 40–48, 50–53; warnings, 143–44, 148, 172–73; during washout period of clinical trials, 239–41
Suicides and Suicide Attempts in FDA Antidepressant Trials, 239–43
Sunday Times, 161

Talbott, Max, 74, 133, 249
Talking Back to Prozac (Breggin), 70
tardive dyskinesia, antipsychotic-induced, 42, 224
Teicher, Martin, 42–45, 50, 62–63, 70, 199–200, 217–19
Temple, Robert, 60–62, 132–33, 248
T.E.N.: The Economics of Neuroscience, 210
test-retest study, 40–45, 47–48, 52, 186. *See also* challenge, dechallenge, rechallenge (CDR)
thalidomide (Contergan, Distaval, Kevadon, Talimol), 224–31
Thase, Michael, 113
Thompson, Leigh, 74, 85, 132–33, 152, 166, 191–92, 203–4, 245, 249–50

Time, 58–59
tobacco companies, 259–62; compared with pharmaceutical companies, 109; funding of medical-scientific research, 262; lawsuits, 237; legal problems with safer cigarette, 261
tobacco products, exposing harmful effects, 234–35, 259–62
Tobias, Marilyn, 85
Tobias, Randall, 70, 259
Tobin v. SmithKline Beecham, 214, 219–22, 235–45; appeal, 253
Tollefson, Gary, 126, 142, 201, 210
Tony L, 40–41, 187, 217
tort cases, balanced in favor of corporations, 233, 272
"Tort Wars," 224
Toxic Psychiatry (Breggin), 70, 138
tranquilizers, 4–7, 81, 281–82; dependence, 28–29. *See also* benzodiazepines
trazodone. *See* Desyrel
tricyclic antidepressants (TCAs), actions of, 167; children and adolescents, 195; compared with SSRIs, 27, 37–39, 79–80, 127; and depression, 214; development, 7–8; lethal in overdose, 22, 79–80
turnover, of employees, 247–48, 256–57
20/20 (ABC-TV), 199

Ugalde, Julie, 131, 139, 147–48
University of Toronto, 371; Healy affair, 215–17, 222–23, 278, 282–83; "Looking Back: Looking Ahead" meeting, 215; Nancy Olivieri affair, 216, 277; safeguards, 283
University of Toronto Bulletin, 277
Unquiet Mind (Jamison), 1
Upjohn Pharmaceutical Company, 24, 32, 57–58, 103–4
USA Today, 211
U.S. News and World Report, 196

Valium, 4–7, 100, 189, 265; effect, 81; marketing, 5–7. *See also* benzodiazepines
van Praag, Herman, 42
van Putten, Ted, 50–51
venlafaxine, 113
Viagra, 265
Vickery, Andy, 88, 129–49, 194, 202–3, 214, 220–22, 238–39, 251–53

von Pettenkoffer, Max, 228
Vratil, Judge Kathryn, 237

Wakelin, Jenny, 23, 207
Waldner, Paul, 129, 252
Wall Street Journal, 59
"war between the sisters," 26
warnings, 148; breast implants, 233–34; hazards of SSRIs, 159, 161, 172–73, 191, 243; of potential drug hazards, 234, 271, 278–79
Warrington, Steven, 189
washout suicides categorized as placebo, 170, 239–43
Weber, Hans, 134, 152, 169
weight loss (Prozac), 3, 31, 37
Weissman, Myrna, 106
Welch, Willard, 25
Wellbutrin, 239–42
Wernicke, Joachim, 33, 131, 248, 250
Wesbecker, Joseph, 64–65
Wesbecker trial. See *Fentress v. Eli Lilly*
West, Ed, 269
Wheadon, David, 62, 204, 209, 220
Whitford, Mervyn, 189
Wilkins, Robert, 13
Wilkinson, Dave, 157
Wirshing, William, 50–51
withdrawal, as cause of dependence, 28–29, 270–72
Wong, David, 16, 30
Wood, Richard, 33, 256
Woods, Robert, 161
World Trade Center, 281
Wyeth Pharmaceutical Company, 113–15

Xanax (alprazolam), 91, 107, 142

Zelmid (zimelidine, H102-09), 18–20; side effects, 19; suicidal acts, 19
Zettler, Nancy, 66–77, 86, 201–2, 249
Zoloft (sertraline), 25; agitation, 194; clinical trials, 36, 239–41, 243; development, 25; dosage, 233, 263; dropout, 188–89; in early stages of treatment, 119, 196–98; ghost-reporting, 116–19; healthy volunteers studies, 174–93; marketing, 25–26; suicidal acts, 119, 239–43; suicidal effects, 152–53, 189–90

About the Author

David Healy is Reader in Psychological Medicine in University of Wales College of Medicine and director of the North Wales Department of Psychological Medicine. He is a former secretary of the British Association for Psychopharmacology and author of over 120 peer reviewed articles and twelve books, including the reference history of antidepressants, *The Antidepressant Era,* and *The Creation of Psychopharmacology.* He has been the lead medical expert in a series of legal cases involving selective serotonin reuptake inhibitors (SSRIs, the group to which Prozac belongs) and is fairly famous in Toronto for his suit against the University of Toronto after they breached his contract following a lecture covering the history of psychopharmacology and the emergence of conflict of interest as a key issue in modern science. The university settled this action and made Dr. Healy a visiting professor.